VOCAL ARTS MEDICINE

The Care and Prevention of Professional Voice Disorders

Michael S. Benninger, MD
Chairman
Department of Otolaryngology-Head and Neck Surgery
Henry Ford Hospital
Detroit, Michigan

Barbara H. Jacobson, PhD
Division of Speech-Language Sciences and Disorders
Department of Neurology
Henry Ford Hospital
Detroit, Michigan

Alex F. Johnson, PhD
Division of Speech-Language Sciences and Disorders
Department of Neurology
Henry Ford Hospital
Detroit, Michigan

1994
THIEME MEDICAL PUBLISHERS, Inc.   New York
GEORG THIEME VERLAG   Stuttgart • New York

Thieme Medical Publishers, Inc.
381 Park Avenue South
New York, New York 10016

VOCAL ARTS MEDICINE: THE CARE AND PREVENTION
OF PROFESSIONAL VOICE DISORDERS
Michael Benninger
Barbara Jacobson
Alex Johnson

Library of Congress Cataloging-in-Publication Data

Vocal arts medicine : the care and prevention of professional voice
    disorders/[edited by] Michael Benninger, Barbara Jacobson, Alex
    Johnson.
        p.   cm.
    Includes bibliographical references and index.
    ISBN 0-86577-439-0.—ISBN 3-13-783101-6
        1. Voice disorders. 2. Voice—Care and hygiene. 3. Singers—
Health and hygiene. I. Benninger, Michael. II. Jacobson,
Barbara, Ph.D. III. Johnson, Alex, Ph.D.
    [DNLM: 1. Voice—physiology.   2. Voice Disorders—diagnosis.
3. Voice Disorders—therapy.   WV 500 V8715 1993]
RF511.S55V63   1993
616.85′5—dc20
DNLM/DLC
for Library of Congress   93-5013
                                                         CIP

Important note: Medicine is an ever-changing science. Research and clinical experience are continually broaden-
ing our knowledge, in particular our knowledge of proper treatment and drug therapy. Insofar as this book
mentions any dosage or applications, readers may rest assured that the authors, editors, and publishers have made
every effort to ensure that such references are strictly in accordance with the state of knowledge at the time of
production of the book. Nevertheless, every user is requested to carefully examine the manufacturers' leaflets
accompanying each drug to check on his own responsibility whether the dosage schedules recommended therein or
the contraindications stated by the manufacturers differ from the statements made in the present book. Such
examination is particularly important with drugs that are either rarely used or have been newly released on the
market.

Some of the product names, patents, and registered designs referred to in this book are in fact registered
trademarks or proprietary names even though specific reference to this fact is not always made in the text.
Therefore, the appearance of a name without designation as proprietary is not to be construed as a representation
by the publisher that it is in the public domain.

Printed in the United States of America.

5   4   3   2   1

TMP ISBN 0-86577-439-0
GTV ISBN 3-13-783101-6

To Our Families
Kathy, Ryan and Kaylin
Gary and Cristina
Linda, David and Jeffrey
for their support, understanding and love

In Memoriam

This book is dedicated to the memory of the late Van L. Lawrence, MD. Dr. Lawrence made unique contributions to the field of voice. He was a humble, gentle, understated otolaryngologist who practiced in Houston. In addition to providing outstanding care for singers, he served as voice consultant to the Houston Grand Opera from 1970 until his death in 1990 and as consultant to numerous music schools. He contributed extensively to otolaryngologic voice literature and was active as a member of the Scientific Advisory Board of The Voice Foundation. However, his greatest contributions were in overcoming boundaries between specialties. His accessible, unassuming style made him a favorite speaker among singers and speech–language pathologists, and a successful author for the National Association of Teachers of Singing. His teaching activities were central to the evolution of our interdisciplinary specialty. His contributions have been innumerable, and the good he has done will be passed on through well-trained, healthy voices and voice care professionals for generations to come.

Contents

Contributors

David M. Alessi, MD
Clinical Assistant Professor of Surgery
University of California, Los Angeles
Cedars-Sinai Medical Center
Los Angeles, California

Michael S. Benninger, MD
Chairman
Department of Otolaryngology-Head and
  Neck Surgery
Henry Ford Hospital
Detroit
Clinical Assistant Professor
The University of Michigan Medical School
Ann Arbor, Michigan

Raymond H. Colton, PhD
Associate Professor
College of Medicine
Department of Otolaryngology and
  Communication Sciences
SUNY Health Science Center at Syracuse
Syracuse, New York

Allan B. DeHorn, PhD
Director, Anxiety Disorders Clinic
Department of Psychiatry
Henry Ford Hospital
Detroit, Michigan

Edith Diggory, PhD
School of Music and Dance
Oakland University
Rochester, Michigan

Charles N. Ford, MD
Chairman, Department of Otolaryngology
University of Wisconsin
Madison, Wisconsin

Wilbur J. Gould, MD
The Center for Care of the Voice
New York
Director, Ames Vocal Dynamics Laboratory
Lenox Hill Hospital
New York, New York

Mary J. Hawkshaw, RN, BSN
Otolaryngology Nurse Clinician
American Institute for Voice and Ear
  Research
Philadelphia, Pennsylvania

Reinhardt J. Heuer, PhD
Speech-Language Pathologist
Voice Research Institute
American Institute for Voice and Ear
  Research
Philadelphia, Pennsylvania

Barbara H. Jacobson, PhD
Division of Speech-Language Sciences and
  Disorders
Department of Neurology
Henry Ford Hospital
Detroit, Michigan

Alex F. Johnson, PhD
Division of Speech-Language Sciences and
  Disorders
Department of Neurology
Henry Ford Hospital
Detroit, Michigan

Carol A. Klitzke, MA
The Voice Center
Minneapolis, Minnesota

Gwen S. Korovin, MD
The Center for Care of the Voice
Attending Physician
Lenox Hill Hospital
Ames Vocal Dynamics Laboratory
Lenox Hill Hospital
New York, New York

Van L. Lawrence, MD
Clinical Assistant Professor
Department of Otolaryngology
Baylor Medical College
Houston, Texas

Howard L. Levine, MD
Director
The Mt. Sinai Nasal-Sinus Center
Cleveland, Ohio

Richard Miller
Professor of Singing
Oberlin College Conservatory of Music
Oberlin, Ohio

Stephen A. Mitchell, MD
Assistant Professor
Department of Otolaryngology
Vanderbilt Voice Center
Vanderbilt University
Nashville, Tennessee

Deborah C. Rosen, RN, MS
Otolaryngology Nurse Clinician
American Institute for Voice and Ear
    Research
Philadelphia, Pennsylvania

Robert T. Sataloff, MD, DMA
Professor of Otolaryngology
Thomas Jefferson University
American Institute for Voice and Ear
    Research
Philadelphia, Pennsylvania

Joseph R. Spiegel, MD
Assistant Professor of Otolaryngology
Thomas Jefferson University
American Institute for Voice and Ear
    Research
Philadelphia, Pennsylvania

R. E. Stone, Jr., PhD
Associate Professor
Department of Otolaryngology
Vanderbilt University
Nashville, Tennessee

Leon Thurman, MS, CCC
The Voice Center
Minneapolis, Minnesota

Harvey M. Tucker, MD
Director, Centers for Otolaryngology
The Innova Medical Group
Beachwood, Ohio

Hans von Leden, MD
Institute of Laryngology and Voice Disorders
Los Angeles, California

John-Paul White
Director, Vocal Program
Oakland University
Rochester, Michigan

Preface

From the first babbles of the infant to the final sigh of the dying, the human voice is mankind's predominant method of communication. It portrays thoughts, emotions, creativity, plans, and expectations. Until relatively recent times, human history has been preserved by the sung or spoken word, with virtually all cultures having oral history.

The technologic and communication explosion over the last few centuries has allowed global dissemination of information but has made little impact on the critical role of verbal communication. The demands of the human voice have actually increased as many societies have rotated toward more service oriented occupations. The singing voice has been a venue of expression of creative thought, emotions, and political commentary. Despite these roles of the voice in human history, the care, development, and protection of the voice have largely been ignored.

With technologic advances for the evaluation of the voice, a strong interest in the performing or professional voice has developed. Objective voice assessment has allowed the expansion of the somewhat limited early interest in laryngology and voice care. The seemingly incompatible disciplines of vocal medical science and vocal arts have begun to merge as the entity of "vocal arts medicine" in an effort to help in the development of the professional voice, prevention of injury while protecting quality, and treatment of vocal dysfunction and pathology.

This book is an effort to bring the art and science of voice care into a format as a reference for all of those who are involved with professional voice care. To this end, otolaryngologists, speech–language pathologists, teachers and performers of music, and psychologists have written this text to introduce the scope of professional voice care, to discuss the need for an understanding of the anatomy, physiology, and art of voice use, to identify the resources available to deliver this care, and to introduce the future of vocal arts medicine. Pro-active preventive measures are emphasized.

The editors believe that it is in an environment of multidisciplinary collaboration and communication, research, education, and creativity that the ultimate care of the performing/professional voice can occur.

Vocal Arts Medicine: Historical and Future Perspectives

WILBUR J. GOULD, MD
GWEN S. KOROVIN, MD

Some of the earliest medical speculation on voice took place in the 5th century BC. At this time, Hippocrates recognized the importance of the lungs, trachea, lips, and tongue in the production of voice. Aristotle in further writings touched on the relationship between the voice and the soul.

Claudius Galen (131–201 AD) can be considered the founder of laryngology and voice science and was the first to distinguish between voice and speech. Further advances in the field of laryngology occurred during the Renaissance. Books and writings on the larynx were published that contained descriptions of voice disorders and hoarseness. Voice production was described, and the importance of both respiratory and voice training was discussed. In the 18th century the term *vocal folds* was first used, and the mechanisms of vocal vibration were elucidated.[1] These all evolved from anatomic visions of the researchers of that time.

In the 19th century Hermann von Helmholtz started acoustic science as a field of study.[1] Benjamin Guy Babington in 1829 was the first to describe a mirror glottiscope for evaluating the larynx indirectly, which prompted Thomas Hodgkin (Hodgkin's disease) to refer to this device as a *laryngoscope*. John Avery developed a reflecting device to add directed illumination, but its use was somewhat cumbersome.[2] Manuel Garcia, a well-recognized opera singer and singing teacher, first used the dental mirror to view the larynx in 1854. He presented this technique before the Royal Society of Medicine in 1855[1] in a treatise he entitled "Physiologic Observations of the Human Voice." He thus popularized indirect laryngoscopy, which has remained a most important part of the laryngeal examination. Shortly thereafter, Johann Czermak of Budapest refined a series of mirrors to allow for a more simplified routine evaluation of the larynx.[2]

With the ability to view the larynx came an interest in the study of voice and the larynx as a specialty. Morrell MacKenzie of England established the first voice hospital in the 1860s and developed a practice of laryngology in which instruments and equipment were designed to support such care.[2]

By the late 1800s, much interest had developed in Europe and the United States in the evaluation and treatment of laryngeal disorders. One of the first major discussions of care of the performing voice occurred in the United States in 1887 at the Ninth Annual Meeting of the American Laryngological Society. The discussions of this meeting were printed in the transactions of the meeting and centered around the "treatment of laryngitis in professionals who can't rest."[3] Many otolaryngologists participated in the discussion. Recommendations included the use of a sharp emetic followed by rest and ice in the mouth and on the neck for acute treatment. Chronic laryngitis was treated by sulfarbolate zinc, inhalation of benzoin or turpentine, or inhalation of terebene and eucalyptol in the longer term. Sprinkling turpentine on the carpet was also suggested. Chloride of ammonia tablets and carbolized spray for acute laryngitis, an astringent solution for chronic problems, and the local use of silver nitrate were mentioned. Although cocaine was advocated to help contract vessels in the nose, most felt that even though cocaine lessened the pain of laryngitis, it did not bring back tone to the vocal cords. Some warned against the use of cocaine and thought that it gave a feeling of a foreign body in the throat, and therefore a singer was unable to use the throat properly.

Some participants thought laryngitis to be caused by disease in the nasal passage or that many cases of acute and chronic laryngitis were due to digestive tract dysfunction for which emetics might be of value. The application of electricity externally to the larynx was recommended. One discussant commented that he did

not believe that there is any method by which the larynx of the professional singer can be put in perfect order while he is at work. Although so many remedies have been found to be sure cures, I doubt if any of the gentlemen have found the condition in question an easy thing to cure at all times.[3]

VOICE EVALUATION

Since the early interest in voice as a subspecialty, the field of voice has undergone amazing changes. Over the years there have been great advances, for instance, in the equipment used for evaluating the voice and visualizing the larynx. Prior to the success of Manuel Garcia, the vocal folds could not be visualized during clinical examination. The treatment of laryngeal disorders therefore were largely based on symptoms rather than direct examination. Indirect mirror laryngoscopy rapidly became the cornerstone of the laryngeal examination. Various light sources and headlights have been developed over the years to be used in conjunction with the mirror, ranging from simple head mirrors and bulbs to fiberoptic headlights.

Although direct operative laryngoscopes were developed early, 113 years passed from the time of Garcia before the next major clinical advance for vocal fold visualization in the office setting was introduced. This was the flexible fiberoptic laryngoscope, which was first introduced by Sawashima and Hirose[4] in 1968. In addition to providing better laryngeal visualization, the fiberoptic laryngoscope was of great use in examining the detailed anatomy of the nasopharynx, oropharynx, and hypopharynx, with pathologic conditions in any of these areas becoming more readily diagnosed and treated.

Although there was experimentation with rigid types of laryngoscopes adapted for visualization of the nose, throat, and larynx, the first specifically designed rigid laryngo-scope to be used in the office setting was described by Andrews and Gould[5] in 1977. This new laryngoscope allowed for closer and clearer views of the vocal folds, arytenoids, and supraglottic structures. Greater details were obtainable. In 1981, a simple method of attaching a rigid scope to a videocamera was described by Yanangisawa et al.[6]

The next significant advance in laryngeal visualization was the introduction of the stroboscope for clinical use in 1979. Earlier work with the stroboscope had been described by Moore[7] in 1937. Timcke et al[8] also published information regarding the stroboscope. However, the instrument was not yet ready for use in the clinical setting. Although the first use of stroboscopic light by the practitioner to evaluate the larynx was in the late 1970s, technologic problems had prevented its wide use.[9] Stroboscopy allowed for simulated slow motion analysis of the vocal folds and their vibratory patterns. Eventually, research advances allowed it to be used with either flexible or rigid laryngoscopes, depending on clinical needs and available equipment. By connecting the laryngoscope to a videocamera and monitor, the clinician could visualize the images and thus perform a more thorough evaluation. In addition, the patient could see his or her vocal folds and more fully understand the problem.

Advances in visual analysis research have been substantially ahead of these clinical advances. The first high speed motion pictures of the larynx were taken at Bell Laboratories in 1937.[10] High speed motion pictures were then advanced to a more quantitative level in the 1950s.[11] This progress can be attributed to the work done by pioneers such as Moore,[7] Timcke et al,[8] and Gould.[10,11]

An efficient means of evaluating these methods of visual analysis was established when Koike and Hirano[12] expounded on their mucosal wave theory in 1973.[12] Digital image processing was subsequently established in 1979, allowing for more accurate and exacting means of collecting and analyzing data from the high speed films.[13] In 1989, Colton et al[14] reported on a small microcomputer for ease and analysis of digital image processing.

In judging the value of high speed films, it became evident that the greatest value was in frame by frame analysis. The presently available processing and digital storage of videoframes digitally makes this much easier than in previous years.

Acoustic analysis, which is used in conjunction with visual analysis, has also undergone great advances over the years. The first and simplest form of acoustic evaluation was that of a skilled listener assessing the quality and characteristics of a patient's voice. Although it was at one time the only means of acoustic evaluation available, listening still remains an important, but too often overlooked, part of the patient's evaluation.

The earliest type of tape recording, or analog recording, is still widely used today. Digital recordings have recently provided more accurate high fidelity tape recordings.[15] Sound spectrograms were developed to provide basic information regarding fundamental frequency. Better devices have paved the way for more accurate measurements, and ratios have been established for quantification and comparison. These include the harmonics to noise ratio, indices of breathiness, and indices of strain.[16] Digital spectrographic instruments allow for on line analysis. Applicable computer algorithms are continually being established and modified. The GLIMPES software package, introduced and used by Scherer et al[17] of the Denver Research Institute, combines acoustic measures and various estimates of vocal fold motion. Furthermore, digital audio tape (DAT) recordings can be stored for accurate analysis at a later date. As more advances occur, these tapes can be reanalyzed to obtain even greater information.[18]

Methods of objective aerodynamic analysis have developed with the goal to determine usable air volume. Initially, basic studies were performed with pulmonary function testing and spirometers. Pneumotachographs allowed measurements of moment to moment speed of air flow.[19] Rothenberg[20] introduced a mask and later filtering techniques to extend the use of the pneumotachometer. The body plethysmograph, which was first described by

Mead[21] in 1960, gave a more accurate and complete evaluation of pulmonary function. As this instrument is cumbersome, it has not been of substantial use in the clinical setting. Hixon[22] developed a kinematic method to look at the respiratory element of vocal production as a two part system consisting of the abdomen and rib cage, with the volume of air displaced from the lungs resulting from the action of both parts. Magnetometers were used to measure volume displacements, and pulmonary functions were then determined.[22]

Researchers have also attempted to relate pulmonary function to utilization of air flow. Different transducers have been developed to determine air flow, and new components are used to measure subglottic pressure. Researchers such as Smitheran and Hixon[23] and Homberg and Leanderson[24] have used subglottic pressure and glottic air flow studies to calculate laryngeal air flow resistance.

Traditionally, sound and air flow had to be measured with separate instruments. A hot wire flowmeter, first introduced in 1980, permitted automatic calculations of the ratio of sound to air flow (AC and DC) and allowed for more rapid determinations of the vocal efficiency index.[25]

Other types of analyses are beginning to change the face of professional voice use. Electroglottography (EGG), which graphs the opening and closing of the vocal folds, is still under investigation. To date, no data show conclusively that the signal generated is actually proportional to the dynamic contact area of the approximating edge of the vocal folds.[26] Differentiated electroglottography (DEGG), photoglottography (PEGG), and echoglottography are also under investigation.[27] Electromyography can now identify the laryngeal muscles in contraction and relaxation.[28] Although the traditional method with needle electrodes is invasive, surface electrodes are being investigated for their accuracy and may be of more use for the professional voice user. Ultrasound with pulse echo ultrasonic images of the vocal folds is being used experimentally.[29]

Most of these advances, made possible by the increased body of research in laryngology, have directly resulted from the work in voice laboratories. Until 1970, there were only three voice laboratories in the United States and Canada. By 1984, there were 35 laboratories. Today there are 93 laboratories registered with the Voice Foundation.[30] Some have simple resources, while others have extensive staff and equipment.[30] The largest laboratory is at Bell Laboratories, which has been producing valuable research over the past 60 years.[31]

Voice laboratories often are affiliated with residency training programs run by attending scientists and trained otolaryngologists. Voice laboratories provide a wide variety of services, including research, diagnostic testing, and treatment planning, as well as pre- and postoperative evaluations. Test results aid in decision making and operative planning. Documentation is valuable for continuity of care and medical legal issues. There appears to be the potential for developing a "voicegram" to examine a voice as the audiogram is used to examine the ear.

The increase in the number of laboratories corresponds to the increase in interest in the field of laryngology. While greater in number, laboratories need to establish cooperation and collaboration to allow greater advances to occur. A centralized computer network could provide a valuable link. The future holds great promise for otolaryngology and the voice laboratory. Most residency training centers are already interested in or are in the process of establishing voice laboratories. This will encourage a greater number of otolaryngologists to become interested in the field. With the greater use of digital systems and a high level of computerization, advances can take place at a much faster rate.

VOICE CARE

In reviewing the history of voice care, one is struck by the similarities of thought and treatment that have prevailed throughout the years. The scientific advances and objective measures mentioned above have in many ways served to support many practices.

Physicians in the 1800s realized the importance of addressing problems of the entire upper respiratory system when treating the voice. They recognized that laryngitis could originate from many sources. In the past, nasal disease had been thought to be the "root" of laryngitis.[3] Although this has not been confirmed, advancements in visual analysis have established associations between nasal pathology and laryngeal dysfunction. Fiberoptic flexible and rigid endoscopic examinations of the nose and nasopharynx have revealed the variety of pathologic conditions that can exist in these areas.

Similarly, digestive problems have been recognized as another source of vocal difficulty. Increasingly, voice care practitioners have become aware of the effect of gastroesophageal reflux on the vocal folds. Recent advances in visual analysis show the extent of arytenoid edema and erythema, cricopharyngeal irritation, and occasional focal fold irritation caused by excessive acid reflux. Even in the late 1800s, it was thought that "digestion derangements" were causes of laryngitis.[3] Rather than the use of emetics as suggested at that time, a wide variety of medical therapies are now available for this condition, including antacids and selective antihistamines. Diagnostic tests such as barium swallows, cine-esophagrams, esophageal manometry, and pH monitoring are now used to confirm the presence of gastroesophageal reflux, hiatal hernia, esophagitis, and other digestive problems.

Many similarities in the beliefs of early laryngologists and those of today have been realized regarding maintenance of good vocal hygiene. In the 1800s, it was observed how difficult it is "to keep the larynx in perfect order" and to "cure laryngitis."[3] The need to rest the voice has been continuously recognized. In the 1800s, physicians mentioned the problems of performers being "pushed by managers."[3] Today, physicians, performers, and management are attempting to work together to maintain good vocal health for performers through communication and education.

As many similarities exist between early and contemporary laryngologists regarding the etiology and prevention of laryngeal disease so too have similarities been identified in the treatment of laryngeal dysfunction. Inhalation of substances has been used throughout time to improve laryngeal hygiene. In the 1800s, solutions used included benzoin, turpentine, terebene, eucalyptol, and perchloride of carbolized and noncarbolized carbons. Today, the value of inhalatory treatment is still recognized. Steam is usually helpful to increase moisture and release excess mucus, while mucolytics, menthol, and steroids are used occasionally.

Cocaine has been a substance of much controversy over the years. Although used more extensively for medical care in the past, the problems of a local anesthetic effect on the throat were addressed early in the history of cocaine use. It was used to contract the blood vessels in the nose and nasopharynx and thus controlled the supposed nasopharyngeal source of laryngitis. It also was used to reduce the pain of laryngeal inflammation in some cases. The foreign body sensation in the throat, however, was thought to alter the tactile sense needed for proper voice use and was thought potentially to injure the voice. Therefore the use of cocaine for treating voice disorders was not generally advocated. Interestingly, no mention of the addictive nature of the drug is made in early laryngologic or voice literature.

The irritation of the respiratory passages from chronic use of cocaine led to other medical problems, including chronic rhinitis, sinusitis, and nasal–septal perforations. With time, both the medical profession and the public have become increasingly aware of these problems. Although of occasional value in the clinical setting, the use of cocaine as a therapeutic agent has significantly decreased throughout the medical field.

With the introduction of new medications, the potential effects of the drugs on the voice have been considered. Local anesthetics, including lidocaine and lidocaine-like solutions, chloraseptic sprays, and anesthetic lozenges are now occasionally used by vocalists. Although these may relieve pain, routine use for the professional voice has been discouraged due to the potential loss of feeling in the throat. This anesthesia can lead to alterations in technique and potentially harm the voice. In addition, certain lozenges contain mentholated ingredients that can cause irritation despite their abilities to moisten the throat.

Antihistamines and decongestants have greatly aided the battle against chronic allergic and nasal disease and enjoy widespread use, although side effects of dryness and drowsiness have been identified. Mucolytic agents have been developed and refined and have been found to be extremely useful in loosening excess or dry secretions.

The use of cortisone by injection or by oral intake has a long-standing role in the care of the voice. In small, carefully controlled amounts, the antiinflammatory properties of these substances have been invaluable, but overuse has been associated with other problems and has been discouraged.

Finally, the development of antibiotics has played a large role in the treatment of the vocal performer. The use of antibiotics for infections of the nose, pharynx, and larynx has prevented many of the problems that often remained untreated in the past. Newer and better antibiotics have provided for quicker and more directed treatment. Overuse, however, has resulted in the development of antibiotic resistance and/or secondary microbial infections.

An area of voice treatment that has remained controversial is that of voice rest. In earlier times, voice rest was advised widely for the treatment of voice problems. With more sophistication in diagnosis and more experience in treatment, voice rest is advised less often. Many problems have been shown to resolve with proper voice training or retraining, while problems that appear to resolve with rest have been found to recur unless the proper use of the voice is learned. The important role of voice rest in some situations is still advocated, with good clinical judgment and appropriate objective evaluations helping in such determinations.

The role of voice training has become more apparent and has undergone some substantial changes over the years. Although the importance of breath control has been long identified, the different theories regarding respiratory, chest, and abdominal support have been debated. Nonetheless, the importance of speaking voice therapy, in addition to singing voice training, in the care of the performing voice has become recognized and is now widely accepted.

Although voice therapy and training have become indispensable and are the framework of the care provided to the vocalist, some vocal problems have not been found to be amenable to voice therapy alone. In such cases, surgery may be necessary. Newer techniques of microsurgery have improved surgical results. Microinstrumentation allows finer precision in the removal of vocal fold lesions. Laser technology has been developed, and the use of CO_2 lasers, when indicated, has improved healing and may help to control bleeding.[32] Newer laryngeal framework surgery to reposition the vocal folds or to change the tension in the vocal folds also has been developed and is valuable in some situations.[33] Surgical procedures have become more exacting because advancements in visual and acoustic analyses have helped in decision making regarding surgical indications and planning (see Chapter 21).

VOICE AS A SPECIALTY

Many organizations have been active in dealing with the assessment and treatment of voice disorders. Spearheaded often separately by otolaryngologists, voice teachers and speech–language pathologists (United States), and phoniatricians (Europe), laryngeal disorders have been evaluated and treated and advancements in care have been made. One of the most important stimuli for the field of voice was the establishment of the Voice Foundation. This organization provided a needed "voice" for the area of "care of the professional voice" and emphasized the importance of collaboration of all those who participate in such care. The Voice Foundation organized its first symposium in 1971. It was held at the Julliard School and was entitled "A Short Course on Basic Concepts of Voice for Teachers of Singing and Speech."[34] The 22nd symposium was recently held in Philadelphia.

Besides organizing the vastly popular annual symposium, the Voice Foundation is responsible for multiple publications, distribution of tapes dealing with the field of voice, and awarding grants to various investigators in the field of research. Until a few years ago, the presentations at the symposium were published as the *Transactions of the Voice Symposium*. In 1987 the *Journal of Voice* was established to publish worthy articles from the symposium along with many other scientific papers. It has become a widely accepted and respected medical journal, showing voice to be a distinct, recognizable subspecialty within the field of otolaryngology.

The Voice Foundation thus was the start of coordinated efforts and teamwork of voice scientists, laryngologists, voice therapists, and singing voice teachers. Through continued efforts, it ensures the recognition of the vocal arts and has been the impetus for worldwide organizations and the formation of satellite symposia devoted to the care of the voice professional.

A number of symposia combining arts and medicine have subsequently occurred. Some of these have been done in association with performing arts centers such as those at Miller Institute in New York, Northwestern University in Chicago, the Arts Medicine Center at Thomas Jefferson University in Philadelphia, and the Center for Evaluation and Treatment of the Performing Artist at Henry Ford Hospital in Detroit. Many hospitals and universities have now established centers dedicated to the care of performers of the arts. These centers not only deal with "vocal arts medicine" but the entire field of arts medicine and its interrelationship with voice.

New noninstitutional organizations combining medicine and the arts such as the International Arts Medicine Association (IAMA), Performing Arts Medical Association (PAMA), and Med Art, which held its first international meeting in New York in February 1992, are helping to promote vocal arts medicine. Through these various symposia and interrelationships of diverse medical fields, the emotional and physical needs of performers have been recognized. Performing arts centers often provide the interdisciplinary care, while individuals specializing in voice care have become sensitive to these needs and can make the proper referrals. These centers and organizations, therefore, have made possible "comprehensive care" of the performing vocalist.

It is interesting to note that only 12 years ago, in 1981, the first extensive article intended to teach clinicians how to approach professional singers was published by Robert Sataloff. Furthermore, the first major textbook of otolaryngology containing a full chapter on care of the professional voice was published in 1986, again written by Dr. Sataloff.[1] With respected journals such as the *Journal of Voice* and, more recently, the *Medical Problems of the Performing Artist*, along with the growing interest in the multidisciplinary aspects of performing voice care, clinical developments and scientific investigation related to the voice will be better heard.

THE FUTURE OF VOICE AS A SPECIALTY

The promotion of voice as a specialty may not have occurred without advances and objective measures. Videoimaging with stroboscopic evaluation has allowed enhanced viewing. The capability to play and replay recordings has produced the ability to pick up subtle changes not seen before. In the future, stereoscopic visualization will give movement in three dimensions, requiring enhanced measurement capabilities. Acoustic analysis developments in the future will depend on extended computer capabilities and further use of digitalization. Aerodynamic analyses will depend on better measurements of air flow, especially subglottic air flow. Further evaluations, including the efficiency of the vocal mechanism and interrelationship to the human vocal potential, are still needed. The role of various diagnostic tests, such as EGG, need to be fully evaluated. Extended use of electromyography, perhaps with wider use of noninvasive surface electrodes, will provide greater information about laryngeal muscular activity.

The view of the voice professional as a "vocal athlete" may be coming toward the forefront. Recent research serving as an initial attempt to look objectively at this hypothesis[35] may open up a new area of study. Just as a great body of research dealing with the training needs of other athletes exists, so may this occur regarding vocal athletes as well.

Newer types of surgery, including laryngeal framework surgery, will increase the current abilities to alter the voice. Intraoperative monitoring and evaluation may provide moment to moment decision making for more exact treatment.

Advancements in instrumentation will provide easier use, potentially less prohibitive cost, and more ready availability to a greater number of clinicians, therapists, and laboratories. Their more routine incorporation into clinical examination should follow. Pre- and postoperative evaluations may then always include objective measures.

Studies of both microscopic vocal folds anatomy and genetics may offer further clues about the normal vocal mechanism and pathologic conditions. Electromicroscopy may help to elucidate such findings further.

The importance of developments of objective measurements and their impact on the future of vocal science as related to the art of speaking and singing cannot be over-emphasized. The development of the stroboscope, stereoscopic enhancement of visualization, digital and other acoustic measures, and aerodynamic studies have all played a contributing role thus far.

The future direction of the vocal arts is directly dependent on objective analysis helping to direct therapy relating to the interplay of art and science. Data obtained can be used to evaluate the performer and to formulate a treatment plan. The effects of voice use and abuse can become more evident. Appropriate therapy can commence and objective measures can be used to guide these treatments. Data can be used to confirm the improvements that were previously described. Artistic experience and subjective evaluations can then be defended with objective findings.

Many of the studies being undertaken today may not seem directly applicable to the professional vocalist. However, results could be extrapolated to include this group. One example is in the study of vocal tremor as related to neurologic disorders. Data obtained from these studies may give useful information regarding vibrato and tremor in the singing voice. Thus, in the future, the benefits of further application of basic research in all areas of laryngology and voice to the field of vocal arts may be realized. While many of the same problems that have forever plagued vocalists still exist today, technologic advances and improved understanding of voice production may result in stronger understanding of nontraditional problems or may identify previously unrecognized conditions.

Although voice has been a topic of study since the 5th century BC, it remains a field in which tremendous growth is still needed. History has given us the foundation. It is a challenge to all who care for the vocal performer both now and in future generations to build upon this solid base.

REFERENCES

1. Sataloff RT: Introduction, in Sataloff RT (ed): *Professional Voice: The Science and Art of Clinical Care*. New York, Raven Press, 1991, pp 1–5.
2. Koltrie PJ, Nixon RE: The story of the laryngoscope. *Ear Nose Throat* 68:494–502, 1989.
3. The Treatment of laryngitis in professionals who are unable to rest, in *Transactions of the Ninth Annual Meeting of the American Laryngological Association*. New York, D. Appleton & Co, 1888.
4. Sawashima M, Hirose H: New Laryngoscopic Technique by Use of Fiberoptics. *J Acoust Soc Am* 43:168–170, 1968.
5. Andrews AH Jr, Gould WJ: Laryngeal and nasopharyngeal indirect telescope. *Ann Otol Rhinol Laryngol* 86:627, 1977.
6. Yanangisawa E, Casuccio A Jr, Suzuki M: Videolaryngoscopy using a rigid telescope and video home system color camera: A useful office procedure. *Ann Otol Rhinol Laryngol* 90:346–350, 1981.
7. Moore GP: Vocal fold movement during vocalization. *Speech Monogr* 4:44–55, 1937.
8. Timcke R, von Leden H, Moore P: Laryngeal vibration: Measurement of the glottic wave, part I: Normal vibratory cycle. *Arch Otolaryngol* 68:1–9, 1958.
9. Oertel MJ: Das laryngoskopische untersuchung. *Arch Laryngol Rhinol* [Berl] 3:11–16, 1895.
10. Gould WJ: The clinical voice laboratory: Clinical application of voice research. *J Voice* 1:304–309, 1988.
11. Gould WJ: The clinical voice laboratory clinical application of voice research. *Ann Otol Rhinol Laryngol* 93:346–350, 1984.
12. Koike Y, Hirano M: Glottal area time function and subglottic pressure variation. *J Acoust Soc Am* 54:1618–1627, 1973.
13. Booth J, Childers D: Automated analysis of ultra high speed laryngeal films. *IEEE Trans Biomed Eng* BME-26:185–192, 1979.
14. Colton RH, Casper JM, Brewer DW, Conture EG: Digital processing of laryngeal images: A preliminary report. *J Voice* 3:132–142, 1989.
15. Baken RJ: Sound spectrography, in Baken FJ (ed): *Clinical Measurement of Speech and Voice*. Boston, Little Brown, 1987, pp 315–392.
16. Yumato E, Gould WJ: Harmonies to noise ratio as an index of the degree of hoarseness. *J Acoust Soc Am* 71:1544–1550, 1982.
17. Scherer RC, Gould WJ, Titze IR, et al: Preliminary evaluation of selected acoustic and glottographic measures for clinical phonatory function analysis. *J Voice* 2:230–244, 1988.
18. Records of Sony Recording Division.
19. Sundberg J: Breathing, in *The Science of the Singing Voice*. Dekalb, Northern Illinois University Press, 1987, pp 24–48.

20. Rothenberg, M. Some Relations Between Glottal Air Flow and Vocal Fold Contact Area, in Ludlow, C, O'Connell, Hart, M (eds): Proceedings of the Conference on the Assessment of Vocal Pathology. *ASHA* 11:48–55, 1981.

21. Mead J: Volume displacement body plethysmograph for respiratory measurements in human speech. *J Appl Physiol* 15:736–740, 1960.

22. Hixon JJ: Speech breathing kinematics and mechanism inferences therefrom, in Gullner S, Lindblom, Lubker J, Pearson A (eds): *Speech Motor Control*. Oxford, Pergamon Press, 1982, pp 75–93.

23. Smitheran JR, Hixon TJ: A clinical method for estimating laryngeal airway resistance during vowel production. *J Speech Hearing Disord* 46:138–146, 1981.

24. Homberg E, Leanderson R: Laryngeal aerodynamics and voice quality, in Lawrence V (ed): *Transcripts of The Eleventh Symposium on the Care of the Professional Voice Medical/Surgical Sessions*. New York, The Voice Foundation, 1983, pp 124–129.

25. Kitajima N, Isshiki N, Tanabe M: Use of a hot wire flow meter in the study of laryngeal function. *Studia Phonol* 25–30, 1978.

26. Karnall MP: Synchronized videostroboscopy and electroglottography. *J Voice* 3:68–75, 1989.

27. Gerratt BP, Hanson DG, Berke GS, Precorda K: Photoglottography: a clinical synopsis. *J Voice* 5:98–105, 1991.

28. Hirano M: *Clinical Examination of the Voice*. New York, Springer-Verlag, 1981, pp 1–98.

29. Hertz, Lindstron, Somesson B: Ultrasonic recording of the vibrating vocal folds: A preliminary report. *Acta Otolaryngol* 69:223–230, 1970.

30. Gould WJ, Korovin GS: Advances in voice laboratory research. *J Voice* 1991, in press.

31. Farnsworth DW: High speed motion pictures of the human vocal cords. *Bell Lab Rec* 18:203–208, 1940.

32. Abitbol J: Limitation of the laser in microsurgery of the larynx, in Lawrence VL (ed): *Transactions of the Twelfth Symposium: Care of the Professional Voice*. New York, The Voice Foundation, 1984, pp 297–301.

33. Isshiki N, Taira T, Tanage M: Surgical alteration of the vocal pitch. *J Otolaryngol* 12:335–340, 1983.

34. Brewer DW: Voice research: The next ten years. *J Voice* 3:7–17, 1989.

35. Saxon KG, Michel JF: The singer as athlete: Lessons from applied and exercise physiology. *J Voice* 1992, in press.

2

Gross and Microscopic Anatomy of the Larynx

HARVEY M. TUCKER, MD

Because of its location at the crossroads of the air and food passages, the larynx serves as a conduit for air to and waste gases from the lungs and as a valve to prevent the passage of secretions, food, and foreign material into the upper respiratory tract. In humans it has also come to serve as an organ of communication—its phylogenetically "youngest" function. The gross and microscopic anatomy of the larynx, which knowledge is essential to an understanding of phonatory disorders and their management, is reviewed in this chapter.

GROSS ANATOMY

Skeletal Support

The structural supports of the larynx include six cartilages and the hyoid bone. Three of the cartilages are bilaterally symmetric and paired. They are connected to each other by membranes and ligaments that are named for the structures to which they are attached.

The hyoid bone (Fig. 2–1) makes up the anterior aspect of the preepiglottic space and is the point of attachment for muscles and ligaments above and below it. It is not part of the larynx proper, but, since it is intimately involved in laryngeal function, it must be considered in any discussion of laryngeal anatomy. It is named for its *U* shape and is situated at the level of the third cervical vertebra (adult), just superior to the thyroid cartilage in the anterior wall of the hypopharynx and anterior and inferior to the base of the tongue. Its parts include the body, bilateral greater cornua, and bilateral lesser cornua. Because it is suspended between the supra- and infrahyoid musculature and articulates with no other cartilaginous or bony structure it can be considered a true sesamoid bone. It produces the concavity between the chin and the anterior neck.

The body is convex forward and from side to side. It is separated by fat and a bursa from the thyrohyoid membrane, which in turn is separated by fat from the anterior surface of the epiglottis. Small tuberosities called the *lesser cornua* are found at either end of the body on its upper surface and serve as points of attachment for the medial ends of the middle

---

This chapter was modified by the author, in part, from Chapter 1 in Tucker HM: *The Larynx*. New York, Thieme Medical Publishers, 1987.

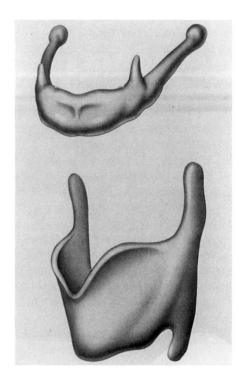

Figure 2–1. Hyoid bone and thyroid cartilage.

constrictor muscles and of the stylohyoid ligaments. The geniohyoid and genioglossus muscles are attached to the upper and inner surfaces of the body, while the mylohyoid muscle inserts upon the anterior surface of the body of the hyoid bone. The greater cornua, which are hornlike structures that extend posteriorly and laterally from the body, give rise to the remainder of the middle constrictor and hyoglossus muscles. The tendon of the digastric muscle is attached to the anterolateral aspect of the body of the hyoid bone by a retinaculum. The remaining muscles attached to the hyoid are the infrahyoid group (sternohyoid, omohyoid, and thyrohyoid muscles). The superior laryngeal nerve, artery, and vein pass in close proximity to the greater cornua of the hyoid bone as they traverse the middle and inferior constrictor muscles to enter the larynx via a hiatus in the thyrohyoid ligament.

The cartilages that make up the laryngeal skeleton include the thyroid, cricoid, and epiglottis and the paired arytenoids, corniculates, and cuneiforms. The thyroid cartilage (Fig. 2–1), which is named for its shieldlike shape when seen en face, is the largest of these and is commonly called the "Adam's apple." It is shaped like a wedge, the sides of which are called the *laminae*. These join each other at the midline to form the laryngeal prominence. These laminae meet at an angle of approximately 90 degrees in males and 120 degrees in females, thus accounting for the more prominent larynx in the male. At their juncture in the midline is a thyroid notch. The superior, greater and the inferior, lesser cornua of the thyroid cartilage are noted bilaterally, at the posterior edges of the laminae. The oblique line is palpable and visible approximately three-fourths of the way from the anterior commissure to the posterior edge of the lamina. It serves as the point of attachment for the major muscles and ligaments in this area. The thyroid cartilage articulates with the cricoid cartilage via the inferior cornua. The inferior border of the thyroid lamina gives attachment to the cricothyroid ligament and along the rest of its inferior margin to the cricothyroideus muscle. The outer surfaces of the laminae give rise to the omohyoid, sternothyroid, and inferior constrictor muscles along the oblique line. The upper border of the thyroid cartilage provides attachment for the thyrohyoid membrane and ligament. The attachment of the ventricular bands and the thyroepiglottic ligament is located on the inner surface, at a point approximately halfway between the thyroid notch and the inferior border in males and at approximately the junction of the superior one-third and inferior two-thirds in females. There is a palpable tuberosity at this point in older larynges. Broyles' ligament, which is the fibrous attachment of the vocal ligaments, penetrates the inner perichondrium of the cartilage and makes contact with the outer perichondrium. The tips of the greater cornua of the thyroid cartilage are attached to the tips of the greater cornua of the hyoid bone by a dense fibrous band that sometimes contains a small sesamoid cartilage (see Fig. 2–6). The thyroid cartilage serves as the point of attachment to the thyroarytenoid muscles on the lower half of its inner surface.

The cricoid cartilage (Fig. 2–2) is shaped like an asymmetric signet ring. Its lower border is horizontal, and the upper border constitutes the signet part of the lamina, which rises above the horizontal between the thyroid laminae posteriorly. The anterior or arch portion is easily palpated immediately below the border of the thyroid cartilage. The cricoid is the only complete cartilaginous ring in the upper airway, since all of the others are deficient in the posterior aspect. It articulates with the thyroid cartilage through the

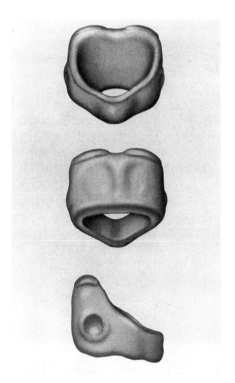

Figure 2–2. Cricoid cartilage. **A**, Anterior view. **B**, Posterior view. **C**, Right lateral view.

cricothyroid joints bilaterally and with the arytenoids, which rest on the upper surface of its posterior or "signet ring" portion. Inferiorly, it is related to the first tracheal ring via ligamentous and musculature attachments only. The cricothyroid ligament and lateral cricoarytenoid muscles are attached anteriorly, along the superior surface of the arch, while its inferior rim gives rise to the cricotracheal ligament. The posterior aspect of the lamina of the cricoid cartilage gives origin to the posterior cricoarytenoideus muscles on either side of the midline. Laterally, the cricoid cartilage receives the lowermost fibers of the inferior constrictor muscle and the semicircular fibers of the cricopharyngeus muscle.

The arytenoid cartilages (Fig. 2–3) are situated bilaterally and shaped like small, three-sided pyramids, the bases of which are concave to provide the articular facets that glide upon the corresponding facets of the posterosuperior aspect of the cricoid lamina. These cartilages are flat on their medial surfaces and are covered only by mucoperichondrium, very tightly applied to the cartilage. The posterior curved surface receives the fibers of the transverse and oblique arytenoideus muscles (sometimes referred to as *interarytenoideus muscles*). The thyroarytenoid muscles are attached to a small tubercle on the posterolateral surface. A prominent muscular process is found at the posterolateral corner, which receives the lateral and posterior cricoarytenoid muscles. The anteromedial, pointed portion is referred to as the *vocal process*. It is the point of attachment for the vocal ligament that is connected to the midline of the inner surface of the thyroid cartilage and forms the structural support of the true vocal folds themselves. The upright process or apex of the arytenoid cartilage is directed anteromedially and serves as the posterior attachment of the aryepiglottic fold.

The corniculate and cuneiform cartilages (Fig. 2–3) are located within the substance of the aryepiglottic fold. They are sesamoid cartilages that serve as battens to prevent the collapse of this membranous structure.

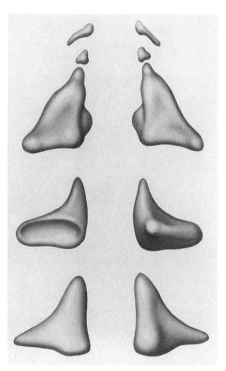

Figure 2–3. Arytenoid cartilages. **A**, Posterior view with cuneiform and corniculate cartilages above. **B**, Inferior view, left; superior view, right. **C**, Anterior view.

The epiglottic cartilage (Fig. 2–4) is the only one of the laryngeal supporting structures composed of elastic cartilage. It is leaf shaped and makes up the skeleton of the epiglottis. It is suspended by a series of ligaments and does not articulate directly with any of the surrounding bony or cartilaginous structures. Its surface is penetrated by multiple small holes that transmit tiny blood vessels and fibrous tissue attachments from its laryngeal surface to the preepiglottic space. The laryngeal surface is covered with tightly adherent mucoperichondrium, whereas the anterior or lingual surface is the posterior wall of the preepiglottic space, which contains loose areolar tissue and fat. Inferiorly, the epiglottis is attached to the inner surface of the thyroid cartilage by the thyroepiglottic ligament. It is attached to the inner surface of the body of the hyoid bone by the midline hyoepiglottic ligament and laterally to the musculature of the base of the tongue by the glossoepiglottic ligaments. The valleculae are bilateral, pouchlike mucosal reflections between the median hyoepiglottic ligament and the lateral glossoepiglottic ligaments. The lateral surface of the epiglottis gives rise to the fibers of the oblique and posterior arytenoid muscles, which send slips into the aryepiglottic fold and ligament. Posteriorly, the mucosa of the aryepiglottic fold separates the laryngeal introitus from the opening to the pyriform sinus. The cuneiform and corniculate cartilages can sometimes be seen as a bulge through the mucosa of the aryepiglottic fold (see Fig. 2–7).

Joints, Membranes, and Ligaments of the Larynx

Only the thyroid, cricoid, and arytenoid cartilages articulate directly with any of the other skeletal structures of the larynx. The cricoid cartilage is the base and support for the entire larynx. It articulates with the thyroid cartilage via the cricothyroid joints and with the

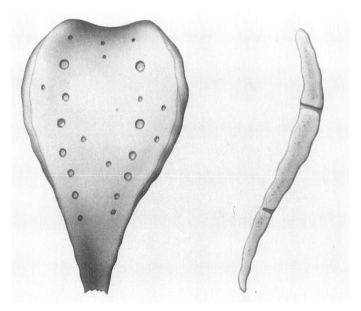

Figure 2–4. Epiglottic cartilage. Note perforations.

arytenoid cartilages via the cricoarytenoid joints (Fig. 2–5). Both of these are true synovial joints.

The cricothyroid joint permits the cricoid cartilage to tilt upward so that the anterior arch can more closely approximate the lower border of the thyroid cartilage. The thyroid cartilage is also able to slide in an anterior and posterior direction along the same joint secondary to the pull of the cricothyroideus muscles (see Fig. 2–12).

The cricoarytenoid joints are located on the posterosuperior aspect of the cricoid lamina. The articular surfaces on the cricoid lamina are oriented in a slightly posterior direction and are biconcave (Fig. 2–5). The articular surfaces on the under side of the arytenoid cartilages are also biconcave, the concavity being directed medially as well as inferiorly. When these joints come into contact with each other, the arytenoid will seek the lowest point of the concavity of both joints, unless there is some muscular pull to the contrary. This accounts for the position assumed by the vocal cords at rest, which is approximately halfway between the midline and full abduction. The movement of the arytenoid cartilages on the cricoarytenoid joints appears to be rotary, but is actually due to the sliding effect in both the anteroposterior and lateromedial directions.

The thyrohyoid membrane (Fig. 2–6) is a broad elastic sheet that stretches from the upper border of the thyroid cartilage, passes beneath the body of the hyoid bone, and inserts on its upper surface. Medially this membrane is thicker and can be identified as the *median thyrohyoid ligament* and laterally as the *lateral thyrohyoid ligament.* A triticeous cartilage is sometimes noted in the lateralmost aspects of this ligament between the tip of the greater cornu of the hyoid bone and the greater cornu of the thyroid cartilage. The membrane is penetrated on each side by the superior laryngeal artery, vein, and internal

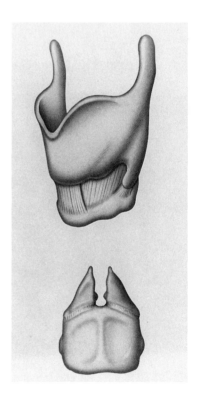

Figure 2–5. Cricothyroid joint, membrane, and ligament, above; cricoarytenoid joints, posterior view, below.

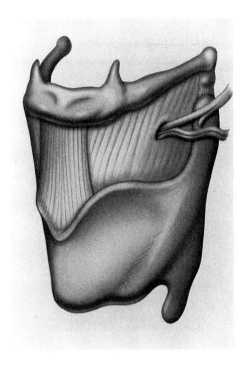

Figure 2–6. Thyrohyoid membrane, ligament, and superior laryngeal neurovascular bundle. Note sesamoid cartilages between greater cornua of thyroid cartilage and hyoid bone.

laryngeal branch of the superior nerve. The outer surface of this membrane is covered by the infrahyoid muscles. With the hyoid bone, it completes the anterior limits of the preepiglottic space (Fig. 2–7).

The cricovocal membrane or conus elasticus (Figs. 2–7, 2–8) arises from the inner surface of the cricoid arch, passing medially and superiorly to insert upon the *vocal ligaments* (see Fig. 2–13), which stretch between the vocal processes of the arytenoid cartilages and the midline inner surface of the thyroid cartilage. The vocal ligaments are condensations of the cricovocal membrane and form the structure of the free margin of the membranous vocal fold. This vocal ligament is surrounded by the medialmost fibers of the lateral thyroarytenoideus muscles, which are sometimes regarded as a separate structure called the *vocalis muscle*.

A less well-defined quadrangular membrane (Figs. 2–7, 2–8) arises from the inner aspects of the epiglottis within the aryepiglottic fold and attaches posteriorly to the arytenoid and corniculate cartilages. Inferiorly it attaches to the vestibular ligament (false cord) and extends inferiorly around the ventricle to the point of attachment of the upper margin of the true vocal folds.

Cavities and Mucous Membrane

The laryngeal introitus (Fig. 2–9) is a roughly triangular-shaped opening in the anterior wall of the pharynx, with its base along the free edge of the epiglottis and its apex at the point between the two arytenoid cartilages. The sides are made up of the aryepiglottic

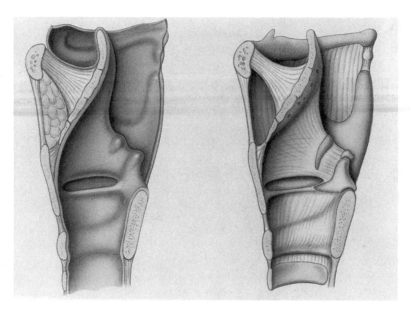

Figure 2–7. Midline cutaway view of larynx. Mucous membrane intact, left; internal membranes exposed, right.

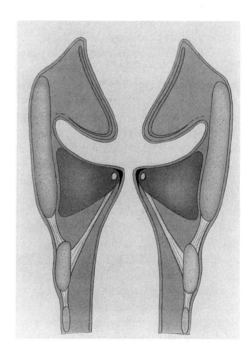

Figure 2–8. Coronal section of larynx (semidiagrammatic).

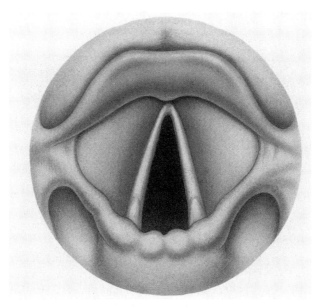

Figure 2–9. Larynx from above. Laryngeal mirror view.

folds of mucous membrane that stretch between the tips of the arytenoid cartilages and the lateral borders of the epiglottis. There are variable aryepiglottic muscle fibers within the aryepiglottic folds.

The vestibule, the glottis, and the infraglottic area make up the internal cavity of the larynx. The vestibule or supraglottic area stretches from the free margin of the epiglottis and aryepiglottic folds inferiorly to the lower margin of the false cords (ventricular bands). The ventricle is the laterally directed sac between the undersurface of the ventricular bands and the upper surface of the true vocal folds. At its anterior end is a small blind sac called the *saccule* or *appendix* of the ventricle. Posteriorly the vestibule abuts upon the fold of mucosa between the arytenoid cartilages and the interarytenoideus muscles. The true vocal folds (vocal cords) form the rima glottidis (glottis, glottic chink) as the space between them. They are approximately 15 mm long in the male and 10 mm in the female. The area within the larynx beginning at the free margin of the vocal folds and extending down to the lower margin of the cricoid cartilage and medial to the cricovocal membrane is referred to as the subglottic or infraglottic area.

The pyriform sinus is a deep recess lateral to the aryepiglottic folds that is closed anteriorly but open posteriorly. It is situated between the inner surface of the upper portion of the thyroid cartilage and thyrohyoid membrane laterally and the lateral surface of the aryepiglottic folds and cricoid cartilage medially (Figs. 2–8, 2–9; see also Fig. 2–13).

The various membranes, ligaments, and skeletal structures of the larynx delineate several potential spaces and compartments. These include the preepiglottic space, the paraglottic space, and the subglottic space.

The preepiglottic space (Fig. 2–7) is bounded by the hyoepiglottic ligament superiorly (valleculae), by the thyrohyoid membrane and ligament anteriorly, and by the anterior surface of the epiglottis and thyroepiglottic ligament posteriorly. It is shaped like an inverted pyramid. It is contiguous with the superior part of the paraglottic space laterally. It contains fat and loose areolar tissue.

The paraglottic space (Fig. 2–8) is bounded laterally by the inner surface of the thyroid cartilage, inferomedially by the conus elasticus, medially by the ventricle, and superomedially by the quadrangular membrane. It communicates superiorly with the space between the thyroid cartilage and hyoid bone, anteriorly with the preepiglottic space near the petiole of the epiglottis, and inferiorly with the space between the thyroid and cricoid cartilages. Posteriorly it is closed off by the reflection of pyriform sinus mucosa. At the level of the vocal fold and ventricle, it is divided by muscular and ligamentous attachments into supraglottic and infraglottic parts.

The subglottic space (Fig. 2–8) is bounded superiorly by the undersurface of Broyles' ligament at the midline, laterally by the medial surface of the conus elasticus, and medially by the subglottic mucosa. Inferiorly, it is continuous with the inner surface of the cricoid cartilage and its mucosa.

The larynx is lined by respiratory, pseudostratified, columnar, ciliated epithelium with goblet cells, except for the vocal folds themselves, which are covered with stratified squamous, nonkeratinizing epithelium that contains no glands or epithelial appendages. Immediately beneath the mucosa of the vocal folds is Reinke's space, which stretches from the tips of the vocal processes to the anterior commissure and overlies the muscles of the vocal fold and the vocal ligament. It contains loose areolar tissue and is essential to the free "flow" of the loose mucosa over the vocal folds during phonation.

Musculature

Extrinsic Muscles

The extrinsic muscles of the larynx are also sometimes referred to as the *strap muscles*. The infrahyoid group includes the omohyoid, sternothyroid, thyrohyoid, and sternohyoid muscles. They are innervated by branches of the descendens hypoglossi portion of the ansa hypoglossi (first to fourth cervical nerves) (Fig. 2–10).

The suprahyoid group includes the digastric, stylohyoid, geniohyoid, mylohyoid, stylopharyngeus, and thyrohyoid muscles, all of which are elevators of the larynx. The middle and inferior constrictor muscles are also extrinsic laryngeal muscles but play their most important role in swallowing and have little or no effect on the intrinsic functions of the larynx. The supra- and infrahyoid groups of muscles meet at the hyoid bone, which serves as a direction-changing point. As a result, their synergistic action is capable of fixing the laryngotracheal complex in any position from its most depressed to its most elevated. The depressor (infrahyoid) group of muscles displaces the larynx downward during the inspiratory phase of respiration, while the elevators lift it during most expiratory cycles. The major displacement of the larynx takes place during deglutition, when the elevator muscles move the larynx both forward and superiorly, which, associated with the downward movement of the base of the tongue, compresses the epiglottis over the laryngeal introitus as one of the major mechanisms to prevent aspiration.

The middle and inferior constrictor muscles (Fig. 2–11) are extrinsic muscles of the larynx but act mostly during deglutition. The cricopharyngeus muscle (Fig. 2–12) may be

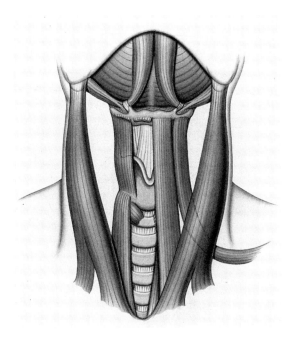

Figure 2–10. Strap muscles.

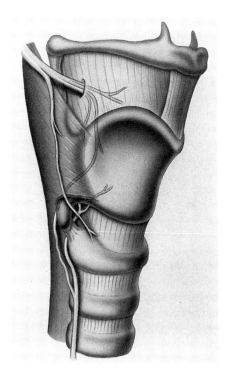

Figure 2–11. Nerve supply of the larynx.
Also note inferior constrictor muscle.

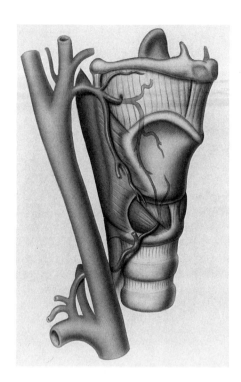

Figure 2–12.   Arterial supply of larynx. Also note cricothyroideus.

regarded as an extrinsic muscle of respiration in that it favors aspiration if it does not function in a timely fashion. The remaining extrinsic muscle of the larynx is the crico-thyroideus (Fig. 2–12). This muscle is innervated by the external branch of the superior laryngeal nerve and is most important during swallowing but also plays a part in increasing tension in the vocal folds, especially at the extreme upper range of pitch or loudness. Its two heads, the oblique and the horizontal, impart a sliding motion in an anteroposterior direction, as well as a rocking motion. The thyroid cartilage is relatively fixed by the strap muscles and the cricoid cartilage moves relative to it. Thus contraction of the crico-thyroideus muscle, which is always bilateral and symmetric under normal circumstances, draws the anteriormost aspect of the cricoid ring upward toward the lowermost aspect of the thyroid ala. This in effect rocks the cricoid lamina posteriorly and applies additional tension to the vocal ligaments, providing that the posterior cricoarytenoid muscle is intact to hold the arytenoid cartilages in position.

Intrinsic Muscles

The intrinsic muscles of the larynx are all innervated by the recurrent laryngeal nerve. They include (1) the posterior cricoarytenoid (the only abductor of the vocal cords); (2) lateral cricoarytenoid; (3) transverse arytenoid; (4) oblique arytenoid; (5) thyroarytenoid (including the vocalis); and the two minor slips of muscle representing (6) the aryepiglottic and (7) the thyroepiglottic muscles (Figs. 2–13, 2–14).

The posterior cricoarytenoid muscle arises from the midline raphe on the posterior aspect of the cricoid lamina. The fibers run superiorly and laterally, converging to insert

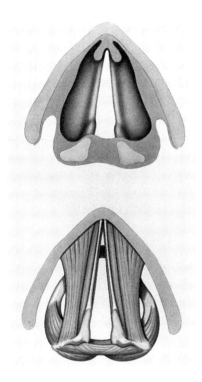

Figure 2–13. Horizontal section of larynx through the ventricles. Mucosa intact, above; mucosa removed to show intrinsic muscles of vocal folds, below.

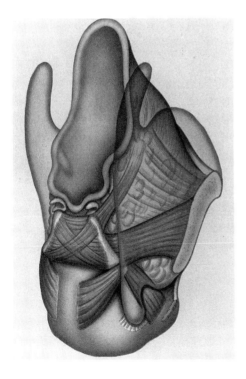

Figure 2–14.   Intrinsic muscles of the larynx.

on the posterior surface of the muscular process of the arytenoid cartilage. As the only abductor of the vocal folds, it serves to open the glottis by a "rotary" motion imparted to the arytenoid cartilages around an apparent axis of the cricoarytenoid joints. Some of the fibers of the muscle then can draw the arytenoid bodies laterally, separating the vocal processes and the vocal folds. During phonation, the posterior cricoarytenoid muscle also serves to tense the vocal fold by acting as an antagonist to the other muscles of the larynx so that the arytenoid cartilage is pulled posteriorly or fixed in position, thus resisting the pull of the other tensor muscles.

The lateral cricoarytenoid muscle has fibers arising from the upper border of the arch of the cricoid cartilage that pass obliquely backward toward the anterior aspect of the muscular process of the arytenoid cartilage. Its action is to close the glottis by adducting the vocal folds, which it does by rotating the arytenoid cartilages medially, bringing the vocal processes together.

The transverse arytenoideus (interarytenoideus) is the only unpaired muscle, and its fibers arise from the muscular process and lateral border of the arytenoid cartilage on each side, crossing the midline. It makes up most of the posterior commissure of the larynx. Its pull approximates the bodies of the arytenoid cartilages, thus closing the posterior aspect of the glottis when the vocal processes have already been brought into apposition.

The oblique arytenoid muscle is made up of diagonal, transverse fascicles that interdigitate between the upright portions of the arytenoid cartilages, in conjunction with the interarytenoid muscles. Its uppermost fibers continue along the aryepiglottic fold, forming the aryepiglottic muscle (Fig. 2–14). The combined action of these two muscles has a sphincteric effect on the introitus of the larynx, closing it down like a purse string during the act of swallowing.

The thyroarytenoideus (Fig. 2–13) is a very broad muscle that arises from the entire inner surface of the inferior half of the thyroid cartilage and also from the conus elasticus. It passes posteriorly and laterally, as well as superiorly, and inserts on the anterolateral surface and vocal process of the arytenoid cartilage. This muscle is usually divided into three parts for anatomic purposes. The first of these are the parallel fibers that arise just lateral to the vocal ligament and sometimes surround it and are usually referred to as the *thyroarytenoideus internus* or *vocalis muscle*. This muscle is classed as an adductor of the larynx, but, once the folds have been brought into close apposition, it is the major tensor of the free edge of the vocal fold. It may also take part in a change in the cross-sectional shape of the free margin, "thinning" the vocal fold as higher pitches are approached. The more lateral and superficial fibers of the thyroarytenoideus are referred to as the *externa*. This is the major adductor of the vocal fold. The third part of the muscle is referred to as the *thyroepiglotticus* and is made up of fibers that pass posteriorly and superiorly to insert into the aryepiglottic fold and along the margin of the epiglottis. Contraction of this muscle draws the arytenoid cartilages forward and downward toward the thyroid cartilage, the result of which is shortening of the vocal ligaments and relaxation of the mucous membrane covering them.

Although each of these intrinsic muscles of the larynx can be assigned an apparent function, it is important to note that the action of these muscles changes, depending on the position of the vocal folds and arytenoids at any given moment. Moreover, the interaction of agonist and antagonist muscles also must be taken into account to understand fully the true function of this exquisitely balanced organ.

Blood Supply

The arterial blood supply of the larynx (Fig. 2–12) is derived from branches of the superior and inferior thyroid arteries and to a small extent from the cricothyroid branch of the superior thyroid artery. The superior thyroid artery is the first branch of the external carotid artery and, in a few cases, actually arises from the bifurcation of the carotid or even the common carotid artery. It passes anteriorly in a superiorly directed loop and, usually near the tip of the greater cornu of the hyoid bone, gives off a small infrahyoid branch. It then goes on a short distance and bifurcates near the tip of the superior cornu of the thyroid cartilage to give off the superior laryngeal artery and continues as the superior thyroid artery on the lateral surface of the middle and inferior constrictor muscles. The superior thyroid artery terminates in the upper pole of the thyroid gland, giving off a small branch to the sternocleidomastoid muscle. The superior laryngeal artery, in company with the superior laryngeal nerves and veins, enters the larynx by penetrating a hiatus in the thyrohyoid ligament, after which it arborizes to supply the area above the vocal folds. There is, however, extensive interconnection with the inferior blood supply of the larynx. The inferior laryngeal artery, which is a continuation of the inferior thyroid artery branch of the thyrocervical trunk, travels superiorly in the groove between the trachea and esophagus in concert with the recurrent laryngeal nerve. It enters the larynx, passing deep to the lowermost fibers of the inferior constrictor muscle with the recurrent laryngeal nerve. It supplies the portion of the larynx inferior to the free margins of the vocal folds, but interconnects freely with its opposite number and with the branches of the superior laryngeal artery. A small cricothyroid artery, which is another branch of the superior thyroid artery, may pass across the upper portion of the cricothyroid ligament and anastomose with its opposite number. Small perforators often enter the cricothyroid membrane from this vessel.

Venous Drainage

Venous drainage (Fig. 2–15) is supplied by the superior and inferior laryngeal veins, which essentially follow the arteries in their course. The superior drainage joins the superior and middle thyroid veins and thence the internal jugular vein. The inferior drainage joins the middle thyroid vein, which is itself emptied into the jugular vein. There is some venous drainage to the inferior thyroid vein, basically a midline structure, and it empties directly into the superior vena cava.

Lymphatic Drainage

The larynx is very well supplied with lymphatics (Fig. 2–16), with the exception of the free margins of the vocal folds themselves. The lymphatics superior to the ventricle cross freely from one side to the other and drain into the superior and middle group of jugular nodes. Drainage from the inferior portion of the larynx, on the other hand, although there is some crossover, tends to be isolated from side to side. The drainage is through the cricothyroid membrane to the middle and inferior jugular group and paratracheal group of lymph nodes.

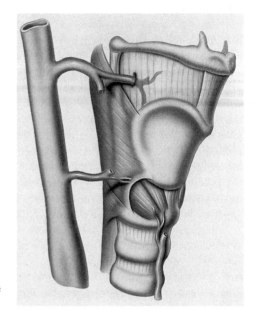

Figure 2–15. Venous drainage from the larynx.

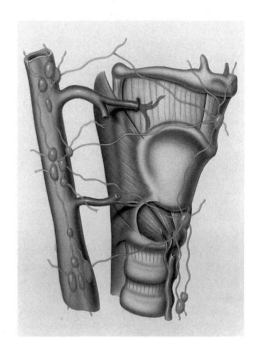

Figure 2–16. Lymphatic drainage from the larynx.

Nerve Supply

The larynx receives its major motor supply and all of the sensory supply below the free margins of the vocal folds via the recurrent laryngeal branch of the vagus nerve (Fig. 2–11). Sensation above the vocal folds is carried by the internal branch of the superior laryngeal nerve, which also has an external motor branch that supplies the cricothyroideus muscle. The larynx likewise receives nerve supply from both the sympathetic and parasympathetic systems.

The superior laryngeal nerve separates from the main trunk of the vagus just outside the jugular foramen at the skull base. It then travels in close proximity to the main trunk, diverging from it above the greater cornu of the hyoid bone. It passes anteromedially on the thyrohyoid membrane where it is joined by the superior thyroid artery and vein. At approximately this level the external laryngeal nerve leaves the main trunk and descends on the surface of the inferior constrictor of the pharynx, deep to the sternothyroid muscles. It sends branches both to the pharyngeal plexus and to the inferior constrictor and finally reaches the cricothyroid muscle, which it supplies. The main *internal laryngeal* nerve continues on the surface of the thyrohyoid membrane in company with and just superior to the superior laryngeal artery and enters the membrane through a hiatus. Immediately within the membrane it divides into three sets of branches: ascending, transverse, and descending. These supply, in the same order, the mucosa of the vallecula and the epiglottis, the pyriform sinus, and the larynx as far inferiorly as the vocal fold. On the medial wall of the pyriform sinus, the descending branches give twigs to the transverse arytenoideus muscle via a plexus and then continue behind the cricoid cartilage as a fine filament that communicates with the recurrent laryngeal nerve. This is referred to as the *ansa galeni*.

Parasympathetic fibers destined for the larynx travel with the superior and recurrent laryngeal nerves from their origin within the jugular foramen. Sympathetic fibers arrive in the larynx in company with the blood vessels, having arisen from the superior cervical sympathetic ganglion near the bifurcation of the carotid.

The recurrent laryngeal nerve is derived as a branch of the vagus nerve, on the left side as it passes the arch of the aorta and on the right side as it passes the subclavian artery. In the latter case the nerve passes from anterior to posterior around the subclavian artery and "recurs" in the tracheoesophageal groove on the right side. As it travels superiorly, it supplies the trachea and esophagus, especially providing fibers to the cricopharyngeus muscle. The left recurrent laryngeal nerve passes lateral to the ligamentum arteriosum behind the arch of the aorta and enters the tracheoesophageal groove. It, too, provides segmental branches to the esophagus and trachea as it ascends. At the lower pole of the thyroid gland it runs between the branches of the inferior thyroid artery and is in intimate proximity to the posterior and medial aspects of the thyroid gland. It reaches the larynx, as does the right recurrent laryngeal nerve, by running under the border of the inferior constrictor muscle of the pharynx, which it also supplies. A communication with the internal laryngeal nerve (the ansa galeni) leaves the recurrent laryngeal nerve some little distance before it reaches the lower margin of the inferior constrictor muscle. The main trunk of the nerve then approaches the larynx at the cricothyroid joint. In the majority of cases the nerve passes posterior to this joint, but in up to 10 to 15 percent of adults it passes either anterior to the joint or splits, sending one trunk posterior and one anterior.

MICROSCOPIC ANATOMY

The mucous membrane lining the larynx is continuous with that of the hypopharynx above and the trachea below. It is mostly respiratory epithelium; that is, it is pseudostratified, ciliated, columnar epithelium with goblet cells (Fig. 2–17). The major exception to this is the vocal folds themselves, which are covered by nonkeratinizing, stratified squamous epithelium with no glandular elements (see Fig. 3–1 in Chapter 3). Stratified squamous epithelium is also found on the anterior surface of the epiglottis, the free margins of the aryepiglottic folds, and in patches here and there in otherwise healthy respiratory epithelium.

The *mucous* and *serous glands*, which provide lubrication and protection for the vocal folds, are largely located within the saccule of the ventricle. Secretions are literally squeezed out onto the upper surface of the membranous vocal fold like toothpaste from a tube. Additional glandular elements are located near the bodies of the arytenoid cartilages, along the free margins of the false vocal cords, and near the posterior commissure.

The epithelium is tightly adherent to the laryngeal surface of the epiglottis and the bodies of the arytenoid cartilages via a true mucoperichondrium. Elsewhere, there is a variable submucosa containing fat and/or loose areolar tissue. The tissues immediately beneath the epithelium can be regarded as a lamina propria consisting of three layers. The most superficial of these is Reinke's space, composed of fibrous tissues and matrix (see Fig. 3–1). It contains very few fibroblasts. This space is critical to the "flowing" movement of the mucous membrane over the underlying ligaments and musculature that is necessary

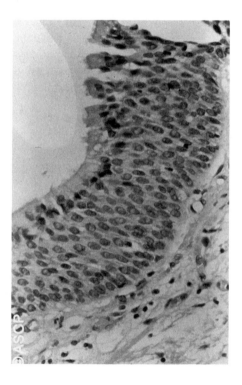

Figure 2–17.   Respiratory epithelium from false vocal fold. Note pseudostratified, ciliated columnar cells and goblet cells.

for normal voice production. The intermediate layer of the lamina propria is made up of elastic fibers and a more dense population of fibroblasts than the superficial layer. The *deep* layer of the lamina propria is composed of dense collagenous fibers and many fibroblasts.

BIBLIOGRAPHY

Abelson TI, Tucker HM: Laryngeal findings in superior laryngeal nerve paralysis: A controversy. *Otolaryngol Head Neck Surg* 89:463–470, 1981.

Broyles EN: The anterior commissure tendon. *Ann Otol Rhinol Laryngol* 52:341, 1943.

Gray H: *The Anatomy of the Human Body*. Philadelphia, Lea and Febiger, 1973.

Hast H: Anatomy of the larynx, in English GM (ed): *Otolaryngology*. Philadelphia, Harper and Row, 1987.

Lockhart RD, Hamilton GF, Fyfe FW: *Anatomy of the Human Body*. Philadelphia, JB Lippincott, 1960.

Tucker HM: *The Larynx*. New York, Thieme Medical Publishers, 1987.

3

Physiology of Phonation

RAYMOND H. COLTON, PHD

Over the past 20 or so years, there has been a resurgence of interest in the voice. Professionals such as speech–language pathologists, physicians, and voice teachers have focused their attention on the voice, producing increased knowledge and understanding of how the voice works. More professional meetings have been devoted to the voice. Foremost among these meetings is the annual Care of the Professional Voice Symposium, held for many years in New York and more recently in Philadelphia. At this meeting, diverse groups from voice science, speech–language pathology, laryngology, singing, and voice pedagogy meet to learn from each other about a wide variety of problems that affect the professional voice user. From these meetings and others (e.g., The Vocal Fold Physiology conferences) have come an expanded research base and the attempt to place into practice the new ideas and concepts emanating from research. Singers and voice teachers in turn have demanded from the researcher and physician relevant studies of the professional voice and methods for its care. In recent years, the desire for the development of standards of voice analysis has increased.

There have been many significant developments in our knowledge about the voice. Among these have been the body-cover model of voice production, computer modeling of vocal fold vibration, and improved and new instruments for the analysis of voice function (e.g., inverse filtered air flow, electroglottograph, stroboscopy) that have greatly aided in the pursuit of knowledge and understanding about the vocal apparatus.

In this chapter, some of these ideas and concepts are discussed in the context of the basic functioning of the voice. First, the physiologic processes involved in the initiation and continuation of the voice are reviewed. Basic concepts as well as newer ideas about the control of vocal pitch are presented. This is followed by a discussion of the physiologic mechanisms for the control of vocal loudness and then vocal quality. Finally, a brief section concerned with the physiology of the voice during singing is presented.

GLOTTAL TONE INITIATION

The Body-Cover Model and Its Implications for Phonation

In the early 1970s, Minoru Hirano[1] reported on his work on the fine anatomy of the vocal folds. He postulated that the vocal folds are a layered structure consisting of a body (the muscle) and a cover (the connective tissue covering the muscle). Anatomically, he

30

demonstrated that the vocal folds consist of epithelium (the outermost layer, like skin), a lamina propria (a middle layer itself consisting of several layers), and the thyroarytenoid muscle (Fig. 3–1). The lamina propria consists of three layers. The superficial layer consists of loose fibrous components and is very pliable. The intermediate layer consists of elastic fibers (also pliable), whereas the deep layer consists of collagenous fibers (more stiff layer). Each of these layers would be expected to exhibit different mechanical characteristics. Many supporting studies by Hirano and his colleagues[2,3] have provided further information on the characteristics of this layered structure and on the mechanical characteristics of the various layers. Vocal pathology affects these layers differently, producing a different effect on vibration.[3]

The body-cover model has many implications for providing explanations about the effect of vocal pathology on vocal physiology and may help to explain some of the phenomena that have been observed in high speed films, during stroboscopy, or in other methods for the study of vocal fold vibration. For example, differences between modal or chest voice phonation and falsetto are easily explained by the degree of coupling between the various layers of the vocal fold. At low pitches, the cover is very loose and can move somewhat independently of the body. Upward displacement of the vocal folds results in a ripple of the cover from below the folds to their upper surface. This ripple helps to produce a sharper acoustic pulse[4] and appears as a mucosal wave when viewed stroboscopically. In the falsetto register, the cover and the body are stretched and move as a unit. This results in a simpler mode of vibration, resulting in fewer harmonics in the tone. One might speculate that singers may learn to use these mechanisms to their advantage, although there are few data regarding layered vibration in singers.

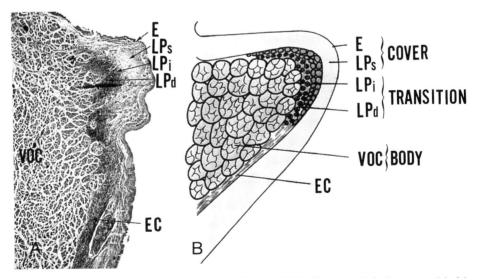

Figure 3–1. Schematic (left) and photograph (right) of the vocal folds illustrating the body-cover model of the vocal folds. (From Hirano.[62] Copyright 1981, American Speech–Language Hearing Association. Reprinted by permission.)

The Bernoulli Effect

Initial Conditions

For phonation, there are several conditions that must be established prior to the initiation of sound. First, the vocal folds must be brought to a partially closed position. (It is also possible to start phonation with the vocal folds completely closed.) This maneuver creates a resistance to the exiting airflow required for phonation. Second, the vocal folds must be tensed using the various muscles of the larynx. Again, this creates a resistance to the exiting airflow. The tension and the mass of the vocal folds also determine the vibrating frequency of the vocal folds.

The Bernoulli Equation

Daniel Bernoulli was an 18th century Swiss mathematician who developed a law that explains how the vocal folds can start oscillation and continue to oscillate. His formula explains how the energy of a fluid redistributes itself as it passes through a conduit. The formula for constant energy is shown below.

$$PE + \tfrac{1}{2}MV^2 = k$$

This equation states that as the velocity (*V*) of a fluid increases, the kinetic energy (expressed as $\tfrac{1}{2}MV^2$) increases; the potential energy or pressure it exerts will decrease provided that the total energy remains constant. Or, since total energy is constant, as kinetic energy increases (the energy due to motion), potential energy (the energy available to perform work) decreases.

A simple and common demonstration of the Bernoulli effect is illustrated in Figure 3–2A. As a person blows across the upper surface of a piece of paper, the paper will rise.

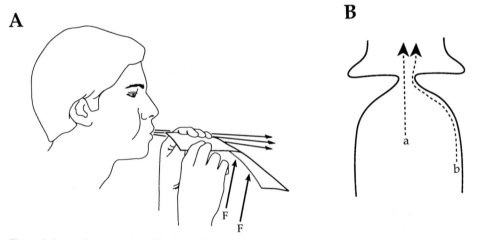

Figure 3–2. **A,** Demonstration of the Bernoulli effect (left) and how it relates to the vocal system (right). Air blown across the upper surface of the paper results in elevation of the paper. **B,** Molecule a has a straight path up the trachea, whereas molecule b has to travel around the vocal folds. If the speed of the airflow remains constant, molecule b must increase its speed to reach the same location downstream as molecule a. Increased speed results in a decrease along the walls of the trachea and the vocal folds.

The airstream across the upper surface represents an increase in kinetic energy. If kinetic energy increases, potential energy must decrease. Therefore the pressure along the upper surface of the paper is less than the pressure beneath the paper. Greater pressure beneath the paper will result in a pushing upward of the paper.

The Bernoulli Effect in Phonation

A cross-sectional view of the airway at the level of the vocal folds is illustrated in Figure 3–2B. Two air molecules are shown. Molecule a is traveling up the center of the airway and meets no obstruction in its path. Molecule b, traveling along the side of the airway, will encounter the partially closed vocal folds. However, molecule b has a longer path to travel than molecule a in order to circumvent the vocal folds. If this molecule is to maintain its position with respect to molecule a, it must increase its velocity. Increased velocity means, according to the Bernoulli equation, increased kinetic energy and, as a consequence, decreased potential energy. Thus the pressure along the surface of the vocal folds is slightly decreased. Since the vocal folds are pliable and moveable, they move in response to this pressure decrease. The process repeats itself until the vocal folds are literally "sucked" together. Once closed, the vocal folds impose an obstruction to the outgoing airstream, causing a pressure buildup beneath them. Eventually, this pressure will be sufficient to overcome the resistance of the vocal folds, and they will be blown open. Simplistically, one might think of vocal fold vibration as consisting of a series of sucking and blowing open of the vocal folds at a rate determined by the degree of muscle activity in the larynx.

The Negative Resistance Model

Conrad[5] and Conrad and McQueen[6] have proposed an alternative to the Bernoulli effect to explain how vocal fold vibration starts and is sustained. Their model depends on the existence of a resistance somewhere downstream from the vocal folds (i.e., in the larynx or vocal tract). Such a resistance, when of sufficient magnitude, will establish conditions that will lead to oscillation.

What Is Negative Differential Resistance?

Aerodynamically, resistance is defined as the ratio of pressure and flow. In simple terms, as air flow through a constriction increases, so does pressure. In a dynamic or vibrating system such as the vocal folds, pressure changes or pressure differences are very important. These pressure differences create differences of resistance that may contribute energy to the vibrating system. Positive resistance occurs when greater flows create greater pressures. Positive resistance is associated with energy loss. But suppose there is a circumstance in which greater flows result in lower pressures! Resistance no longer increases, but decreases and is associated with energy increase. It is possible for a negative resistance to occur associated with differences of pressure created in the vocal tract. Technically the name of such resistance should be *differential negative resistance*. However, in this discussion the term *negative resistance* is used.

Is such a phenomenon of negative resistance common in the real world? Yes, and it is more common than at first thought. Tubes, when clamped appropriately, will exhibit negative resistance and will oscillate. This may be a problem in water pipes, air tubing, or ventilation shafts (provided the proper resistance, flow, and pressures are created). Negative resistance may also be found in blood vessels in the human body. Negative resistance must be created in order for some electronic oscillators to function. Special electronic components have been developed to create such negative resistance.

Oscillation in Tubes

Tubes will oscillate if a resistance is created and the walls of the tube are sufficiently pliable to permit oscillation. An easy demonstration of this fact can be created by using a piece of flexible tubing (soft walled), two small clamps, and a compressed air source: Connect the tube to the air source, and position the clamp near the end of the tube. Start the airflow at a moderate flow rate. Gradually tighten the clamp until a low frequency oscillation starts. Some experimentation may be required, depending on the type of tubing and air source used.

Possible Resistances in the Human Airway

For negative resistance to be established, it is important to create a resistance to flow somewhere downstream in the vocal tract. This resistance may consist of the vocal folds themselves, the false vocal folds, the aryepiglottic sphincter, the pharyngeal walls, or the velum or the tongue. In reality, resistances not within the larynx itself are probably impractical, since structures in the vocal tract are needed for articulation and would not remain constant. The most likely possible source of the supraglottal resistance may be the vocal folds themselves.

It is well known that the vocal folds vibrate in parts and not as a single solid mass. From high speed films, it can be observed that there are two points of initial contact during the vibratory cycle (for frequencies produced in the modal or chest voice). During closure, the first contact occurs at the bottom margin of the vocal folds, followed shortly thereafter by contact at the upper margins. Schematically this is shown in a cross-sectional view of the larynx as in Figure 3–3A. The bottom portion of the vocal folds appears to move independently of the

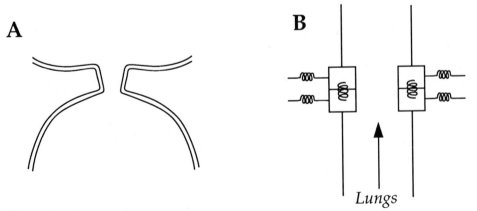

Figure 3–3.   Two-mass model of the vocal folds. **A,** Schematic cross section of the vocal folds. Note the upper and lower lips that appear to act independently. **B,** Model of the vocal folds that would simulate the somewhat independent action of the upper and lower portions of the vocal folds.

portion above the vocal folds. This behavior can be modeled by considering the upper and lower portions of the vocal folds as two masses (Fig. 3–3B).[7-9] When the vocal folds open, the lower mass opens first, followed by the upper mass. It is possible that while the lower mass is opening, the still closed (or partially closed) upper mass acts as a downstream resistance creating a negative differential resistance necessary for oscillation.

The Vocal Folds: A Negative Differential Resistance Oscillator?

How can the negative resistance model explain vocal fold oscillation? In theory, all of the necessary components for the model exist in the larynx and vocal tract: oscillator, air flow, and downstream resistances. A very simplistic, one mass model of the vocal folds is shown in Figure 3–4A. Above the folds is the supraglottal resistance. Pressure beneath the vocal folds is greater than the pressure above the vocal folds. As the vocal folds open, these pressure relationships change dynamically. As the vocal folds move, they may create subglottal and supraglottal pressure changes as a function of airflow as shown in Figure 3–4B. It is important to note that it is the pressure differences that are important for vocal fold oscillation. As the vocal folds start to open and airflow increases, subglottal pressure increases. In the early stages of vocal fold opening, the pressure above the vocal folds (supraglottal pressure) rises at a slow rate. This results in a positive resistance as shown by the positive slope change in the left portion of Figure 3–4B. With further vocal fold opening and increased airflow rate, subglottal air pressure rises at a slow rate or not at all because of the magnitude of the vocal fold opening. However, supraglottal pressure continues to rise. The pressure difference (supraglottal–subglottal) is reduced, creating a decrease of resistance. This region of negative differential resistance creates an unstable aerodynamic condition that may result in oscillation of the vocal folds.

A recent in vivo experiment[10] has been reported in which canine larynges were used to test the negative resistance model. A pressure/flow pattern very similar to that shown in

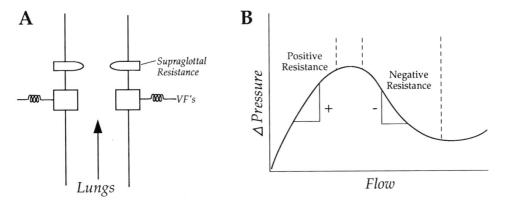

Figure 3–4. Negative differential resistance. **A,** Simple one-mass model of the vocal folds with the addition of a supraglottal resistance. **B,** Derivation of differential negative resistance. As the vocal folds open, the pressure difference between the space beneath the vocal folds and the space above the vocal folds is large and increases with increases of airflow rate. This relationship is shown as a rising curve and is positive resistance. When the vocal folds become more open, the pressure difference across the vocal folds decreases, partly due to the decrease in subglottal pressure and partly to the increase in supraglottal pressure. This pressure decrease results in decreased resistance as shown in the right portion of the curve. This is negative resistance that results from the differential pressure changes occurring during a vibratory cycle.

Figure 3–4B was found, providing evidence of possible negative differential resistance as a potential mechanism for the initiation and continuation of phonation. Future work may provide further evidence showing that the negative resistance model warrants careful consideration in any explanation of vocal fold function.

MECHANISMS OF PITCH VARIATION

The human voice can potentially span a range of vocal pitch as large as seven octaves, although it is doubtful that an individual could produce such a range. The vocal pitch or frequency (the acoustic correlate of pitch) range in a typical nonsinger for everyday speaking conditions may encompass about two octaves; during singing the range may reach four octaves. Although variable, it is apparent that the human voice can achieve a large variation of vocal pitch. In this section, some of the significant physiologic mechanisms for the control of vocal pitch are reviewed. Some attention is given to newer ideas about pitch variation and the role of nonmuscular properties of the vocal folds and larynx in the control of pitch.

Determinants of Pitch Variation by the Vocal Folds

The String Model

In the past, much was written comparing the vocal folds to common string instruments such as the violin, guitar, or bass. Anatomically, the vocal folds were often pictured as stringlike, which may have been responsible for the term *vocal cords*. We know that the vocal folds are folds of tissue and do not necessarily have the same physical shape as a string. Nevertheless, the vocal folds are often compared with strings, with the implication that the physical mechanisms to control pitch or frequency in the vocal cords are similar to the physical mechanisms known to control pitch or frequency in a string.

Three properties of string are related to its pitch or basic vibrating frequency: (1) the mass of the string, (2) the length of the string, and (3) the longitudinal tension applied to the string. The relationships between the three variables are summarized in the classic formula for determining the vibratory frequency of a string:

$$\text{Freq} = \frac{1}{2\text{I}} \sqrt{\frac{\text{Tension}}{\text{Mass/length}}}$$

Basically, this formula shows that the vibrating frequency of a string is inversely related to the length of the string, directly related to the tension exerted on the string, and inversely related to the mass (or thickness) of the string. In many stringed instruments, the player alters the length of the string and therefore achieves frequency variation. The mass of the string is selected by selecting different strings. Tension plays a role in tuning the instrument to the desired pitch.

The vocal folds also have a length and a mass or thickness. Furthermore, their tension can be altered by variations in muscles attached to or that makeup the vocal folds. In the next three sections, the relationships between each of the three parameters and vocal pitch are explored.

Vocal Fold Length and Pitch

In a string, pitch is indirectly related to the length of the string. Simply speaking, the longer the string, the lower the vibrating frequency and vice versa. What about the vocal folds?

There have been several studies[11,12] in which the length of the vocal folds has been measured, as speakers produce fundamental frequencies over a wide range and in different vocal registers. The results of one of these studies are shown in Figure 3–5.[11] These data were obtained from six male subjects producing fundamental frequencies within their modal register frequency range. (*The modal register* refers to that range of frequencies produced during everyday speech activities.) Although there is variation, all subjects increased the length of their vocal folds as they increased fundamental frequency. A later study[12] confirmed these results in female subjects. It is apparent that, for phonation in the modal register, subjects increase the length of their vocal folds. This relationship is exactly the opposite of the effect of length on the frequency of vibration in a string. In falsetto, however, the relationship between vibrating frequency and length is similar to that of a string. In fact, Rubin and Hirt[13] have shown that in falsetto the vibrating length of the vocal folds is systematically shortened as frequency is increased.

Vocal Fold Thickness and Pitch

The relationship between length and frequency in the vocal folds makes sense if one considers the vocal folds more like an elastic band with which vibrating frequency is dependent on the mass of the band and the tension exerted on it. The vocal folds are similar in that increases in length produce decreases in the mass (or thickness) of the vocal folds, thus permitting higher vibrating frequencies. Such a relationship between vocal fold mass and fundamental frequency was demonstrated by Hollien and Colton.[14] The results of that study are shown in Figure 3–6. The systematic decrease in vocal fold mass continued until about the start of falsetto frequencies. Thereafter the mass remained constant as higher fundamental frequencies were produced in falsetto. This is analogous to stretching the elastic band until it can be stretched no longer. At this length the thickness of the band will remain about the same. It is possible, of course, to continue to exert tension until the elastic band breaks.

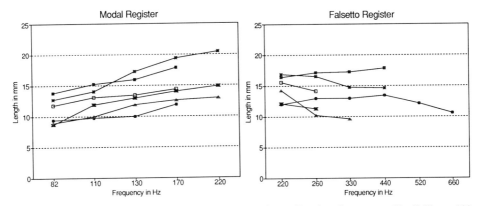

Figure 3–5. Vocal fold length in the modal and falsetto registers. (Based on data presented by Hollien and his colleagues.[11,12])

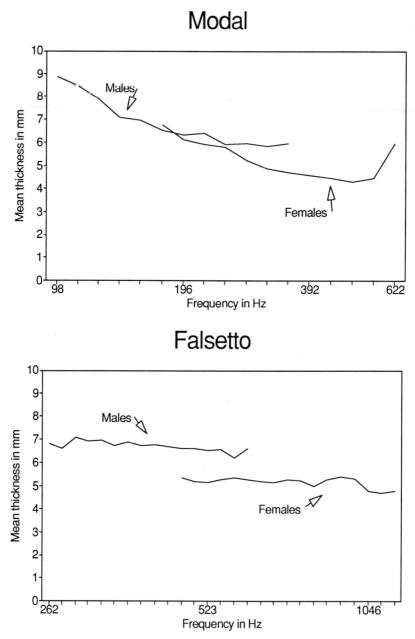

Figure 3–6. Vocal fold thickness in the modal and falsetto registers. (Based on data presented by Hollien and Colton.[14])

Vocal Fold Tension and Pitch

Fortunately, it is not possible physiologically to produce enough tension in the vocal folds to produce a breaking of the vocal folds, although excessive tension may produce damage to the fine structures in the vocal folds and perhaps cause pain. Tension can be varied over a considerable range and according to van den Berg[15] is responsible for variation of fundamental frequency in the falsetto register. van den Berg reported that in chest voice (similar to modal register) a small amount of tension produces a fairly large amount of elongation. For frequencies produced in so-called mid-voice, a moderately large range of tension produces a small amount of elongation whereas in falsetto voice large increases of tension produce very little elongation. Thus tension on the vocal folds is much more dominant in producing fundamental frequency change than in the chest or modal voice in which there are large changes of vocal fold length.

The role of tension in controlling vocal pitch has been investigated by Titze,[16,17] Perlman et al,[18] and Titze and Durham.[19] They have hypothesized that some of the pitch variation produced in everyday speech utterances, as well as pitch variation in more demanding endeavors like singing, may be explained by the tension changes that occur as a result of the lateral movement of the vocal folds during vibration or by the increasing stress placed on the vocal folds as a result of increased longitudinal tension. For example, during production of a vowel, there is a tendency for fundamental frequency to decrease slightly as phonation is sustained. This slight decrease may be explained, according to Titze and Durham,[19] by the slight decrease in tension that results after the initial application of a force to a structure. Of course during speech there are several variables that may change, resulting in a possible change in vocal frequency (e.g., subglottal pressure, vocal fold mass, and so forth). Tension may also change during the aging process.[20] Nevertheless, the roles of tension, both active and passive, must be considered in an explanation of vocal frequency variation by the human voice.[21]

In summary, there are three physiologic parameters that control the fundamental frequency of vibration in the vocal folds. These are (1) length, (2) mass, and (3) tension. Length is least important in this process, and mass may be more dominant at low fundamental frequencies, especially those produced in modal (and pulse) register, and tension much more dominant at frequencies produced in the falsetto register. Further information about the factors that affect and contribute to the development of tension in the vocal folds can be found in several publications.[15-21]

MECHANISMS OF LOUDNESS VARIATION

Vocal loudness is determined by several factors, including the intensity of the sound produced by the vocal folds. In this section, the contribution of the vocal folds to vocal loudness is considered. Loudness is a perceptual attribute of sound; its physical correlate is the sound pressure level of the sound. Consequently, this discussion is concerned with the production of sound pressure level variations by the vocal folds.

Air Pressure and Sound Pressure Level

Sound is the variation of air pressure at a rate to be audible. The sound pressure level of sound produced by the vocal folds is directly dependent on the air pressure driving the vocal folds into vibration. The greater the air pressure, the greater the sound pressure level of the sound. This relationship between air pressure and sound pressure has been reported by several investigators[22-25] and the basic relationship, based on the work of Ladefoged and McKinney,[22] is illustrated in Figure 3–7. What are the mechanisms for producing this increase in air pressure and the subsequent increase in sound pressure level?

There are two basic mechanisms that can be used to produce greater air pressures. First, the thorax can increase the flow of air and create a greater force beneath the vocal folds. Second, the vocal folds can remain closed for a greater proportion of their vibratory cycle and produce a greater pressure beneath them even when the force from the lungs remains constant. Both mechanisms are used during phonation, although one might expect that greater thoracic pressures are used to achieve large changes in sound intensity, and variations in vocal fold closed time are responsible for small variations of sound intensity, such as might be found during the production of a sentence.

Glottal Resistance and Vocal Intensity

Greater closed time of the vocal folds produces a greater resistance to vibration, which appears to be the major physiologic parameter controlling vocal intensity for phonations produced in the modal register. Resistance is defined as the ratio of the air pressure divided by the airflow. Isshiki[23,24] reported that for frequencies produced in chest voice (or the modal register) increases in airflow were less than the increases in air pressure, with increases in sound intensity. Consequently, glottal resistance increased with increases in

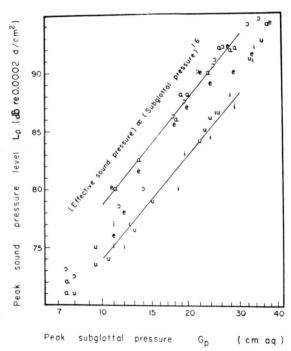

Figure 3–7. Relationship between subglottal air pressure and the pressure level of the sound produced. (From Ladefoged and McKinney.[22])

sound intensity. He concluded that glottal resistance was the major controlling parameter of vocal intensity for low pitched phonations (i.e., those within the chest or modal register).

To increase glottal resistance, there must be increased contraction by muscles of the larynx, especially those that will force the vocal folds to the midline.[25,26] Increased muscle activity, especially in those muscles that close the vocal folds, will increase vocal fold resistance, requiring greater pressures beneath the vocal folds in order to sustain vibration. When the vocal folds open, the air pressure released into the vocal tract will be greater, producing greater sound pressure levels.

Phonations produced in falsetto voice do not show systematic changes in glottal resistance with changes in vocal fold intensity. In this register, airflow is related to increases in vocal intensity. There is considerable muscle activity in falsetto[26] that would produce high levels of glottal resistance even at low intensity levels. Additional increases in glottal resistance may be difficult to achieve in this register. Airflow rate may be more important to produce variation in vocal intensity.

The range of vocal intensity is much smaller in falsetto than in the chest or modal register. In modal, one can produce ranges of vocal intensity between 40 and 50 dB (from about 60 to about 110 dB sound pressure level [SPL]). In falsetto, the range of vocal intensity is about 15 to 20 dB (from about 60 to 75 or 80 dB SPL). When phonations are produced at equivalent fundamental frequencies in both registers, those produced in modal register have a range from 25 to 32 dB, whereas those produced in falsetto have a range from 9 to 20 dB.[27] Apparently the change in the physiologic mechanism responsible for controlling vocal intensity in falsetto results in a smaller range of intensity, especially the maximum intensity that can be produced.

The relationships between vocal intensity, air pressure, air flow, and glottal resistance have been accepted by many authors (see, e.g., Zemlin[28] for a review of these data). However, Colton,[29] in a preliminary experiment with one subject, reported little difference in airflow rate for phonations produced in the modal and falsetto registers at different vocal intensity levels. Air pressures and glottal resistance were also similar for phonations produced in the two registers. The data were obtained from inverse filtered air flow waveforms and indirect estimates of air pressure below the vocal folds. It is possible that procedural differences account for some of the discrepancies between these and other data. The results suggest that, at the very least, we should continue to explore the relationships between air flow, air pressure, and vocal intensity to elucidate more clearly the physiologic mechanisms that control vocal intensity.

MECHANISMS OF QUALITY VARIATION

Voice quality, like voice intensity, is not solely determined by the vocal folds. Resonance affects the quality of the voice emitted at the lips. In this section, discussion is focused on the contribution of the vocal folds to voice quality and the physiologic mechanisms that can be important for its control.

Vocal Fold Spectrum and Voice Quality

The major acoustic correlate of voice quality is acoustic spectrum. Spectrum is usually depicted by plotting the amplitude of a component of the tone with respect to its frequency.

Variations in the amplitude of a frequency and even the existence of a specific frequency will alter the quality of the tone.

During everyday speech, the vocal folds produce a tone with a spectrum similar to the one shown in Figure 3–8.[30] However, the spectrum may be altered according to the needs and wishes of the individual. Singers and actors learn to make these variations in order to convey emotions, effect, or beauty of tone. Examples of some of these variations are shown in Figure 3–9, which is a plot of the average spectrum of four voice qualities produced by five subjects phonating the vowel /ah/.[31] Each of these qualities is very distinctive, which is evident in their spectrum differences. Within a quality, the spectrum differences are less marked, although there are differences in spectrum shape at different fundamental frequencies. Figure 3–10 illustrates the spectrum of modal register quality produced at five different fundamental frequencies.[31] As fundamental frequency is increased, there will be little or no energy in those frequencies below the fundamental. Conversely, as fundamental frequency is increased, there will be greater energy in the higher frequencies, simply because the harmonics of the tone will be shifted upward in frequency.

The Vibratory Cycle and Vocal Tone Spectrum

Given that voice quality is directly determined by the spectrum of the vocal fold tone, how does one vary the spectrum of the vocal fold tone? The simplest explanation is based on an analysis of the vibratory cycle of the vocal folds. Typical vocal fold vibratory cycles are

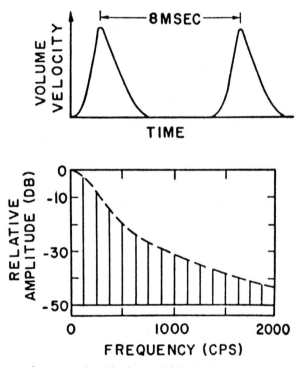

Figure 3–8.   Spectrum of a tone produced by the vocal folds during everyday speech. (From Stevens and House.[30])

Spectrum of Four Voice Qualities

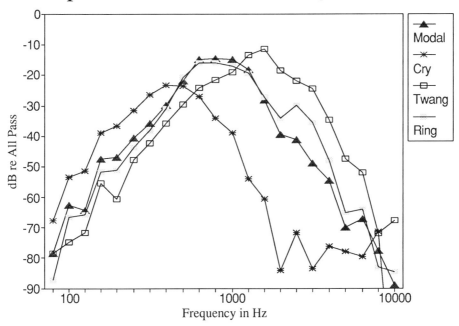

Figure 3–9. Spectrum of four voice qualities. These data were produced by five singers. (Based on data reported by Colton et al.[31]).

illustrated in Figure 3–11 for phonations produced in the modal (Fig. 3–11A) and the loft or falsetto (Fig. 3–11C) registers. Modal register phonations are produced with a faster closing phase of the vocal folds producing greater energy in the higher frequencies, whereas in falsetto the closing slope is more gradual, producing little energy in the upper harmonics. The speed of closing of the vocal folds has a great effect on the energy produced in the higher frequencies. Thus the details of the vibratory cycle are important to consider in predicting the energy distribution of the frequencies present in the vocal fold tone. Note also the larger airflows in falsetto and the very brief time when the airflows are at a minimum.

It is possible to observe the effects of the vocal fold vibratory cycle by observing the area waveform between the vocal folds (Fig. 3–12). In this example, the waveform drawn with the solid line was produced at a normal loudness level, whereas the second waveform was produced with greater loudness. There is an increase in the time of the closed phase, producing greater vocal intensity. There is also an increase in the speed at which the vocal folds close. Faster closure rates result in the production of greater high frequency energy. Increased vocal loudness will change the spectrum of the vocal fold tone with a resultant change in voice quality.

The Vocal Tract as a Determinant of Voice Quality

The focus of this chapter is on laryngeal physiology and the focus of this section has been on the role of the vocal folds in determining the quality of a person's voice. However, an

Modal Spectrum
Over Five Fundamental Frequencies

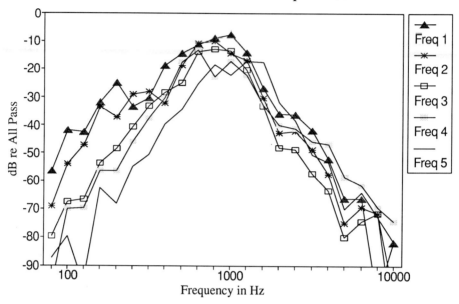

Figure 3–10. Spectrum of phonations produced in the modal register at different fundamental frequencies by five singers. (Based on data reported by Colton et al.[31])

individual's voice quality is not solely determined by the tone produced by the vocal folds. The vocal tract or the tube connecting the vocal folds with the lips also affects voice quality. The vocal tract is an acoustic resonator, and much is known about its effects on sound.[33–35] Much of the data on the effects of the vocal tract have been concerned with the acoustic characteristics of specific vowels and consonants. However, the vocal tract may also determine the overall quality of a person's voice. For example, Coleman[36,37] has shown that some of the difference between a male and a female voice is determined, in part, by differences in the size and shape of the vocal tract. Colton and Estill[38] reported data showing vocal tract differences when phonations were produced in different voice qualities. Kitzing[39] and others have shown how vocal tract features may reflect abnormal voice qualities.

The vocal tract is the resonator of the tone produced by the vocal folds. The size and shape of the vocal tract determines the precise frequencies that will be affected. Each speaker possesses a unique vocal tract, and the sound produced by the vocal folds will be altered in a unique way for that speaker. A speaker's vocal tract configuration in combination with the unique vocal fold tone will determine the speaker's voice quality.

PHYSIOLOGY OF PHONATION DURING SINGING

In this section, some acoustic and physiologic characteristics of singing are reviewed briefly. Considerable research has been accumulated on the singing voice, and it is not

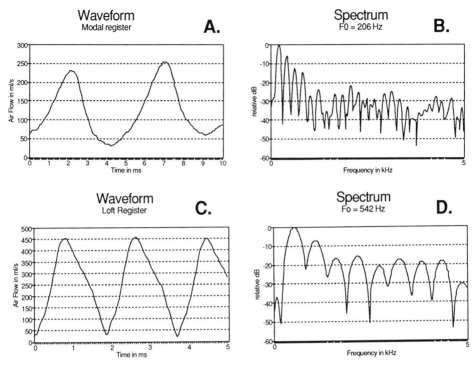

Figure 3–11.   **A,C,** Glottal waveforms and **B,D,** spectra for phonations produced in the modal (**A,B**) and falsetto (loft) (**C,D**) registers.

possible to review all the pertinent findings in this section. The reader is referred to an excellent text by Johann Sundberg[40] for further information.

Some Acoustic Characteristics of Singing

Three topics are discussed in this section: (1) vocal differences between singers and nonsingers, (2) acoustic characteristics of voice types, and (3) vocal registers.

Singer/Nonsinger Differences

During singing, trained professional singers produce phonations with acoustic characteristics different from those of nonsingers. However, many of these differences may be attributed more to the training and practice than to inherent (or genetic) anatomic differences. For example, singers and nonsingers exhibit very similar physiologic frequency ranges (ranges produced without regard to the musicality of the tone) and very similar dynamic ranges (range of intensity produced). On the other hand, singers produce a larger range of musically acceptable tones than nonsingers and typically have much greater control of the intensity they produce.

The glottal source spectra appear to be different in singers. These differences are

Glottal Time Waveforms

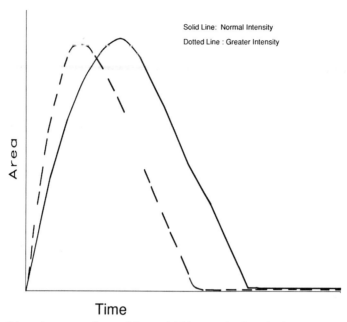

Figure 3–12.   Schematic area waveforms of the vocal folds at two loudness levels.

illustrated in Figure 3–13, which is a plot of the differences from an ideal spectrum in which the component energy decreases at a rate of 12 dB per octave. This type of display helps to emphasize the differences in spectra of the singers and nonsingers. The greatest difference occurs in the first partial, which is the fundamental frequency of the tone. Singers produce about a 5 dB greater level of the first partial than do nonsingers. Singers also tend to produce greater energy in the seventh to ninth partials.

Singers also produce energy in a greater number of partials. That is, they produce more energy in the higher frequency components of the tone. The average number of partials with significant energy (greater than 2 dB above the noise in the signal) at three different frequency levels in the modal register is shown in Figure 3–14.[43] (These frequencies were chosen because they overlap the lower part of the falsetto register. Characteristics of tones produced in this area of overlap were the main focus of the study.[43]) At the lowest fundamental frequency, the singers only produced a tone with one more partial than a tone produced by the nonsingers. At the highest frequency, however, the singers produced phonations with an average of three more partials than the nonsingers. A greater number of partials is associated with a larger frequency bandwidth of the glottal tone, which may partially account for the "richer" timbre of a singer's tone.

There are other ways in which singers differ vocally from nonsingers, including the extent of the musical singing range, the consistency of the spectrum produced by the vocal folds across different pitches, the ability of the singer to produce pitch changes without concomitant changes in vocal loudness, and differences in the control of breathing and

Spectrum Differences
Untrained vs Trained Singers

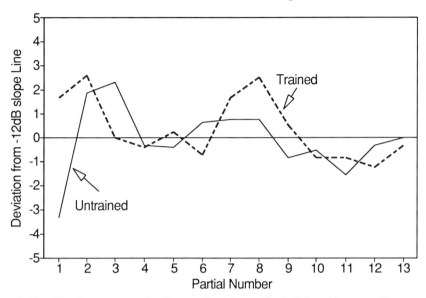

Figure 3–13. Glottal source spectra for singers and nonsingers. The deviation of the spectra from a spectrum with a slope of −12 dB/octave is shown. (Redrawn from Sundberg,[40] Carr,[41] and Cleveland.[42])

formant frequencies. These have been documented in a number of publications and provide good evidence that singers are "special."[44]

Spectral Characteristics of Voice Types

Each singer is usually classified into one of several major voice types. Typically these include (but are not limited to) bass, baritone, tenor, alto, and soprano. Subclassifications of these major types are also possible. Some of the acoustic differences for these various voice types include singing range, formant frequencies (resonances), and spectrum of the glottal tone.

The spectral deviation from an ideal −12 dB per octave spectrum for alto and tenor singers is shown in Figure 3–15. These data are based on work by Agren and Sundberg[45] and show that both voice types exhibit major deviations from the ideal voice source spectrum. Altos tend to have greater energy in the first two or three partials of the tone, whereas tenors show greater energy in the fifth and sixth partials. Note also that the spectrum of the tenors is lower than that of the altos in the highest partials of the tone. It appears that part of the difference between alto and tenor singers (who share a considerable portion of the fundamental frequency range) are spectral.

In another study,[46] minor spectral differences were reported for a small sample of singers with bass, tenor, alto, and soprano voice types. Only in extreme cases was there a noticeable difference in the source spectrum. This is illustrated in Figure 3–16, in which the spectral deviations (from the ideal −12 dB/octave) for a bass and a tenor singer are shown.

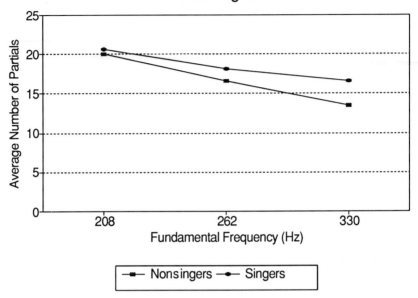

Figure 3–14.   Number of partials produced in modal register phonations produced by singers and nonsingers. (Based on data reported by Colton.[43])

These spectra were obtained from phonations produced at one of the extremes of the singers' ranges (130 Hz for the tenor and 329 Hz for the bass). Thus these are probably not representative of the true spectral characteristics of basses and tenors. Both Cleveland and Sundberg conclude that, although some spectral differences exists among voice types, they are minor and probably of little importance to voice type classification.

Spectral Differences Among Vocal Registers

There is little agreement on exactly how many vocal registers exist in the singing voice. However, most writers discuss three or four registers. A vocal register is a series of consecutive vocal tones with approximately equal vocal timbre or quality.[47] Registers usually reside in a certain frequency range. The lowest register on the frequency scale is referred to as vocal *fry* or *pulse register*. It is little used in singing and appears infrequently in speaking. Above pulse register on the frequency scale is what Hollien[47] called *modal register*. This is the range of frequencies used most often in speaking and singing. Above modal is falsetto or loft register. Males may use this register in singing in the upper portions of their range, although the timbre of falsetto is not usually desirable in a musical performance. Finally, some female singers may be able to produce tones in the whistle register, a very high frequency register.

  Inherent in the definition of a vocal register is the concept of voice quality. As has been discussed previously, the major acoustic correlate of voice quality is spectrum. Thus one would expect differences in the glottal source spectrum among the various vocal registers.

Spectrum Differences
Altos and Tenors

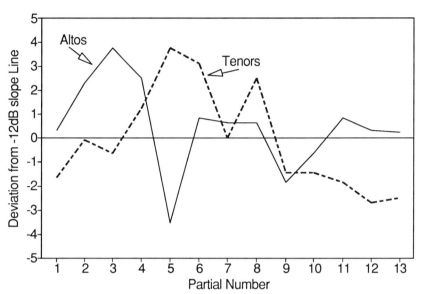

Figure 3–15. Glottal source spectra for alto and tenor singers. The deviation of the spectra from a spectrum with a slope of −12 dB/octave is shown. (Redrawn from Sundberg.[40])

Spectrum Differences
Tenor and Bass

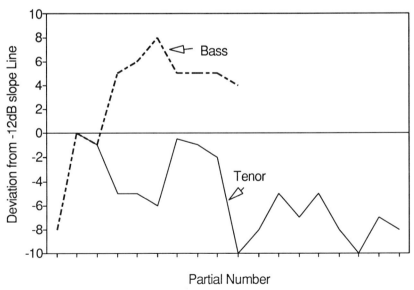

Figure 3–16. Glottal source spectra of a tenor and a bass voice. The deviation of the spectra from a spectrum with a slope of −12 dB/octave is shown. (Drawn from data presented by Cleveland.[46])

Most of the available data, especially for singers, exists on the spectral characteristics of the modal and falsetto registers.

Figure 3–17 shows the average numbers of partials (frequency components) in phonations produced at identical fundamental frequencies in the modal and falsetto registers by a small group of singer subjects.[43] Note the greater number of partials in the modal register than in the falsetto register. The number of partials in falsetto for the three frequencies studied was constant. Another way of viewing these data is that the frequency bandwidth (range of frequencies present in the glottal tone) is much smaller in falsetto than in modal register productions. This acoustic difference may account for the perceived "lighter" quality of falsetto productions.

Colton[48] has shown that even when the spectra of modal and falsetto phonations are identical, listeners can perceive differences in voice quality. This suggests that there are differences in the relative energy in the lowered number partials between the two registers. Observe the 5 dB difference in energy in the first partial (or fundamental frequency) between the two registers. There is also a minor difference in the third partial. Colton[48] also reported differences between the modal and falsetto registers among the first five to seven partials.

In summary, there are spectral differences between the modal and falsetto registers. Falsetto has a smaller bandwidth and tends to have greater energy in the fundamental frequency than modal phonations (Figs. 3–17, 3–18).

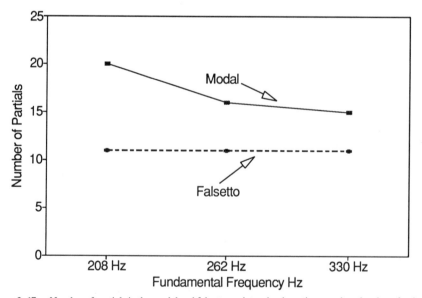

Figure 3–17.   Number of partials in the modal and falsetto registers in phonations produced at three fundamental frequencies by singers. (Drawn from data of Colton.[43])

Spectrum Differences
Modal vs Falsetto

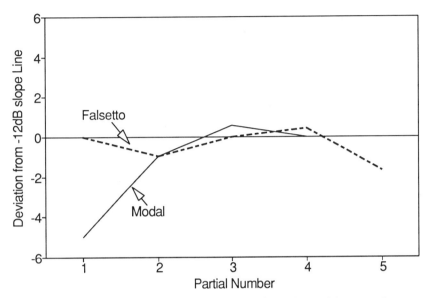

Figure 3–18. Glottal source of the modal and falsetto registers. The deviation of the spectra from a spectrum with a slope of −12 dB/octave is shown. (Redrawn from Sundberg.[40])

Some Vibratory Characteristics of Singing

In this section a brief review of some of the vibratory characteristics of singing is presented. These vibratory characteristics include: (1) informal observations about vocal fold vibration as seen in videostroboscopic recordings of singers, (2) characteristics of singing as viewed in high speed motion pictures of the vocal folds, and (3) vibratory characteristics of singers using the indirect measurement technique of the flow glottogram.

Informal Observations About Vibratory Characteristics of Singing as Shown With Videostroboendoscopy

Over the past few years, we have had the opportunity to observe singers using videostroboscopy. Most of these had been referred with complaints such as a break within the middle of the range or an inability to reach their high notes.

Stroboscopically, singers tend to show more rapid closure of the vocal folds. This is manifested by a small number of frames during the closing phase of the vibratory cycle. Furthermore, singers tend toward slightly longer closed phases with little or no leakage of airflow during this phase. Closure is complete from the anterior to the posterior ends of the vocal folds. In some singers, the height of the larynx appears lower than for nonsingers, although this probably depends on the pitch, loudness, and style of singing. Of course, singers can control the various parameters of the voice (such as pitch, loudness, and quality), permitting much better visualization of the vocal folds and other structures in the larynx.

We have also made observations about the vocal fold vibratory characteristics of singers (professional as well as students) whose chief complaint was a chronic or acute problem in a certain part of their phonatory range.[49] The second most frequent complaint was vocal fatigue, pain, or discomfort when they phonated. The majority of the singers were rated as possessing normal voice quality, at least during the examination. In addition to finding nodules or other growths on the vocal folds, we found that many signers exhibit vibratory problems: problems such as low amplitude of vibration of the vocal folds, a predominantly open (or closed) phase, phase asymmetry, and abnormalities of mucosal wave propagation. The strobe examination was valuable in detecting these abnormalities and assisted in selection of the proper treatment.

Vibratory Characteristics of Singers as Viewed With High Speed Motion Pictures

Several studies have been reported in which singers or various singing techniques have been investigated with high speech motion pictures of the vocal folds.[13,50] Rubin and Hirt[13] investigated the mechanism of falsetto voice production in singers, including the infamous "falsetto break." During the maneuver from chest voice to falsetto, there are numerous irregular movements of the vocal folds and the picture is of "complete chaos." After the break, the vocal folds achieve regular vibration but with a mode more characteristic of falsetto (thin, elongated vocal folds with a small amplitude of vibration). Rubin and Hirt[13] also reported several modes of falsetto voice production, including the "open-chink" mechanism, in which the vocal folds hardly ever touch each other, and the "closed-chink" mechanism, in which the main bulk of the vocal fold muscle shows little movement. These authors also reported that some singers achieved a delicate balance between these two kinds of falsetto mechanisms. A third kind of falsetto mechanism involved "damping" of the vocal folds. In this mode of falsetto vibration, a portion of the vocal folds stopped vibrating, producing the appearance of a very short vibrating segment. This type of mechanism appeared most often at the upper frequencies of falsetto voice production.

About 25 years after the classic Rubin-Hirt films, Hirano[50] reported on the vibratory characteristics of one singer as he produced different kinds of singing maneuvers (many of which involved differences of voice quality). Measurements of glottal width, open quotient, speed index, airflow rate, and fundamental frequency were made along with the film recordings. Among the different voice qualities and singing techniques investigated there were differences in closed time, closing rate of the vocal folds, airflow, and the speed of opening and closing. When the singer produced a phonation in what was apparently chest or modal register, there was a fairly long closed time and rapid vocal fold closure. However, at the same pitch the singer could produce another type of phonation that had a gentler rate of vocal fold closure with less airflow and produced a soft and gentle sound with little energy in the higher harmonics. Falsetto was investigated, showing little or no vocal fold closure, a slow rate of closure, and moderately high airflow rates. Other types of singing techniques were also investigated, but they were not identified. Consequently it is difficult to determine exactly what kind of phonation was produced or was intended to be produced.

Unfortunately there are no other studies of the singing voice using high speed motion pictures. Of interest would be the pattern of vocal fold vibration during classic opera singing as well as other forms of classical singing and singing in other styles such as broadway (belting),[51,52] country–western, pop, and rock. Classical singers appear to produce phonation characterized by rapid closure of the vocal folds, slightly longer closed times, and more complete closure along the total length of the vocal folds than do speakers or singers with different singing styles.

Vibratory Characteristics of Singers From Inverse Filtering of the Oral Airflow Waveform

Inverse filtering of the airflow waveform produced at the lips is an indirect technique for investigating the pattern of airflow modulation by the vibrating vocal folds. It is postulated that the airflow waveform emitted at the lips is the product of the airflow pattern by the vocal folds and the resonant effects of the vocal tract. If the resonant effects are removed from the recorded waveform, what remains is the pattern of airflow variation through the vocal folds. To a large extent, this model of speech production appears valid, although not for all conditions. Sundberg has labeled the results of this technique as the *flow glottogram* and has reported on several studies concerned with singers.[53–56]

Some waveforms recorded in different types of phonation by singers are shown in Figure 3–19.[40] A normal speech waveform is shown in the second panel of Figure 3–19, depicting a gentle onset of airflow until it reaches its peak and then a more rapid decrease of airflow associated with the closing of the vocal folds. Note the small amount of airflow existing even when the vocal folds are supposedly closed. This small leakage flow is typical for normal speakers and may be associated with a small gap between the posterior portions of the vocal folds, especially in women. Pressed phonation is produced when the vocal folds are more tightly closed with the result that the vocal folds have less lateral excursion and less airflow can pass between them. Perceptually, it is associated with a strained voice production. Nonsingers tend to produce this kind of phonation at their higher pitches, thus distorting the quality of their phonation. Sundberg calls phonation when there is greater than normal airflow but with nearly complete closure *flow* phonation. It might be perceived as slightly breathy. Breathy phonation is often associated with a leakage of airflow between the vocal folds even during their closed phase. Finally, during a whisper there is little modulation of the airstream by the vocal folds in addition to a high airflow rate. Some of these phonation types may occur during singing, although the appearance of breathy and whisper phonation during performance is and should be infrequent.

Colton and Estill[38] obtained flow glottograms while three singers produced phonations in four different modes of production. Examples of waveforms produced by one of the singers are shown in Figure 3–20. The normal flow glottogram (Fig. 3–20A) is very similar to those reported by Sundberg and others. Peak flow rate is about 200 ml/s, and there is a very gradual decline of airflow during the closed portion of the vocal fold vibratory cycle. We have noted this characteristic in many phonations produced by singers and nonsingers. We interpret this phenomenon as the result of a slow closing motion of the vocal folds from the front to the back. Figure 3–20B shows a waveform obtained during the production of cry or sob phonation. This kind of phonation is very soft and might be used during quiet passages or in a lullaby. Note the extremely short closed portion of the vocal folds as manifested by the brief period of minimum airflow. The rise and fall of the airflow waveform is slow, suggesting a simple, slow opening and closing motion of the vocal folds. In spite of the softness of the sound, there is considerable airflow and very little leakage

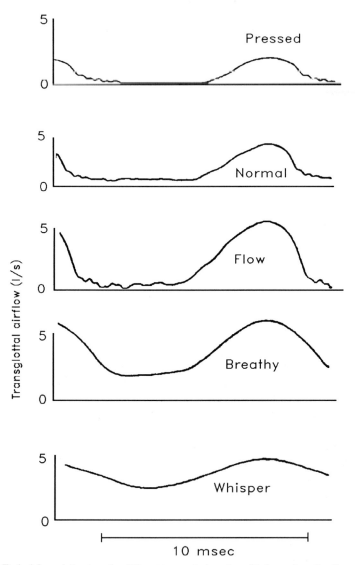

Figure 3–19. Typical flow glottograms for different types of phonation. (Redrawn from Sundberg.[40])

flow. A phonation typical of country–western singing is shown in panel C of Figure 3–20C. It is clear that little egressive air escapes during the closed period of the vocal folds, and the closed phase is rather long compared with the entire cycle. Finally, a phonation produced with a quality typically heard during western operas or on the concert stage is shown in Figure 3–20D. The falling phase of the airflow waveform is somewhat faster than the rising phase, and there is a long period of no airflow during the closed phase.

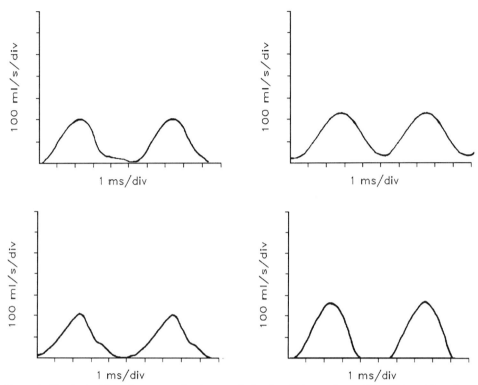

Figure 3–20. Typical flow glottograms of a singer producing four different voice qualities. (Adapted from data reported by Colton and Estill.[38])

Muscle Activity During Singing

Various muscles within the larynx contract during phonation to control various aspects of the tone such as pitch, loudness, and quality. These muscles have both of their connections to structures within the larynx and thus are referred to as *intrinsic laryngeal muscles*. The intrinsic laryngeal muscles are (1) arytenoideus, (2) lateral cricoarytenoid, (3) posterior cricoarytenoid, (4) cricothyroid, and (5) thyroarytenoid. In many texts and articles, the term *vocalis muscle* is used. This refers to the portion of the thyroarytenoid muscle that is adjacent to the airway. It is that part of the thyroarytenoid that vibrates most of the time during phonation.

The activity of intrinsic laryngeal muscles is investigated using the technique of electromyography. Briefly, very thin needles or hooked wire electrodes are placed within the muscle, and the voltage activity of the muscle is amplified, displayed, and recorded. The electrical activity recorded actually represents the sum of many individual muscle fibers. However, in general, as the level of muscle activity increases, the level of the electromyogram also increases. An example of an electromyogram is shown in Figure 3–21.

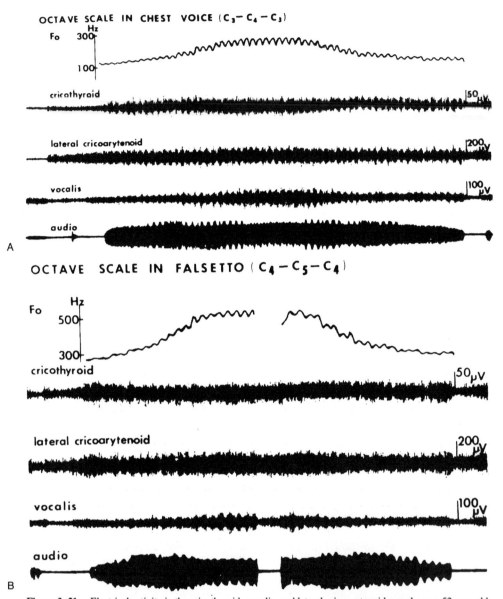

Figure 3–21.   Electrical activity in the cricothyroid, vocalis, and lateral cricoarytenoid muscles as a 52-year-old male bass singer produced an octave scale in chest voice (top) and in falsetto (bottom). (From Hirano et al.[57])

There have been numerous studies concerned with the activity of the intrinsic laryngeal muscles during speech and singing. In this section, a brief review of studies concerned with intrinsic muscle activity during singing is presented.

Laryngeal muscle activity in singers has been investigated by Hirano et al.[57,58] They reported differences in activity among the vocalis, lateral cricoarytenoid, and cricothyroid for different registers, fundamental frequencies, and intensities. For example, in the chest register all three muscles increased their activity as fundamental frequency was increased (see Fig. 3–21). However, in falsetto there was little variation of activity in the cricothyroid muscle, a somewhat unusual finding considering that the cricothyroid is the major muscle for pitch control. Activity in the vocalis muscle increased with increases in fundamental frequency but with overall lower levels.

Increased loudness of phonation was accompanied by steady or slightly decreased activity in the cricothyroid muscle and increased activity in the lateral cricoarytenoid and vocalis muscle. In the falsetto register, the lateral cricoarytenoid decreased or remained steady, the vocalis was unchanged, and the cricothyroid decreased with increasing loudness. Similar results were reported by Hirano and colleagues[58] with four professional singers performing a variety of vocal tasks.

Sometime later, a report on the muscle behavior in William Vennard, a well known singer and singing teacher, was published.[59] Some of the major findings of this study are reported in Table 3–1. For this singer, phonations produced in the chest register were accompanied by high levels of electrical activity in the vocalis muscle. Electrical activities in the cricothyroid and lateral cricoarytenoid muscles were at moderate levels. All three muscles showed moderate electrical activity when phonations were produced in head voice and low levels of activity for phonations produced in falsetto. Laryngeal height also affected the amount of electrical activity in these muscles. The cricothyroid muscle showed much greater than normal levels of activity for phonations produced with a low larynx, the lateral cricoarytenoid showed greater than normal levels, and vocalis activity was normal. Two muscles showed less electrical activity when phonations were produced with a high larynx.

The finding of increased muscle activity with increased pitch in the modal (or chest or heavy) register is consistent with electromyographic findings during phonation by non-singers.[26] However, nonsingers also showed increases in cricothyroid activity even when they produced tones in the falsetto registers. On the other hand, singers did not show any systematic changes in cricothyroid activity with increases in fundamental frequency in falsetto phonations. This discrepancy may reflect a fundamental difference between singers and nonsingers, not necessarily in the way they are built but rather in the manner in which they use their instrument. A more obvious example of this difference is that singers, when

**Table 3–1   Levels of Electromyographic Activity in the Vocalis (VOC),
Cricothyroid (CT), and Lateral Cricoarytenoid (LCA),
in a Singer Producing Phonations in the Different Vocal Registers
and at Different Laryngeal Heights***

	VOC	CT	LCA
Register			
Chest	High	Moderate	Moderate
Head	Moderate	Moderate	Moderate
Falsetto	Low	Low	Low
Larynx height			
Low larynx	=	++	+
High larynx	−	+	−

Key: ++, much greater than normal; +, greater than normal; =, equal to normal; −, less than normal.
*Based on data presented by Hirano.[59]

they increase their pitch, do not also increase their vocal intensity, whereas in nonsingers increases in loudness accompany increases in vocal pitch. Furthermore, singers are able to sing tones with the same vocal quality throughout much of their pitch range, whereas nonsingers will break into falsetto as they increase their fundamental frequency. One might conclude that singers finely adjust their intrinsic laryngeal muscle activity as they increase pitch, with the result that when falsetto frequencies are produced there is little change of activity in the cricothyroid muscle.

With increases in vocal loudness, singers increase activity in the lateral cricoarytenoid and vocalis but hold constant or decrease activity in the cricothyroid. Why? One possibility is that in order to produce the greater subglottal air pressures associated with increased vocal intensity they adduct their vocal folds more firmly. However, increased adductory forces may result in increased tension along the length of the vocal fold and thus an increase in vocal pitch. Contraction of the vocalis (which tends to shorten the vocal folds) will reduce that tension and keep the proper vocal frequency. If needed, the singer could slightly decrease activity in the cricothyroid to achieve the same end. According to Isshiki,[24] vocal loudness in falsetto is controlled by variations in airflow rate. Consequently there is little need to change activity in these three intrinsic laryngeal muscles in falsetto.

Little has been said about the posterior cricoarytenoid. This muscle is the only intrinsic laryngeal muscle that opens the vocal folds. As such, one would expect to find increases in electrical activity at the end of phonation when the vocal folds open and normal breathing is resumed. However, there may be considerable activity in this muscle during speech for a variety of reasons, including opening the vocal folds to produce nonvoiced consonants, producing a pause in the ongoing speech, or acting as an antagonist to the lateral cricoarytenoid so that fine control of the vocal fold vibration can be achieved. Martin et al[60] reported considerable activity of the posterior cricoarytenoid in supported and nonsupported singing, falsetto, vibrato, and when the loudness or the pitch of the phonations was varied. In fact, the posterior cricoarytenoid appeared very similar in its behavior to both the cricothyroid and vocalis muscles. These authors attribute their findings to the concept of agonist–antagonist pairs. According to this concept, there is a reciprocal relationship between the vocalis and cricothyroid in which one is responsible for increases in vocal pitch whereas the other is responsible for decreases in vocal pitch. Even that statement may not be entirely true. Titze et al[61] showed in two singers that, depending on the relative level of contraction of the cricothyroid and vocalis muscles, increases in activity in the vocalis muscle could produce increases or decreases in vocal pitch.

Muscles rarely act alone. Muscles when they contract shorten the length of the muscle. Some other muscle must restore the original length of the muscle. Reciprocal relationships among muscles are necessary to produce an action as well as to restore that muscle in order that it might perform again. Activity in all muscles of the larynx is necessary in order to control phonation.

SUMMARY

In this chapter, a brief review of the basic physiologic mechanisms involved in phonation have been presented. In addition, some new thinking about the anatomy of the vocal folds, the manner in which the vocal folds start and sustain vibration, and how we change pitch, loudness, and quality have been discussed. Finally, some acoustic and physiologic characteristics of the singing voice have been reviewed.

The human vocal instrument is unique anatomically and physiologically. It possesses considerable range and fine control. It can be used to stimulate, soothe, inform, please, and excite. Much of our understanding about how it functions and how we can control it is very elementary. Considerable effort is being expended and progress is being made toward a greater understanding of the voice be it for everyday speech activities or acting or public speaking or singing. The next decade should produce greater knowledge about the voice and how more effectively to correct problems that affect the voice should be gained in the next decade.

Acknowledgment—Bill Conrad was kind enough to review the material on differential negative resistance and offered suggestions to improve the clarity and accuracy of the discussion.

REFERENCES

1. Hirano M: Morphological structure of the vocal cord as a vibrator and its variations. *Folia Phoniatr* 26:89–94, 1974.
2. Hirano M: *Clinical Examination of Voice*. Wein, Austria, Springer-Verlag, 1981.
3. Hirano M, Matsuo K, Kahita Y, et al: Vibratory behavior versus structure of the vocal fold, in Titze I, Scherer R (eds): *Vocal Fold Physiology*. Denver, Denver Center for the Performing Arts, 1983, pp 26–40.
4. Fujimura O: Body-cover theory of the vocal fold and its phonetic implications, in Stevens K, Hirano M (eds): *Vocal Fold Physiology*. Tokyo, Japan, University of Tokyo Press, 1981, pp 271–288.
5. Conrad WA: A new model of the vocal cords based on a collapsible tube analogy. *Med Res Eng* 13:7–10, 1980.
6. Conrad WA, McQueen DM: Two mass model of the vocal folds: Negative differential resistance oscillation. *J Acoust Soc Am* 83:2453–2458, 1988.
7. Flanagan JL, Landgraf L: Self-oscillating source for vocal tract synthesizers, in *Conference on Speech Communication and Professions*. Boston, MIT, 1967.
8. Ishizaka K, Matsudaira M: *Fluid Mechanical Considerations of Vocal Cord Vibration*, in Speech Communications Research Laboratory, SCRL Monograph No. 8. Santa Barbara, 1972.
9. Ishizaka K, Matsudaira M: What makes the vocal cords vibrate? in Kohasi Y (ed): *The 6th International Congress on Acoustics*, Vol II. New York, Elsevier, B9–B12, 1968.
10. Berke GS, Green DC, Smith ME, et al: Experimental evidence in the in vivo canine for the collapsible tube model of phonation. *J Acoust Soc Am* 89:1358–1363, 1991.
11. Hollien H, Moore GP: Measurements of the vocal folds during changes in pitch. *J Speech Hear Res* 3:157–165, 1960.
12. Hollien H, Brown WS, Hollien K: Vocal fold length associated with modal, falsetto and varying intensity phonations. *Folia Phoniatr* 23:66–78, 1971.
13. Rubin HJ, Hirt C: The falsetto: A high speed cinematographic study. *Laryngoscope* 70:1305–1324, 1960.
14. Hollien H, Colton R: Four laminagraphic studies of vocal fold thickness. *Folia Phoniatr* 21:179–198, 1969.
15. van den Berg JW, Tan TS: Results of experiments with human larynges. *Pract Oto-Rhinolaryngol* 21:425–450, 1959.
16. Titze I: On the mechanics of vocal fold vibration. *J Acoust Soc Am* 60:1366–1380, 1976.
17. Titze I: Comments on the myoelastic-aerodynamic theory of phonation. *J Speech Hear Res* 23:495–510, 1980.
18. Perlman AL, Titze IR, Cooper DS: Elasticity of canine vocal fold tissue. *J Speech Hear Res* 27:212–219, 1984.
19. Titze I, Durham P: Passive mechanisms influencing fundamental frequency control, in Baer T, Sasaki C, Harris K (eds): *Laryngeal Function in Phonation and Respiration*. San Diego, College Hill Press, 1986, pp 304–319.
20. Damste PH, Wieneke GH: Experiments on the elasticity of the vocal cords. *J S Afr Speech Hear Assoc* 20:14–21, 1973.
21. Colton RH: Physiological mechanisms of vocal frequency control: The role of tension. *J Voice* 2, 1988.
22. Ladefoged P, McKinney NP: Loudness, sound pressure and subglottal pressure in speech. *J Acoust Soc Am* 35:454–460, 1963.
23. Isshiki N: Regulatory mechanism of voice intensity regulation. *J Speech Hear Res* 7:17–29, 1964.
24. Isshiki N: Vocal intensity and air flow rate. *Folia Phoniatr* 17:92–104, 1965.
25. Koyama Y, Kawaski M, Ogura J: Mechanics of voice production. I: Regulation of vocal intensity. *Laryngoscope* 79:337–354, 1969.

26. Shipp T, McGlone R: Laryngeal dynamics associated with voice frequency change. *J Speech Hear Res* 14: 761–768, 1971.

27. Colton RH: Vocal intensity in the modal and falsetto registers. *J Speech Hear Res* 25:62–70, 1973.

28. Zemlin WR: *Speech and Hearing Science: Anatomy and Physiology*, 3rd ed. Englewood Cliffs, NJ, Prentice Hall, 1990.

29. Colton RH: Glottal waveform variations associated with different vocal intensity levels, in Lawrence V (ed): *Transcripts of the Thirteenth Symposium: Care of the Professional Voice*. New York, The Voice Foundation, Part I, pp 39–47, 1984.

30. Stevens KN, House A: An acoustical theory of vowel production and some of its implications. *J Speech Hear Res* 4:303–320, 1961.

31. Colton RH, Estill JE, Gertsman L: Identification of four selected voice qualities by spectral analysis. Paper presented at Vocal Fold Physiology Conference, Madison, WI, 1981.

32. Fant G: Descriptive analysis of the acoustic aspects of speech. *Logos* 5:3–17, 1962.

33. Fant G: *Acoustic Theory of Speech Production*. The Hague: Mouton; 1970.

34. Stevens KN, House AS: Development of a quantitative description of vowel articulation. *J Acoust Soc Am* 27:484–493, 1955.

35. Stevens KN, House AS: Studies of formant transitions using a vocal tract analog. *J Acoust Soc Am* 28:578–585, 1956.

36. Coleman RO: Male and female voice quality and its relationship to vowel formant frequencies. *J Speech Hear Res* 14:565–577, 1971.

37. Coleman RO: Speaker identification in the absence of inter-subject differences in glottal source characteristics. *J Acoust Soc Am* 53:1741–1743, 1973.

38. Colton RH, Estill J: Elements of voice quality: perceptual, acoustic and physiological aspects, in Lass N (ed): *Speech and Language: Advances in Basic Research and Practice*. New York, Academic Press; 5:311–403, 1981.

39. Kitzing P: LTAS criteria pertinent to the measurement of voice quality. *J Phonetics* 14:477–482, 1986.

40. Sundberg J: *The Science of the Singing Voice*. DeKalb, IL, Northern Illinois University Press, 1987.

41. Carr PB, Trill D: Long-term larynx excitation spectra. *J Acoust Soc Am* 36:575–582, 1964.

42. Cleveland T: *The Acoustic Properties of Voice Timbre Types and Their Importance in the Determination of Voice Classification in Male Singers*. Ph.D. Dissertation, University of Southern California, 1976.

43. Colton RH: Spectral characteristics of the modal and falsetto registers. *Folia Phoniatr* 24:337–344, 1972.

44. Sundberg J: What's so special about singers? *J Voice* 4:107–119, 1990.

45. Agren K, Sundberg J: An acoustic comparison of alto and tenor voices. *STL-QPSR* 1:12–16, 1976.

46. Cleveland T: Acoustic properties of voice timbre types and their influence on voice classification. *J Acoust Soc Am* 61:1622–1629, 1977.

47. Hollien H: On vocal registers. *J Phonetics* 2:125, 1975.

48. Colton RH: Some acoustic parameters related to the perception of modal-falsetto quality. *Folia Phoniatr* 25:302–311, 1973.

49. Woo P, Brewer D, Colton R, Casper J: Videostroboscopy: Its multiple roles in the management of singers. Presented at the *Symposium on Objective Voice Measurements and Standards*, July 1991, Philadelphia, PA.

50. Hirano M, Miyahara T: Vocal fold vibration vs singing voice quality. *Acta Phon Lat* 8:169–176, 1986.

51. Lawrence V: Laryngeal observations on belting. *Int J Res Singing* 2:26–28, 1979.

52. Estill J: Belting and classic voice quality: Some physiological differences. *Med Prob Perf Art* 37–43, 1988.

53. Sundberg J, Gauffin J: Waveform and spectrum of the glottal voice source, in Lindbolm B, Öhman S (eds): *Frontiers of Speech Communication Research*. London, Academic Press, 1979, pp 301–320.

54. Gauffin J, Sundberg J: Data of the glottal voice source behavior in vowel production. *STL-QPSR* 2:61–70, 1980.

55. Sundberg J, Rothenberg M: Some phonatory characteristics of singers and nonsingers. *STL-QPSR* 4:65–77, 1986.

56. Gauffin J, Sundberg J: Spectral correlates of glottal voice source characteristics and wave form characteristics. *J Speech Hear Res* 32:556–565, 1989.

57. Hirano M, Ohala J, Vennard W: The function of laryngeal muscles in regulating fundamental frequency and intensity of phonation. *J Speech Hear Res* 12:616–628, 1969.

58. Hirano M, Vennard W, Ohala J: Regulation of register, pitch and intensity of voice. *Folia Phoniatr* 22:1–20, 1970.

59. Hirano M: Behavior of laryngeal muscles of the late William Vennard. *J Voice* 2:291–300, 1988.

60. Martin F, Thumfart WF, Jolk A, Klingholz F: The electromyographic activity of the posterior cricoarytenoid muscle during singing. *J Voice* 4:25–29, 1990.

61. Titze I, Luschei E, Hirano M: Role of the thyroarytenoid muscle in regulation of fundamental frequency. *J Voice* 3:213–224, 1989.

62. Hirano M: Structure of the vocal fold in normal and disease states, in *ASHA Report 11*, Proceedings of the Conference on the Assessment of Vocal Pathology, December 1981. Rockville, MD, ASHA, 1981.

4

The Mechanics of Singing: Coordinating Physiology and Acoustics in Singing

RICHARD MILLER

ESTABLISHING PHYSIOLOGIC AND ACOUSTIC RELATIONSHIPS IN CLASSICAL SINGING

Efficient vocal technique facilitates artistic communication and vocal health. Since singers must portray textual and dramatic ideas as well as produce musical sounds, there is a frequent misconception that the art of singing is based almost entirely on imagination and intuition. The singing voice, as with any musical instrument, can communicate adequately only when there exists the technical means to do so. The singer may be highly artistic and imaginative, but if the tools of technique are not available, those attributes cannot be demonstrated. An imaginative personality given to strong emotive expression may be lacking in analytical technical skill.

A major reason why the problems of singers are different from those of other musicians is that the voice is considered "the hidden instrument." One can press keys, find finger positions, and apply motor skills to visible instruments. Musical instruments other than the voice exist separately from the bodies of the performers and therefore can be externally observed. The vocal mechanism, on the other hand, is part of each person. Singers have the advantage of not needing to buy the instrument. Because the body is also the instrument case, no one can steal the instrument or sit on it. The vocal instrument cannot be exchanged for a better model, nor can it be sold to the instrument shop for money when one has finished with it.

Since the voice is considered to be "the hidden instrument," techniques of singing often are shrouded in speculation and false assumptions. Imaginative theories have developed as to what takes place during singing. In some instances, singing techniques project a human physiology unknown to the rest of mankind. Pseudophysiologies might be quite harmless, except that the singer may try to make the instrument work in accordance with mistaken physiologic assumptions.

These "vocal mythologies" have given rise to a number of opposing techniques of singing in the areas of breath management, resonation, and articulation. Many idiosyncratic systems of vocal instruction ignore the fact that physical and acoustic functions tend to follow universal patterns in voicing. Although individual morphology plays a contributing role in singing, all singers function as members of the same species.

This being the case, it would appear logical to base vocal instruction on two fundamental principles: (1) The voice functions as a *physiologic* instrument; vocal instruction should not violate efficient physiology. (2) The voice is an *acoustic* instrument; vocal instruction should not violate efficient acoustic function.

These principles are founded on the premise that what is functionally most efficient in the singing voice produces what is esthetically most pleasing. A singing voice that does not violate physical or acoustic functions realizes its full capacity for beauty. The question for the singing artist is not how differently from other voices can the individuality of the instrument be manifested, but how best can inherently unique qualities of the instrument be disclosed. A great singer does not originate interesting vocal timbre solely through the imagination; a great voice is remarkable because of its inherent beauty, the result of the body's coordinated response to mental concepts. The artistic imagination then makes use of a well-functioning instrument. Vocal coloration should not be achieved through malfunction.

Allowing the voice to function freely as an instrument in no way diminishes artistry. Technical proficiency frees the singer from production concerns of the instrument so that artistic communication may occur.

COMBINING MOTOR, VIBRATOR, AND RESONATOR SOURCES IN THE SINGING INSTRUMENT

A number of historic techniques of singing are based on documentable principles of acoustic and physiologic function. Some others are not. One of the reasons to investigate functional aspects of the singing voice is to identify which of the historic techniques induce good function and which inhibit it.[1]

The manner by which sound is initiated is important in most methods of singing. A centuries-old technique, the *attacco del suono* (attack of the sound), concerns itself with how inspiration for phonation takes place, with the coordination of vocal fold approximation and airflow in the phonation itself and with the termination of the sound: The glottis is fully opened through silent inhalation; subsequent onset (vocal fold adduction) is precise, being neither pressed nor breathy; the conclusion of the sung phonation (vocal fold abduction) is the result of new inhalation. In pedagogic terms, "the release is the new breath." The coordination of clean vocal fold occlusion (vocal fold approximation that avoids either pressed phonation or breathy phonation) and subsequent silent breath renewal can be developed through series of phonations known as *onsets*.

Singing tasks require coordination that goes beyond normal speech needs. The singer's ability to open the glottis completely and to renew the breath silently demands an acquired high level of coordination between laryngeal action and the mechanism of breathing. Superb coordination is developed between the laryngeal abduction/adduction muscles and the respiratory muscles. During a complete inspiration, sudden glottal opening results from widely abducted vocal folds. This ensures efficient inspiration with sufficient air for easy subsequent voicing. The singer's perception is one of remaining near the inspiratory position throughout the cycle of onsetting (the commencement of phonation), releasing (the termination of phonation), and renewing the breath (inspiration).

The technique of combining good "attack" and good breath management can be verified in studies dealing with subglottic pressure measured through esophageal pressure, because esophageal pressure varies in response to changing lung volume. (An esophageal balloon is suspended in the subject and registers changes in pressure during phonation.) At inspiration, the subglottic pressure lowers. In the trained singer, during a phonation of continuous intensity, an almost constant mean subglottic pressure can be found (Fig. 4–1).[2,3] Consequently, air is supplied to the larynx from the lungs in a slow, controlled fashion.

In Figure 4–1A, esophageal pressure is shown as measured by means of a small balloon suspended in the esophagus during a series of slow onsets on the vowel [e], concluded by a sustained phonation. The lower portion of the graph displays the variation of sound intensity over a span of 25 seconds, indicated by the time measurement bar at the top of the graph. Peaks correspond to voicing and spaces between them to inspiration. Precision in both onsetting and releasing ensures zero sound during the inspiratory phases.

The upper portion of Figure 4–1A displays corresponding levels of esophageal pressure. As in the lower half of the figure, the peaks relate to voicing and the spaces to inspiration. The esophageal pressure is nearly constant during each voiced segment and subsequently constant during intervening silences. Because these levels of esophageal pressure correspond to levels of subglottic pressure, long-held assumptions regarding efficiency in breath management for singing are verifiable.

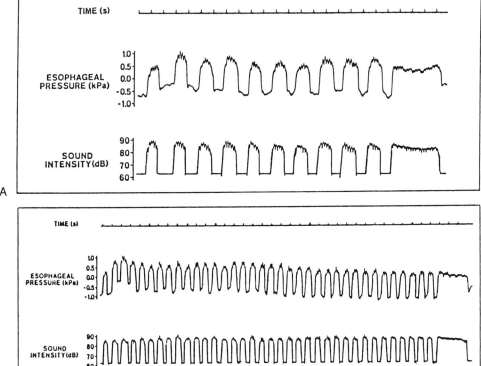

Figure 4–1.   Registration of esophageal pressure. **A,** Simultaneous registration of esophageal pressure, measured by means of an esophageal balloon, and the produced sound intensity of vowel [e] at E3 (165 Hz), in repeated onsets, with a breath between voicings. **B,** Simultaneous registration of esophageal pressure, measured by means of an esophageal balloon, and the produced sound intensity of vowel [e] at E3 (165 Hz), in quickly repeated onsets, with a breath between voicings.

The jagged peaks in both upper and lower halves of the graph indicate vibrato in each phonation. In a well-trained classical singer, vibrato begins immediately with the onset of sound and continues to the point of termination unless purposely suppressed.

Figure 4–1B graphs the same vocal task at quicker tempo, with 36 onsets being sung within 25 seconds. The precision of onsets and releases is indicated by the regularity of the peaks and valleys of both graphs. The more rapidly occurring phonations do not cause changes in relationships of sound intensity and esophageal (subglottic) pressure. The singer is able to perform this exercise for long periods of time. In so doing, a high degree of coordination between the mechanisms of breathing and the mechanisms of phonation is established. Speed of breath emission is determined by the degree of resistance on the part of the inspiratory musculature to the opposing expiratory collapse of the organs of breathing.[4]

Good singers retard the normal rate of collapse of the thoracic cavity that occurs in speech by remaining for extended periods of time near the inspiratory posture. The term *appoggio* (from *appoggiare*, meaning to be in contact with, to lean against, or to support) has been applied to this breath-emission management. The technique for quick, silent breath renewal learned for introducing the brief onset can be applied as preparation for sustained phrases. The singer then can either continue series of brief onsets or can maintain a long sustained phrase. Short onsets and sustained phrases may be alternated in rapid, silent breath renewal exercises. Such technical studies prepare the singer for the tasks encountered in "classical" vocal performance literature. They are crucial in establishing the physiologic and acoustic relationships that comprise the *appoggio* breath management technique of the historic international Italianate school, which dominated serious vocalism in the 19th century and which remains today the main route of "breath support" for major "classical" singers.

Subjective descriptions of the *appoggio* include the concept of maintaining the inspiratory posture for as long as possible, thereby delaying expiratory activity. Subglottic pressure, airflow, glottal abduction and adduction (vocal fold opening/closing), and frequency and amplitude levels combine in appropriate measure to accomplish the requirements of artistic singing.

RESONANCE BALANCING IN THE SINGING VOICE

Sounds generated at the larynx are complex tones composed of frequencies that are exact multiples of the lowest frequency, the fundamental. Frequencies other than the fundamental are overtones or harmonic partials of the fundamental frequency. The sound spectrum includes acoustic energy peaks known as *formants*.

Vowel Formants

Each vowel has its own distinct pattern of acoustic energy that differentiates it from other vowels. The shape of the vocal tract resonator tube produces prominent patterns of acoustic energy that define vowels.[5]

The vocal tract resonator system consists of the pharynx, the mouth, and, at times, the nasal passages. Postures of the lips, tongue, jaw, velum (soft palate), and pharynx filter the laryngeally generated sound. Vocal tract configurations result from degrees of constriction between tongue and velum, length of the tongue with regard to constriction points in the vocal tract, as well as the degree of lip separation or rounding, extent of jaw opening, velopharyngeal aperture, and pharyngeal widening. Resulting vocal tract configurations produce acoustic energy peaks known as *vowel formants*.

In speaking or in singing, clear enunciation is achieved by maintaining vowel integrity, which is accomplished by "tracking" the laryngeally produced vowel with appropriate resonator tube configurations. When singers are inaccurately taught to produce all vowels through one "ideal" buccopharyngeal (mouth/pharynx) shape, it becomes difficult to track vowel formants; vowel distortion is characteristic of such vocal productions. Although the acoustic principles of speaking and singing are similar, classical vocalism demands finely honed control over the source of the sound and the manner by which it is filtered. In the singing of high frequencies, space between adjacent harmonics in the source is large and may not exactly correspond to the formants of the filtering process so that there is not sufficient energy to excite them. The singer, then, as a result of pedagogic training to which the ear has become accustomed, makes adjustments to maintain consistent timbre in the mounting scale.

In singing, the number of possible shapes achieved through combinations of the pharynx, mouth cavity, and nasal chambers are nearly incalculable. Lips, tongue, jaw, and mandible can be, to some extent, controlled by the singer. The complexity of supraglottic factors largely determines the quality of the singing voice. Concern for supraglottic resonation during singing is centuries old. The history of vocal pedagogy is replete with examples.

The Singer's Formant

Singers are frequently taught to depend on "resonance" sensations. The quest for resonance balance gives rise to pedagogic terminology that mystifies not only the scientific community but performers as well. Colorful terms confuse sensation with source. The most frequently encountered expressions come from the four historic schools of Western classical vocalism: *l' impostazione della voce* (also *imposto*) (Italian); *place* (French); *Sitz* (German); *voice* or *tone placement* (English).[1]

These terms subjectively describe relationships among fundamental frequency, vowel formants, and a clustering of harmonic partials required for a "resonant" voice. "Placement" can be explained scientifically as including the acoustic phenomenon known as the *singer's formant*.

In singing, when the male voice is properly "placed," strong spectral energy is displayed in the region of approximately 2,500 to 3,300 Hz, regardless of changes in either vowel or fundamental. Thus, in a sung phonation, spectrum analysis shows both the formants that define the vowel and (if the vocal technique permits) the singer's formant. Although each vowel has its own distinct formants, the well-trained singing voice shows a continuous area of independent acoustic energy beyond that of vowel definition.

A vowel sequence [i e ɑ o u] is shown in a spectrographic display in Figure 4–2A, which describes the distribution of acoustic energy (indicated by degrees of darkness) in a frequency range from 0 to approximately 4,000 Hz (vertical axis) during an 8 second phonation (horizontal axis). The fundamental, perceived as pitch, is represented by the lowest "line" of the spectrogram, in this case 220 Hz (A3). Lines lying above the fundamental frequency indicate harmonic partials, which are multiples of the fundamental.

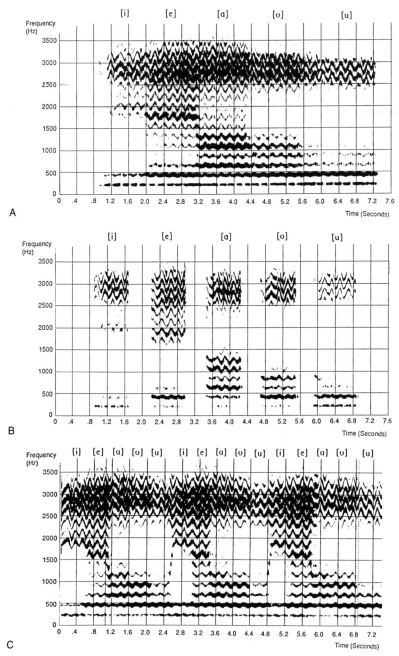

Figure 4–2. Spectrographic displays of sung vowel sequences. **A,** Sustained sung phonation, showing spectral relationships of fundamental frequency and harmonic partials during the changing vowel sequence [i e ɑ o u]. **B,** Detached brief sung phonations (onsets) on the vowel sequence [i e ɑ o u]. **C,** Repeated series (three) of the vowel sequence [i e ɑ o u] in a sustained phonation of approximately 7 seconds.

It should be remarked that, in phonations by trained male singers, there is limited acoustic energy beyond 4,000 Hz. Furthermore, there is little acoustic energy between any two partials. This verifies the absence of intrusive "noise."

Regardless of the vowel being sung, the singer's formant is visible as in Figure 4–2A, beginning at 2,500 Hz. In skillful singing, this concentration of acoustic energy remains relatively constant. (On the contrary, a sequence of front to back vowels [/i/ to /u/] at normal speech levels tends to show gradual downward shift in all acoustic energy.)

In the trained singing voice, as represented in the separate phonations of Figure 4–2B, acoustic strength remains constant in the region of the singer's formant, regardless of vowel differentiation. However, a descending steplike vowel formant pattern occurs as the singer progresses downward from front to back vowel, but without loss of the singer's formant.

A repeated [i e ɑ o u] sequence is shown in Figure 4–2C, beginning at the left margin. The front vowel [i] has acoustic strength in the upper half of the spectrum, quite apart from the singer's formant; the front vowel [e] at a somewhat lower position in the spectrum; the more neutral vowel [ɑ] in the bottom half of the spectrum, the back vowels [o] and [u] at increasingly lower levels.

The wavy nature of the lines in phonations of Figure 4–2A–C records the presence of vibrato. The constancy of vibrato in changing from one vowel to the next is an important factor in maintaining equalized timbre. Each of the harmonic partials mirrors the vibrancy rate of the fundamental. (Vibrato is not perceived as a pitch variation but rather as a parameter of vocal quality.)

When singers speak of a "resonant" voice as opposed to one lacking in "resonance," they refer to a quality of sound that incorporates several equally important factors: (1) acoustic tracking of the vowel by proper adjustment of the vocal tract, (2) balancing of the formants within the spectrum, (3) presence of the singer's formant, and (4) presence of vibrato.

As long ago as 1934, Bartholomew[6] identified several characteristics of good solo voice quality on which most admirers of classical vocalism still agree. He included (1) vibrato, (2) the ability to produce tones of considerable intensity, (3) the strengthening of a low partial at around 500 Hz in the male voice, and (4) a relatively large amount of energy centering around 2,800 Hz (with a span of about 2,400 to 3,200 Hz). His assumptions correspond with recent spectrographic evidence that vocal intensity can be increased by tuning the formants (which are produced by shapes of the vocal tract) to the laryngeal source.

It is generally conceded that vibrato provides "life" or "warmth" to the sound, that the strong low formant provides "roundness" or increased sonority, and that the high formant brings "ring" to the timbre as well as making it possible to produce a powerful tone. Thus much of the mechanical work of a well-produced sung phonation involves "vowel tracking" and "formant tuning," what might best be termed *resonance balancing*. Traditional vocal pedagogies speak of a "well-placed" voice. Such subjective terminology relates to identifiable sensations; they are now scientifically verifiable.[7]

REGISTRATION FACTORS IN THE SINGING VOICE

A vocal register is made up of a series of consecutive voice tones of similar quality. Changes in quality of the singing voice are related to the presence or absence of proprioceptive sensations. These sensations result from alterations in frequency levels (registers). It is possible to "tune" the fundamental and the formants throughout the scale, in a variety of ways. Although there may exist a multitude of possible overtones in a spectrum generated by the laryngeal source (see above), it is chiefly the presence of three or four formants and (depending on the register) a number of contributing harmonics that determine good vocal quality in the singing voice.[8] The manner in which the singing voice is "registered" depends, in part, on the relationship of the overtones to the fundamental. These relationships in turn produce varying sensations as the performer sings at different frequency levels. Phonations that are strong in the lower portion of the spectrum (frequencies that often correspond to speech range) induce subglottic sensations in the chest. A vibratory rumble is felt in the hand if the hand is placed on the sternum when speaking or singing in this register. As the singing voice is inflected upward, that sensation gradually diminishes. In the upper ranges of the voice, vibratory sensations shift to supraglottic areas and are located in the head. In an intermediate range between "chest" and "head," sensations may partake of both locations. Most accomplished singers testify to unifying the entire scale through retention of sensations in the frontal head regions, especially in the face.

Researchers often remain mystified at the persistence in vocal pedagogy of *three* main register designations, because they tend to recognize only two. But the singer depends on the perception of identifiable sensations of "chest," "mixture," and "head." These sensations result from laryngeal activity involving changes in frequency levels, as well as from formant and fundamental frequency relationships.

Skilled singers can keep consistent quality throughout the vocal range. As pitch ascends, the vocal folds elongate and their mass diminishes. In accomplishing highly skilled dynamic muscle balance that permits an evenly sung scale (unmarked by pivotal registration points), the following events occur at the level of the larynx: (1) contraction of the vocal folds (which changes the quantity of the vibrating mass and the degree of vocal fold stiffness), (2) longitudinal tension of the vocal folds (largely in response to action by the cricothyroid muscles), (3) medial compression of the vocal folds (chiefly a result of action of the lateral cricoarytenoid muscles), and (4) laryngeal positioning (effect of the external frame musculature and the laryngeal elevator and depressor muscles on the larynx).[3]

Evenly accomplished vocal registration originates in the esthetic desire to produce uniformity of sound over an extended range. Mechanically, it results from skillful coordination of laryngeal action and vocal tract acoustic adjustments.

Register pivotal points (in traditional vocal pedagogy known as *passaggi*) identify vocal categories more accurately than do range limitations. (Limitations of range are frequently due to technical faults, not to the structure of the instrument itself.) Pivotal points, also termed *register breaks* or *lifts* in some pedagogies, are dependent on the customary frequency level of the speaking voice. The first such pivotal registration point in the male voice occurs near the end of the speech–inflection range, just prior to pitches that require calling or shouting because of the need for increased breath energy. The speaker could continue to call for approximately an additional four musically notated whole tones, but such phonation would be forced and even painful. Most males cannot speak or call above those pitches, but trained singers can sing those pitches and a number of higher ones. "Mixed" voice begins at the termination of the comfortable speech–inflection range and continues to the end of the "calling" range.

These two pivotal points (*primo passaggio, secondo passaggio*) are located for the several male vocal categories as follows:

> *tenore leggiero*: E-flat4 to A-flat4
> *tenore lirico*: D4 to G4
> *tenore spinto*: C-sharp4 to F-sharp4
> *tenore drammatico*: C4 to F4
> *heldentenor*: C4 to F4; B3 to E4
> *baritono lirico*: B3 to E4
> *baritono drammatico*: B-flat3 to E-flat4
> *basso cantante*: A3 to D4
> *basso*: A-flat3 to D-flat4
> *basso profondo*: G3 to C4

The descending levels of frequencies indicated above for the several categories of male voice present the same registration phenomena at corresponding pivotal points from highest to lowest male vocal category. In traditional vocal pedagogies, the register below the *primo passaggio* is termed *chest voice*; the region between the two *passaggi* is designated as *voce mista*, *voix mixte* (mixed voice), or *voce media* (middle voice). This middle area comprises the *zona di passaggio*, the passage zone between "chest" and "head." The range above the *secondo passaggio* is termed *head voice*.

From a purely functional standpoint, the short middle-voice range with its overlapping of "chest" and "head" is largely a proprioceptive response generated by the unconscious gradual elongation of the vocal folds and by acoustic factors. *Voce media* is an area where the singer makes choices as to how he will "mix" physiologic and acoustic events that produce the two chief vocal registers.

A number of voice researchers distinguish only two registers, termed *modal* and *falsetto*. At times the terms *heavy mechanism* and *light mechanism* are similarly used to designate two kinds of register activity. Although useful, these terms imply two distinct and separate functions, whereas the aim of good singing is to avoid sudden shifts in timbre; two separate mechanisms for the production of pitch do not exist. Rather, there are graded laryngeal changes dependent on vocal fold elongation and the diminution of vocal fold mass.

To the singing community, *falsetto* refers almost exclusively to the imitative sound of the female voice for effects or for countertenoring. Much of the confusion in applying registration research from nonsingers to singers stems from a lack of shared terminology among the scientific and the performance communities with regard to the term *falsetto*.

Structural differences exist between male and female larynges. Events of puberty are more radical in the male than in the female. The membranous portion of the adult male vocal fold is longer than that of the female. Cartilaginous portions of the male fold are proportionately shorter than in the female fold.

Female speech habits may include heavy reliance on "chest" or on both "chest" and "head" for speech inflection or may be restricted almost entirely to "head." E-flat4 is the traditional point for the soprano voice, above which chest timbre is considered inappropriate. The corresponding point for the mezzo-soprano is at F4; for the contralto at F-sharp4 or G4. This pivotal point is the *primo passaggio* of the female vocal instrument, generally referred to as the *lower passaggio*. (The *secondo passaggio* is then termed the *upper passaggio*.) The long middle ranges of female singing instruments are as follows:

> *soprano lirico*: E-flat4 to F-sharp5
> *soprano drammatico*: F4 to F-sharp5 (or F5)

> *mezzo-soprano*: F-sharp4 to F5
> *contralto*: G4 to E5 (or A-flat4 to D5)

Pitches above the upper register points are said to be in "head." The overlapping of registers means that a number of pitches can be sung in several kinds of registration. The singer makes artistic choices. The female singer can "mix" register timbres at will in the lower portion of the scale.

Investigative studies of both males and females confirm functional differences that occur throughout the scale in singing; these events are termed *vocal registers* in traditional pedagogies. It is generally conceded that carrying chest voice too far up the ascending scale violates the processes of vocal fold elongation and vocal fold mass diminution and may lead to unhealthy voicing in both males and females.

VOWEL MODIFICATION IN SINGING

Covering is a subjective term used in some pedagogies to describe adjustments of the spectra to achieve greater uniformity of the scale in mounting pitch. The purpose of "cover" is to avoid blatant or "white" voice that results from the joining of high fundamental frequencies to high-lying formants, especially in the lateral front vowels. This adjustment is both laryngeal and acoustic.

Accomplishing uniformity of timbre from the lowest to the highest note of a singing voice is the aim of most pedagogies. This process involves a subtle adjustment of the harmonic partials as they relate to rising pitch and vowel formation. In general, singers tend to "modify" vowels toward neighboring vowels in order to reduce the conjoining of high frequencies and vowels that have acoustic strength in the upper portions of the spectra. This technique is also known as "vowel migration."[9]

To avoid blatant timbre, the larynx must remain in a relatively low posture. External frame support offered by the musculature of the neck helps to maintain low laryngeal position. The volume of the pharynx is enlarged when the larynx is so positioned. If the larynx mounts with the ascent of pitch, pharyngeal space is diminished.

However, in good singing techniques, the larynx remains stable, without elevating for rising pitch; any need for suddenly induced laryngeal lowering is avoided by proper initial laryngeal positioning, the result of external frame support by the neck musculature.

Equalization of vocal registers is accomplished through coordinating gradual modification of the laryngeal configurations (which generate vowel definition) with the corresponding vocal tract resonator shapes. This is the technique of vowel modification by means of which natural "covering" is accomplished without radical laryngeal adjustment.

THE LANGUAGE OF IMAGERY VERSUS
THE LANGUAGE OF FUNCTION

It is *not* the case that in the past vocal pedagogy relied entirely on the language of imagery. A strong case can be made that major singing teachers of the past two centuries used the scientific and medical information available to them. It should be recalled that Manuel Garcia, perhaps the most important voice teacher of the past century, invented and used a precursor of the modern laryngoscope. Interest in applying the findings of science to vocal pedagogy is not a recent development.

On the other hand, it cannot be claimed that modern-day vocal pedagogy has abandoned the language of imagery in favor of the language of function. Without doubt, however, professional organizations from both performance and scientific communities, through symposia and publications, have done much to bring about an awareness of the functional aspects of the singing voice. Although that impact has not resulted in complete victory for the language of function, the increasing availability of instrumentation for examination and analysis of the sounds of singing is changing the nature of American vocal pedagogy. Today's teacher of singing is expected to be informed on how the voice functions.

This situation is due in part to contemporary interdisciplinary approaches in caring for the professional voice user. The voice teacher is no longer dependent on unverifiable assumptions as to how the "hidden" instrument functions physiologically and acoustically, nor must he or she any longer be alone in diagnosing problems in vocal technique. There is at hand a complete battery of instrumentation for both acoustic analysis and clinical examination.

In meeting the strenuous demands of singing, the most efficient vocal production is the most viable. If the vocal instrument functions well from a mechanical standpoint, the singer has the means by which to communicate artistically.

It is presupposed that the teacher of singing possesses the ability to diagnose technical problems and to prescribe corrective measures. This can take place only if there is comprehension of vocal acoustics and physiology. Modern vocal pedagogy is based on specificity of information, not on mythology. Historical schools of singing are not always in accord with regard to pedagogic practices; some are more efficient than others. Conflicting viewpoints on vocal technique should be examined in light of information regarding healthy vocal function.

REFERENCES

1. Miller R: *English, French, German, and Italian Techniques of Singing*. Metuchen, NJ, Scarecrow Press, 1977.
2. Schutte HK: *The Efficiency of Voice Production*. Groningen, the Netherlands, Groningen University Hospital, 1980.
3. Schutte HK, Miller R: Breath management in repeated vocal onset. *Folia Phoniatr* 36:225–232, 1984.
4. Winckel F: *Music, Sound, and Sensation: A Modern Exposition*. Translated by Thomas Binkley. New York, Dover Publications, 1968.
5. Sundberg J: *The Science of the Singing Voice*. Dekalb, IL, Northern Illinois University Press, 1987.
6. Bartholomew WT: A physical definition of "good voice" quality in the male voice. *J Acoust Soc Am* 6:25–33, 1934.
7. Miller R: *The Structure of Singing*. New York, Schirmer Books/Macmillan, 1986.
8. Titze I: Rules for modifying vowels. *NATS J* 40:30–31, 1984.
9. Appelman R: *The Science of Vocal Pedagogy*. Bloomington, IN, Indiana University Press, 1974.

5

Professional Voice Users: Obtaining the History

ROBERT THAYER SATALOFF, MD, DMA
JOSEPH R. SPIEGEL, MD
MARY J. HAWKSHAW, RN, BSN
REINHARDT J. HEUER, PhD

As in all areas of medicine, a penetrating history provides information that is invaluable in caring for professional voice users. Professional voice users include not only singers and actors, but also clergy, attorneys, politicians, teachers, sales people, telephone receptionists, and other people whose ability to earn a living is affected by voice impairment. However, professional voice users (especially singers) are particularly interesting because of their extreme vocal demands and astute self-analysis. This chapter concentrates on singers and actors because mastering their care prepares the laryngologist and speech–language pathologist to care for virtually any professional voice patient.

A great deal of historical information is needed for thorough evaluation of the professional voice. It is often useful to augment the verbal history with information gathered by questionnaire. Questionnaires for singers and nonsingers have been published in several languages and have proven most useful in helping patients to organize their thoughts, directing the physician's inquiry, and obtaining comprehensive information consistently on all voice patients.[1] (see Appendix A: Patient History Questionnaire for the Professional Voice User.)

AGE

For most patients, one of our first questions is "How old are you?" Extensive voice use may start in early childhood and continue throughout life. Voice abuse during laryngeal development may produce vocal habits and muscle contour that underlie problems throughout a lifetime. Some of these may be difficult to correct in later life. Many people advocate avoidance of serious singing during childhood, although it appears that childhood voice instruction and performance is safe as long as attention is paid to gradual voice development and to avoidance of voice abuse. Most experts still believe that singing during puberty should be minimized or avoided, especially in males.

The vocal tract changes during normal aging, as discussed in Chapter 17. With advancing age, lungs lose elasticity, the thorax loses distensibility, muscle tone and strength often decrease, the mucosa of the vocal tract atrophies, secretions change character,

72

neuromuscular functions differ, and the cricoarytenoid joints may become arthritic. Hormonal and other changes also occur. Changes in vocal efficiency, slightly decreased range, and increased breathiness are among the common aging changes. However, the pitch inaccuracies, vocal "wobble," loss of dynamic control, and other problems frequently encountered among professional singers and actors may not be inevitable consequences of aging, but rather reversible alterations in pulmonary and muscular conditioning and control. Physicians should be most cautious about ascribing marked voice problems to inevitable aging changes alone.

THE VOICE COMPLAINT

It is essential to separate acute from chronic problems in professional voice users and to glean specific information about parts of the body outside of the head and neck. As will be explained in Chapter 14, virtually all body systems affect voice performance and must be taken into account. Often an accurate description of the voice complaint helps to localize the problem. Voice patients use the term *hoarseness* like disequilibrium patients use the term *dizziness*. A more articulate description of the problem often provides helpful insights.

Hoarseness is a coarse, scratchy sound usually caused by abnormalities on the vibratory margin of the vocal folds, such as laryngitis, scar, or mass lesion. It is caused by turbulence secondary to impaired vibration. *Breathiness* is caused by excessive loss of air due to failure of glottic closure. It is often due to improper technique, but any condition that prevents full approximation of the vocal folds can be causative. Such conditions include a mass lesion separating the vibratory margins, paralysis or paresis, vocal fold scarring, atrophy, and cricoarytenoid joint dysfunction. *Fatigue* is the inability to phonate for extensive periods of time without change in vocal quality. It is often caused by hyperfunctional voice abuse, but it may also be associated with generalized fatigue, myasthenia gravis,[2-5] or other serious health problems. *Volume disturbance* may arise as an inability to phonate loudly or softly. In young vocalists, this is usually a training deficit. However, in established voice professionals, superior laryngeal nerve paralysis, fluid retention in Reinke's space, and other causes must be considered. *Prolonged warm-up time* is most commonly caused by gastroesophageal reflux laryngitis that produces temporary vocal fold edema. *Tickling* or *choking* during phonation is suggestive of pathology on the vibratory margin. Extensive voice use should be stopped immediately when this occurs until after the vocal folds have been examined. *Pain* in the neck while singing or speaking is most commonly associated with hyperfunctional voice abuse, although vocal fold lesions, arthritis, reflux, infection, and neoplasm occasionally cause similar complaints.

DATE OF THE NEXT IMPORTANT PERFORMANCE

Singers and actors frequently seek medical care within days or even hours of important performances. Otolaryngologists must recognize that this does not imply hypochondriasis, neurosis, or stage fright. In the young singer, illness occurs shortly before performances because of the enormous physical and emotional stress caused by pre-performance rehearsals, publicity commitments, and other professional demands. These problems are compounded when the performance is not in the vocalist's home city. In this case, the performer is exposed to new allergens, an unfamiliar bed and hotel room, and other factors that can impair vocal performance. For established professionals, performances are nearly a daily occurrence. Consequently, *any* time they get sick is likely to precede a performance.

To provide optimal advice, the physician must appreciate the importance of a performer's voice and his or her career plans, the importance of upcoming commitments, and the consequences of canceling specific performances. Improper prescription of voice rest can be almost as damaging to a career as injudicious performance. Canceling a concert at the last minute may seriously damage a performer's reputation and may have enormous financial implications. Certainly no one should be permitted to perform when there is serious risk of permanent vocal fold injury. However, in the more frequent borderline cases, the condition of the vocal folds must be weighed along with other factors affecting the professional voice user in the context of his or her profession.

AMOUNT AND NATURE OF VOCAL TRAINING

It is important to establish how long a singer or actor has been studying voice and performing. Extensive voice use without training is often responsible for vocal difficulty. The number of years of training is only a partial guide to vocal proficiency. Physicians must also assess the nature of the training, whether it has been continuous or interrupted, how many teachers have been used, and how recently lessons occurred. These factors are important not only in singers, but also in actors. In assessing singers, it is also important to learn whether a trained singer has had any formal instruction on speaking technique. Most have not, and vocal problems in excellent singers are often caused by abuses during speaking.

TYPE OF SINGING AND ENVIRONMENT

Singers, actors, and other professional voice users are often required to work under circumstances that adversely affect voice function. Background noise is particularly troublesome. Trained singers learn to compensate for the Lombard effect (tendency to speak more loudly in the presence of background noise) by learning to control vocal volume "by feel" rather than "by ear." Such training often fails early in a career, especially during the first performances in large or outdoor theaters, and with loud amateur orchestras. Pop musicians have greater auditory feedback problems unless they use monitor speakers correctly. Choral and amateur singers and actors in large rooms not designed for voice performance, stock traders, telephone users in an open office pool, and others also tend to abuse their voices through excessive volume, increased neck and tongue tension, and other technical deficiencies. Voice fatigue and hoarseness are common, and nodules may also result.

REHEARSAL

Practice is as important to the vocalist as exercise is to the athlete. Effective vocal practice involves scales and specific exercises designed to develop strength, agility, and endurance.

Physicians must establish whether a professional voice user practices regularly. Both warm-up and cool-down exercises are important in training routines. "Warming-up" the voice before extensive voice use is analogous to stretching and "limbering up" before running a marathon. "Cooling-down" following heavy voice use involves similar vocal exercises and is analogous to other athletic cool-down procedures. Many people neglect warm-up and cool-down exercises and consequently develop minor technical errors to compensate for loss of strength and control during initial vocalization. These lead to vocal strain, fatigue, and decreased range.

VOICE ABUSE

An extensive discussion of vocal technique in speaking and singing is beyond the scope of this chapter. These items are discussed elsewhere in this book. However, it is essential for physicians to be familiar with common vocally abusive behavior. Physicians must be alert for them in order to establish accurate diagnoses and to be familiar with them in order to counsel voice patients on vocal hygiene. This is especially imperative when allowing a professional voice user to perform with mild laryngitis or other health impairments.

GENERAL HEALTH

Optimal voice use requires well-coordinated interaction of a myriad of physical functions. Phonation, especially professional singing and acting, is highly athletic. Pulmonary and abdominal muscle conditioning is especially important, but maladies anywhere in the body can be reflected in the voice. The otolaryngologist must consciously attend to problems outside the head and neck, as well as regional otolaryngologic concerns.

The history must include questions that elicit symptoms of medical problems throughout the body, as discussed in Chapter 14. These include inquiries about weight and weight changes, exercise, and general aerobic conditioning, all problems that can interfere with effective support. One must also seek subtle signs of pulmonary disease, particularly occult asthma, which may present with hyperfunctional technique.[6] A history of prolonged warm-up time, morning hoarseness, halitosis, excessive phlegm, cough, or other symptoms of reflux laryngitis is important to detect this common condition, particularly since classic "heart burn" is often absent. Reports of otalgia, pain, or tension in the jaw or neck may lead to a diagnosis of temporomandibular joint dysfunction or cervical dysfunction, which may impair performance. Any condition that interferes with effective abdominal and back muscle function may undermine support and result in dysphonia and voice fatigue. Constipation, diarrhea, muscle spasm, abdominal cramps, lack of exercise, and similar problems may be responsible for the complaint that brings the patient to an otolaryngologist's office.

The human voice is extremely sensitive to psychological factors, which accounts for the unique beauty and communicative ability of the voice. When stress becomes uncontrolled, alterations in autonomic function or in fine motor control may be disabling to the professional voice user. When such problems occur routinely before vocal commitments, they are known as pre-performance anxiety. When this is incapacitating, training, counseling, and therapy are usually the best course; but self-medication is more common. A careful history of alcohol and drug abuse must be obtained.

The voice is also affected greatly by even slight changes in hormone levels. Special attention must be paid to the symptoms of hypothyroidism and sex hormone dysfunction. Even a mild degree of hypothyroidism can produce muffling of the voice. Loss of vocal efficiency in the premenstrual period is common. Similar problems occur during menses. Lowering of the fundamental frequency of the voice and other undesirable changes occur routinely following menopause and may be forestalled by hormone therapy. However, androgen administration must be avoided whenever possible. Even relatively small amounts of androgen, such as those used to treat endometriosis, can cause coarsening of the voice and lowering of fundamental frequency.

EXPOSURE TO IRRITANTS

Any substance that alters the character of mucosal secretions can impair voice performance. Allergies to dust and mold are common problems in rehearsal and performance halls. Cold air conditioning and dry heat produce similar problems. The symptoms are aggravated in the presence of nasal obstruction. Nasal breathing permits warming, filtration, and humidification of inspired air. When the nasal airway is partially occluded, an individual is forced to breathe cold, unfiltered, unhumidified air, which further irritates and dehydrates the vocal mucosa.

These problems can be ameliorated by use of a protective mask such as those worn by carpenters or surgeons. Masks that contain fiberglass should be avoided. The use of a mask is especially helpful when set construction is going on in the rehearsal area.

A history of airplane travel is also suggestive of mucosal irritation. Airplanes are noisy and dry.[7] Certain cities (especially Las Vegas) are also notorious for their irritant effects. The deleterious effects of tobacco smoke on mucosa are indisputable. Even in voice professionals who do not smoke, secondary smoke may produce similar problems, especially for performers working in nightclubs.

DRUGS

A history of alcohol or drug abuse suggests the probability of poor technique. These substances interfere with fine motor control, the fundamental goal of voice training. In addition to seeking a history of alcohol, narcotic, and sedative medications, physicians should also inquire about abuse of common over-the-counter and prescription drugs. These are discussed in the chapter on "Medications and Their Effects on the Voice" (Chapter 15). Abuse of antihistamines, antibiotics, diuretics, and beta blockers is especially common. Cocaine and marijuana are also abused commonly, especially by pop musicians.

FOOD

Various foods can have adverse effects on the voice. Milk and milk products are troublesome for many people. They can increase the viscosity of mucosal secretions. Casein and allergy have been implicated as causes. Problems associated with milk products are well known to otolaryngologists, who are accustomed to restricting these products from the diets of patients who have undergone supraglottic laryngectomy. Vocalists complaining of "increased phlegm" may have a milk-related problem. Chocolate can produce similar effects. Highly spiced foods tend to aggravate reflux, as do caffeine and alcohol. Other dietary habits may also have a bearing on voice complaints. Physicians should inquire not only about the specific foods consumed, but also the time of eating in relation to voice performance.

SURGERY

The voice can also be affected by surgical procedures outside the larynx, including tonsillectomy, neck surgery (thyroidectomy), thoracic surgery, abdominal surgery, surgery on the extremities, and intubation for any procedure performed under general anesthesia.[1] It is important to determine the relationship between the dysphonia and the surgery, especially whether the voice complaint occurred before the operation, immediately after surgery, or days to weeks following surgery. It is also important to ask when speaking and singing were resumed after surgery.

These historical facts can provide very useful diagnostic information. For example, a history of voice fatigue, decreased range, difficulty singing softly, and increased neck tension occurring weeks after abdominal surgery often lead the physician to discover that the patient began singing shortly after the operation, some times even in the recovery room. Voice use during the healing period when abdominal support is impaired by pain and surgical weakness lead to changes in singing technique, usually with compensatory hyperfunction in the neck and tongue. Similar problems can result when performance is impaired by abnormal posture following extremity surgery.

SUMMARY

A comprehensive history frequently reveals the nature of a voice problem even before a physical examination is performed. The history must include information not only about head and neck disorders, but moreover about the function of all bodily systems. Additional information about relevant medical conditions, and about the subsequent specialized physical examination, are given in the following chapters.

Acknowledgments—The authors express their appreciation to Raven Press for permission to republish material from the book *Professional Voice: The Science and Art of Clinical Care*, 1991; to W.B. Saunders for permission to republish material from "Professional singers: the science and art of clinical care," *Am J Otolaryngol* 2:251–266, 1981; to Raven Press for permission to republish material from "The professional voice: part I," *J Voice* 1:92–104, 1987; "The professional voice: part II," *J Voice* 1:191–201, 1987; and "The professional voice: part III," *J Voice* 1:283–292, 1987; and to the *Journal of Otolaryngology* for permission to republish material from "Physical examination of the professional singer," *J Otolaryngol* 12:277–382, 1983.

REFERENCES

1. Sataloff RT: *Professional Voice: The Science and Art of Clinical Care*. Raven Press, New York, 1991.
2. Aronson AE: Early motor unit disease masquerading as psychogenic breathy dysphonia: A clinical case presentation. *J Speech Hear Dis* 36:116–124, 1971.
3. Ball JRB, Lloyd JH: Myasthenia gravis as mysteria *Med J Aust* 58:1018–1020, 1971.
4. Neiman RH, Mountjoy JR, Allen EL: Myasthenia gravis focal to the larynx. *Arch Otolaryngol* 101:569 570, 1975.
5. Wolski W: Hypernasality as the presenting symptom of myasthenia gravis. *J Speech Hear Dis* 32:36–38, 1967.
6. Cohn JR, Sataloff RT, Spiegel JR, Fish JE, Kennedy K: Airway reactivity-induced asthma in singers (ARIAS). *J Voice* 5:332–337, 1991.
7. Feder RJ: The professional voice and airline flight. *Otolaryngol Head Neck Surg* 92:251–254, 1984.

6

The Multidisciplinary Voice Clinic

MICHAEL S. BENNINGER, MD
BARBARA H. JACOBSON, PhD
ALEX F. JOHNSON, PhD

The evaluation of the professional with a voice disorder has been discussed in previous chapters. In this chapter we discuss the role of the voice clinic as the central focus in the global evaluation and management planning of the professional voice user.

ROLE OF THE VOICE CLINIC

The specialized demands on the professional voice user can result in vocal dysfunction, which can require the expertise of several individuals for evaluation and treatment. In minimal or mild dysfunction without significant laryngeal pathology, a thorough history and physical examination may readily yield an etiology of the problem, which may be modified through simple behavioral, social, or vocal techniques. Under these circumstances, a formal voice clinic evaluation may not be indicated for appropriate recommendations and follow-up. This scenario occurs infrequently. The more typical patient is one who has multiple factors that interact and may complicate treatment planning. A complete physical examination, appropriate objective testing, and speaking and singing voice assessment are necessary to diagnose and treat such a patient appropriately and thoroughly.

The expanding role of performing arts medical centers and multidisciplinary evaluation and treatment groups in many other areas of medicine have supported the importance of the input of individuals with expertise in pertinent areas of diagnosis and treatment. This is particularly true in vocal arts medicine. The bridging of what at first may seem to be the unrelated areas of medicine and art have allowed the voice teacher, physician, speech–language pathologist, voice scientist, and other medical specialists to join together to best understand, evaluate, and treat the professional voice user.

With this interdisciplinary approach has come the development of clinics directed at treating patients with voice-related disorders. As refinement of diagnostic skills has occurred and a greater appreciation of the special needs of the professional voice has evolved, such general voice clinics have been developed into professional voice clinics to treat specific voice dysfunction.

There are many different approaches to the professional voice clinic. The primary components are knowledgeable professionals experienced in the science and art of performing voice care, appropriate objective diagnostic capabilities, and a network for referrals for individuals who need to receive a portion of their evaluation and treatment outside of the physical confines of the voice clinic. Diversity of approach and organization of such clinics will vary depending on the knowledge and experience of those who treat the individuals. Themes that seem to be universal are the ability of the voice clinic to continue to evolve and develop as experience, technology, and patient needs change and the role of the clinic in standardization of evaluation and treatment for specific patient groups.

With a multidisciplinary approach, the voice clinic serves as a center to focus the creative energy of the professionals who are involved in the treatment of the professional voice user. This provides an environment of collaboration and standardizes the nomenclatures so that all members of the voice team are fluent in the terms of otolaryngology, speech–language pathology, and vocal pedagogy. Ongoing information is made available to all members of the team regarding modalities of assessment and treatment. Often, formal training in medicine, speech–language pathology, and vocal pedagogy lack the breadth of exposure to the relevant fields necessary to manage the professional voice user appropriately. Finally, the voice clinic becomes a central point for ongoing education and instruction for both members of the voice team and residents and fellows in training. The availability of such a specialized group of patients also provides an excellent environment for ongoing clinical research.

APPROACHES TO THE PROFESSIONAL VOICE CLINIC

The practice environment and the previous experience of the voice team members will likely determine the specific organization of the voice clinic. In the voice clinic in which the otolaryngologist has extensive experience in vocal performance, professional voice use, and voice training, he or she may include general instruction on voice production and voice care and may implement such suggestions alone, under the proper circumstances. This would be used to augment traditional medical and surgical evaluation. The help of the speech–language pathologist, however, would still be available and in the more frequent circumstances be used.[1]

In a different scenario, described by Rammage et al,[2] the voice clinic team includes an otolaryngologist, speech–language pathologist, psychiatrist, and voice teacher. A standardized protocol for assessment with joint initial interview occurs with a psychiatrist and voice teacher participating "if information on the patient obtained previously indicates that a more comprehensive assessment is advisable from the onset." After assessment, the otolaryngologist and speech–language pathologist confer on diagnosis and management prior to discussion with the patient, with management decisions possibly being deferred until evaluation by a voice teacher is obtained.

A third possible clinic model is one in which the clinical voice laboratory team includes a laryngologist, speech–language pathologist, voice teacher, nurse clinician, and voice scientist. The laryngologist completes the history (with the aid of a questionnaire) and performs a physical examination and a limited evaluation of the speaking and singing voice as applicable. The patient then undergoes objective special procedures such as electroglottography and strobovideolaryngoscopy testing, which is in part performed by the laryngologist and at least one other member of the team. This is followed by objective voice analysis. The patient is then evaluated by the speech–language pathologist and subsequently by the voice teacher. At the conclusion of the examination process the team members share their findings and the laryngologist provides the patient with a comprehensive treatment plan.[3]

Many other permutations are possible, depending on facility resources and patient demand. For staff who are involved, basic requirements are a commitment to the professional voice user and a knowledge of the issues and needs that are particular to this patient group. While extensive staffing is not necessary at one site to provide adequate care, it is imperative that there be accessibility to other professionals (e.g., psychologists, pulmonary physicians) whose levels of interest mirror those of the voice clinic team.

THE PROFESSIONAL VOICE CLINIC AT HENRY FORD HOSPITAL

The Professional Voice Clinic at Henry Ford Hospital meets on a routine basis to utilize the multidisciplinary approach for both the evaluation and treatment of the performing vocalist with vocal dysfunction. The otolaryngologist, speech–language pathologist, and voice teacher are all present at the time of evaluation. For patients who require neurologic intervention or electromyography, a neurologist is also incorporated into the team. Referrals are made to the Professional Voice Clinic through a variety of sources, including outside otolaryngologists, internal physicians within the Henry Ford Health System, individual patients of the speech–language pathologist or otolaryngologists, and directly through the Center for the Evaluation and Treatment of the Performing Artist at Henry Ford Hospital. Ideally, the initial assessment is in the formal Professional Voice Clinic. On occasion a patient is evaluated by the attending otolaryngologist or speech–language pathologist first and then is referred to the clinic for multidisciplinary input.

Patients are staggered for their appointment time by approximately 30 minutes, and the entire assessment process takes approximately 2 hours per patient. If patients are referred from outside speech–language pathologists, otolaryngologists, or voice teachers, these professionals are encouraged to attend the clinic so that continuity of care may be maintained.

Upon arrival at the Professional Voice Clinic and after registration, the patient fills out appropriate informational data and a historical questionnaire. Subsequently, four separate assessments are accomplished in four separate areas. There is no specific direct sequence for the assessment to allow team members to evaluate more than one patient at any given time. In general, however, it is preferred that the otolaryngologist, speech–language pathologist, or voice teacher perform clinical assessment and that objective voice analysis conclude the session.

The otolaryngologist sees patients with a resident in training in otolaryngology. A thorough history is taken to supplement and to complete the historical data that is either present from previous evaluation or from the questionnaire. A complete otolaryngologic, head, and neck examination is then accomplished, with laryngeal examination normally occurring with indirect laryngoscopy. If the larynx is poorly visualized using indirect technique, then flexible laryngoscopy is accomplished. A general impression of the speaking voice and occasionally the singing voice (as applicable) is undertaken. In this group setting, however, no in-depth evaluation of the speaking and in particular the singing voice is performed during the otolaryngology evaluation. A form is utilized to objectify data both for ongoing evaluation and continuity and for correlation between the laryngologic and objective voice evaluations.

CLINICAL VOICE ASSESSMENT

During clinical voice assessment at Henry Ford Hospital, a speech–language pathologist completes a standard voice examination following a protocol developed specifically for professional voice users. The complete protocol consists of three components: (1) a detailed description of voice use, analysis of rehearsal patterns, careful delineation of vocal difficulties, and identification vocal irritants; (2) a complete speech production examination; and (3) audio and video recording of speech and singing samples as appropriate.

Detailed description of the various components of the clinical voice assessment are described in Chapter 8. It should be emphasized, however, that it is this component of the voice clinic appointment that allows for careful recognition of the functional causes and effects of the patient's disturbed vocal behavior. The availability of sophisticated technology for the purpose of documenting the status of the vocal mechanism does not replace the need for a detailed understanding of the patient as a "user" of voice. In the clinical voice assessment, the patient's attitudes about the voice problem, performance goals, and motivation for behavioral change are all assessed through interaction with a skilled examiner.

SINGING VOICE ASSESSMENT

In the comprehensive clinic, the role of the voice teacher is to evaluate the singing voice of the patient. By necessity, this assessment is brief, but it is possible for the skilled voice teacher to observe basic singing technique and to identify singing behaviors which contribute to vocal difficulties. The assessment may include observation of warm-up and cool down routines, singing range, aesthetics, and singing technique within the patient's vocal repertoire. In addition, the voice teacher elicits a singing history including amount of voice training and current singing voice use. Chapter 9 outlines a comprehensive voice assessment which may be adapted for use in the multidisciplinary voice clinic.

OBJECTIVE VOICE ANALYSIS

Ideally, the objective voice analysis occurs last in the sequence. Specific instrumentation to be used depends on the complaints reported by the patient, as well as on particular problems noted by other team members. Clinical voice laboratory instrumentation is addressed elsewhere in this text (Chapter 10). At the minimum, we recommend video-stroboscopy. It is especially important to look at the specific range of voice production that is problematic for the patient. We observe and record as many extremes of phonatory behavior as possible in addition to phonation at habitual or comfort levels of pitch and loudness. We also include acoustic and aerodynamic analyses. While some measures may not be sensitive to dysfunctional phonatory behavior, voice production at physiologic extremes often may illuminate problems.

Date _____

Voice Evaluation Results

Name_____ **Age** _____
Otolaryngologist _____
Speech-Language Pathologist _____
Referred by_____

I. Our impression of your voice problem is:
    ___ vocal swelling or nodule
    ___ vocal cord polyps
    ___ contact ulcer
    ___ vocal cord weakness
    ___ normal physical structure, abnormal voice
    ___ normal physical structure, normal voice

II. Clinical Results

    Vocal Pitch _____

    Vocal Loudness _____

    Vocal Quality _____

III. Vocal Laboratory Summary

    Acoustic Analysis_____

    Aerodynamic Analysis _____

    Stroboscopic Analysis _____

    Hearing Screening Results_____

    Other Results _____

IV. Recommendations _____
_____
_____
_____
_____
_____
_____

Figure 6–1. Final page of the voice clinic brochure. Information is recorded for patient education and documentation for comparison with post-treatment assessment and to improve communication with others who may have to treat the vocalist in the future.

In addition to this triad of analyses, we may elect to include electroglottography or resonance analysis, again depending on the patient's complaint. Although these measures may provide less substance to the final diagnosis, they produce a record for use in comparing pre- to posttreatment status.

During this segment of assessment in the voice laboratory, an attempt is made to explain the rationale for objective testing and to teach the patient some basics of vocal behavior measurement. The highly visible aspect of this type of testing is very appealing to the patient and can be very motivating in terms of understanding the final diagnosis and learning concrete ways of measuring behavioral changes in the speaking and singing voice as treatment progresses. If time permits, instrumentation may be used to document effects of various treatment techniques.

Upon completion of the voice evaluation, the members of the clinical voice team meet, review the results of the testing, and view the videostroboscopic evaluation. Since members of the team have taken separate histories, the historical data are used to assess the etiology of the voice disorders and to plan treatment. Subsequently, a diagnosis is made and a framework is established for treatment.

The members of the voice treatment team then meet with the patient (and, if present, the patient's voice teacher, speech–language pathologist, or otolaryngologist) as a group. The otolaryngologist, speech–language pathologist, and voice teacher discuss with the patient the etiology, diagnosis, and treatment plan. The objective voice data and videostroboscopic tape are reviewed with the patient to illustrate these findings. The patient is encouraged to ask for clarification to increase understanding of the diagnostic process as well as future management. All recommendations are given to the patient via the voice clinic brochure, which lists subjective and objective results (see Fig. 6–1).

This interdisciplinary approach to the patient with a professional voice disorder allows for a framework through which all aspects of the patient's voice are evaluated and considered. Formalized objective voice analysis is obtained that can be utilized for treatment response assessment and further planning. It also provides an environment ideally suited for voice research and for voice education. Finally, it establishes an environment that optimizes the patient's understanding of his or her disorder and, if attended by outside speech–language pathologists or voice teachers, their ongoing involvement with the person's voice care. This approach is well appreciated by patients and referring professionals and improves the visibility and potential referrals to the voice clinic. If there are medical disorders that seem to be playing a major role in the voice dysfunction, referrals can be made through the voice clinic to other medical professionals for their input and treatment.

Perhaps one of the greatest benefits of the multidisciplinary voice clinic is the opportunity to share and understand the diverse perspectives brought to the process by each professional. In addition, the different approaches to treatment planning, while often specific to each discipline, can be useful in expanding one's repertoire of treatment methods. This knowledge gained from the clinic is easily applicable to other models for diagnosis and treatment.

The multidisciplinary voice clinic may be used for follow-up after therapy to confirm effects of treatment or to redirect treatment goals during the therapy process. Often, an abbreviated version of the diagnostic process is sufficient to answer diagnostic questions or to modify a treatment plan.

CONCLUSION

Although there are many approaches to the professional voice clinic that are largely determined by the experience and background of the participating voice team members, all seem to focus on the role of a multidisciplinary approach to the voice professional. The voice clinic provides an environment for a thorough assessment of all the variables that may interact to result in vocal dysfunction and for objectification of data and is ideally suited for diagnosis and treatment planning. It allows involvement of referring speech–language pathologists, voice teachers, and otolaryngologists. In addition to achieving primary goals of diagnosis and treatment, this approach provides an environment for prevention, research, and education.

REFERENCES

1. Bastian RW: Factors leading to successful evaluation and management of patients with voice disorders. *Ear Nose Throat* 67:411–420, 1988.
2. Rammage LA, Nichol H, Morrison MD: The voice clinic: An interdisciplinary approach. *J Otolaryngol* 12: 315–318, 1983.
3. Sataloff RT, Spiegel JR, Carroll LM, et al: The clinical voice laboratory, in Sataloff RT (ed): *Professional Voice: The Science and Art of Clinical Care*. New York, Raven Press, 1991, pp 101–136.

7

The Medical Examination

MICHAEL S. BENNINGER, MD

An in-depth history (see Chapter 5) sets the stage for the physical examination of the vocalist. Without a thorough understanding of the patient's complaint and history of voice use, the physical examination becomes difficult and unfocused. Although an otolaryngologist is generally the first person to assess the patient with a vocal complaint, a number of medical and nonmedical professionals contribute to the delineation of the patient's problems. These individuals may include internal medicine physicians, pulmonologists, neurologists, endocrinologists, speech–language pathologists, and nutritionists. In many cases, when the otolaryngologist is the initial contact person for medical care, he or she will coordinate the assessment process although may not be the primary therapist for treatment of the voice disorder.

THE HEAD AND NECK EXAMINATION

A comprehensive head and neck evaluation should be completed in all vocalists who have a voice-related complaint. Although it always seems reasonable to focus on the site of most common pathologies such as the larynx, it is important to make sure that no potential sources of dysfunction are excluded because of an inadequate evaluation. The chapter on medical problems in the vocalist (Chapter 14) provides more detail about various medical conditions that affect the voice. During the initial interview, an assessment of normal facial movement, obvious deformities, and skin lesions can usually be identified.

An otologic examination is critical in the evaluation of the vocalist. Hearing loss may interfere with the prominent role of auditory feedback necessary for fine-tuning the vocal mechanism. The external ear or auricle should be examined for any skin lesions, particularly in fair-skinned individuals, and for evidence of lateral external auditory canal inflammation. With an otoscope, the external auditory canal, tympanic membrane, and middle ear can be well visualized. In some cases impacting cerumen may need to be removed and is best achieved with small ear curettes, although under some circumstances irrigation of the ear may be necessary to remove impacting cerumen. Visualization of the drum should reveal an opaque structure, and the normal malleus and incudostapedial area should be able to be identified through the tympanic membrane. Pneumatic otoscopy will give information regarding the mobility of the tympanic membrane and determination of any fluid in the middle ear space. In some cases an operating microscope can be utilized for better binocular visualization of the external and middle ear.

Nasal examination should begin with the external nose. Marked external deformities can result in internal derangements in breathing. In addition, significant external nasal deformities may be cosmetically displeasing to the individual, and the possibility of corrective surgery can be raised at that time. The nasal speculum has been in use for internal nasal examination for over two centuries.[1] With adequate over-the-shoulder light and binocular visualization with the use of a head mirror (Fig. 7–1), most of the internal structures of the nose can be seen. If the individual has a nasal complaint and has redundant turbinates or the posterior aspects of the nose cannot be well visualized, a small amount of 0.25% Neosynephrine can be sprayed into the nose for decongestion. Gross lesions such as nasal polyps, marked septal deviation, or turbinate hypertrophy should be noted. Special attention should be paid to the middle meatal complex, where thick mucus, polypoid changes, or gross purulent drainage would indicate the possibility of chronic nasal sinus inflammation.

In some cases, despite adequate anterior rhinoscopy, the more posterior aspects of the nose and particularly the area under the middle turbinate may not be well visualized. Recently the importance of the ostiomeatal complex and the middle meatus has been emphasized in the pathophysiology of many chronic nasal–sinus disorders.[2] Rigid nasal endoscopy has been shown to be effective in diagnosing disorders and blockage in the area of the sinus ostia, which could not be visualized with anterior rhinoscopy.[3,4] Rigid rhinoscopy can be performed easily without discomfort in the office, with a small amount of topical anesthetic such as 4% xylocaine being sprayed in the nose. Photographic or video documentation can allow the physician and patient to better assess the nasal–sinus problem and to determine which treatment is most efficacious.

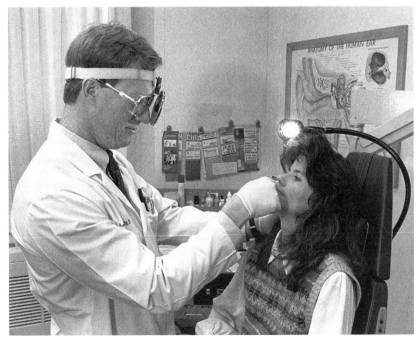

Figure 7–1.   Anterior rhinoscopy with head-mirror-directed light.

Either with an over-the-shoulder light or preferably with a head mirror, the oral cavity can then be examined. All mucosal surfaces of the oral cavity, particularly the buccal mucosa and the lateral aspects of the tongue, which are sometimes difficult to visualize, should be seen. At that time an assessment of teeth stability and dental caries can be made. The physician must be careful to look for evidence of chronic mucosal irritation, which may be caused by dental problems, utilization of irritating substances such as alcohol or cigarette smoke, or benign mucosal lesions. Most otolaryngologists and oral surgeons use two tongue blades simultaneously to be able to visualize all areas of the oral cavity or use their gloved fingers to help manipulate the cheek and gums. The patient then should be asked both to protrude the tongue and to allow the tongue to touch the hard palate to assess normal tongue mobility.

Once the oral cavity examination has been completed, the two tongue blades can then be utilized to compress the tongue gently. If the tongue blades are used anterior to the circumvallate papillae, in general the patient does not experience any gagging sensation and normally the oropharynx can be well seen. On some occasions the tongue blades need to be passed more posteriorly to see the entire oropharynx. The tonsils should be observed for tonsillar hypertrophy, crypts, or evidence of inflammation or infection. The soft palate can now be seen, and, by asking the patient to pronounce the letter /k/, the palatal movement can be addressed. Asymmetry of the plate should be noted, and in a rare circumstance a bifid uvula may be seen, and the palate should be palpated to exclude a potential submucous cleft palate. The lateral aspects of the posterior tongue are often difficult to visualize unless the tongue is manipulated from one side to the other.

Visualization of the nasopharynx is particularly difficult. A small nasopharyngeal mirror with light directed from a head mirror will allow the otolaryngologist to observe the nasopharyngeal structures. After compressing the tongue with tongue blades, the mirror can generally be used to visualize the entire nasopharynx. If the palate interferes, the patient can be asked to breathe through the nose or make an /ŋ/ (ng) sound during examination. Attention should be placed on good observation of the eustachian tube orifices, the posterior aspect of the nose, or choana, and the color and appearance of the posterior aspects of the nasal turbinates. Adenoid hypertrophy is uncommon in adults but may be present in children or teenagers. A general assessment of nasality can be achieved at this time by having the individual pronounce the nasal consonants /m/, /n/, and /ŋ/ (ng) to assess hyponasality and oral consonants and vowels to see if there is any hypernasality.

Although the tendency is to wish to observe the laryngeal structures quickly, the examiner should follow a regimented pattern of examination in every patient. Examination of the larynx can be accomplished in a number of ways. Indirect laryngoscopy with a head mirror is recommended for initial assessment, as this gives an excellent global view of the hypopharynx and larynx (Fig. 7–2). Sitting comfortably in a chair at the physician's eye level, the patient is asked to open the mouth and protrude the tongue. A 4 × 4 cotton is then used to grasp the tongue, which is firmly (but not too firmly) pulled forward. As the tongue is pulled forward a heated laryngeal mirror is brought into the back of the mouth and positioned near, but preferably not touching, the palate to prevent elicitation of a gag response. The patient is then asked to breathe gently and with direct observation is then asked to pronounce the letter e, /i/. Different vowel sounds will allow the epiglottis to assume a more anterior position, which can allow better visualization of the laryngeal structures.[5] Other vowel sounds can be utilized, depending on the portion of the larynx wished to be seen. In general, the letter e /i/ is best for visualization of the anterior portion of the larynx.

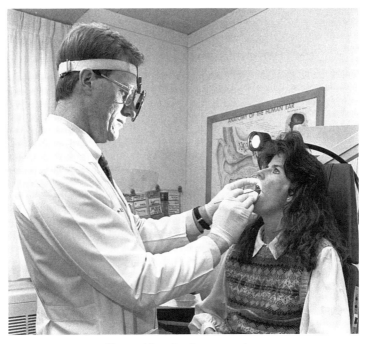

Figure 7–2. Indirect laryngoscopy. Note position of patient to examiner.

The epiglottis should be seen, looking for epiglottic cysts or abnormalities in epiglottic movement. The hypopharynx and posterior pharyngeal areas including the pyriform sinus can be visualized during phonation. The author prefers to look at the false and true vocal folds last so that other abnormalities are not overlooked. In most cases the entire larynx can be well visualized by this technique. For individuals with hyperactive gag reflexes, a small amount of topical xylocaine sprayed into the back of the throat is usually enough to diminish the reflex so that an adequate view can be obtained. In unusual circumstances, the entire larynx cannot be well visualized due to a posterior sitting epiglottis or a large base of tongue or because the patient has a hyperactive gag reflex. Under such circumstances flexible laryngoscopy should be utilized.

Throughout the pharyngeal and nasal examination attention should be placed on observing the quality, amount, and characteristics of the mucus. Evidence for decreased mucus or general mucosal atrophy may indicate either inadequate hydration or a disorder of mucus production.

Palpation of the salivary glands and neck structures are very important to the complete examination. Palpation of the temporomandibular joint and sternocleidomastoid muscles, as well as the strap (paralaryngeal) musculature, will give information regarding musculotension-related syndromes. Neck lymphadenopathy or masses should be noted. Careful palpation of the thyroid gland should reveal any hypertrophy such as noted with a goiter or thyroid masses. This is often best accomplished from behind the patient while asking him to swallow small sips of water. The thyroid gland will elevate in the neck with swallowing. Palpation of the laryngeal cartilages for tenderness and lateral movement of the cartilages should reveal crepitance, which is normally felt. A complete absence of crepitance should raise suspicion of an inflammatory or neoplastic lesion.

THE NEUROLOGIC EXAMINATION

An assessment of most of the cranial nerves is easily achieved by just observing the patient throughout the interview process. Whether or not the patient wears glasses or contact lenses gives information about the second cranial nerve. Extraocular motility and range of motion will assess the third, fourth, and sixth cranial nerves. A wisp of cotton or a clothespin is valuable for assessing the fifth cranial nerve and facial sensation. The seventh nerve controls facial animation and movement. Problems with facial movement are generally apparent although smiling and grimacing will allow for exaggerated facial movement for assessment of movement.

In general, questions about hearing and the person's ability to respond to questions during the interview are satisfactory for hearing assessment. However, if there is any concern of hearing loss, a formal audiogram should be recommended. An appropriate gag sensation would indicate normal ninth nerve function, while normal vocal fold mobility on laryngoscopy would suggest a normal tenth nerve. A shift of the posterior aspect of the larynx to one side with asymmetry in the level of the vocal folds despite otherwise normal movement of the folds may be indicative of a superior laryngeal nerve paralysis.[6] This can be confirmed by electromyographic testing of the cricothyroid muscle. An assessment of sternocleidomastoid muscle and shoulder shrugging ability is used to assess the eleventh cranial nerve, and normal tongue mobility would verify normal input from the twelfth cranial nerve.

A generalized neurologic examination is normally not indicated in a singer who has a focused head and neck or laryngeal complaint. However, if there is any evidence by history that there might be a neurologic disorder, a complete neurologic examination should be accomplished and, if necessary, a neurology consultation obtained. Evaluation with finger to nose and heel–shin tests, a Romberg test, and tandem gait will all give information regarding the vestibular cerebellar system. If there is a history of vertigo or dizziness, these evaluations should be performed, and Hallpike maneuvers would allow the detection of benign paroxysmal positional vertigo. Objective balance testing might be indicated.

THE HEART, LUNGS, AND ABDOMEN

A routine heart and lung examination is not necessary in most singers. Frequently, patients are followed by general internists who are kept well abreast of any cardiopulmonary disorders. However, on some occasions the vocal arts physician may be the first to detect a cardiopulmonary disorder, and therefore a thorough history is recommended for all vocalists.

Similarly, an abdominal examination would generally not be performed unless there was evidence of difficulty with the support mechanism or symptoms referable to the abdomen. A history of an irritable stomach and heartburn would be suggestive of gastroesophageal reflux, which may be noted on physical examination of the larynx with posterior glottic erythema and edema, occasionally with cherry red arytenoids.

ASSESSMENT OF POSTURE, VOICE SUPPORT, AND THE MUSCULOSKELETAL SYSTEM

The support of the voice is critical for controlled phonation and respiration. By examining the singer's posture, assessments as to difficulties with support can often be made.[7] Whether this is done by the examining physician, speech–language pathologist, teacher of music, or all three is dependent on the expertise of the evaluator. Some otolaryngologists have sufficient voice training to be able to assess adequately the technical aspects of voice support; however, if the otolaryngologist does not have such expertise, this may be better accomplished by the speech–language pathologist or singing teacher. A general assessment of posture and breath support, however, is an important part of the physical examination. The importance of an appropriate evaluation of speaking and singing voice cannot be overemphasized. These are discussed in more detail in subsequent chapters.

FLEXIBLE DIRECT NASOPHARYNGOLARYNGOSCOPY

The flexible pharyngolaryngoscope (Fig. 7–3) has become a very important part of the evaluation of the pharynx of any individual with an ear, nose, and throat related complaint. This is particularly true in the performing vocalist in whom what may seem like a minor abnormality may have a significant effect. The ability to visualize the pharynx adequately may be somewhat limited with a standard technique such as mirror evaluation. With the

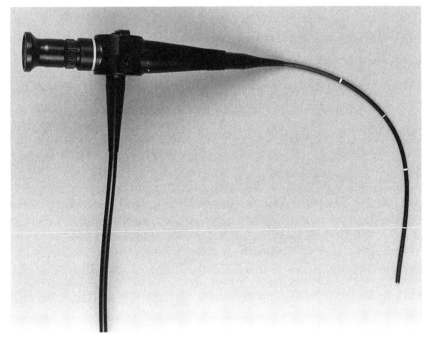

Figure 7–3.   Flexible pharyngolaryngoscope.

advent of flexible fiberoptics, the inability to visualize all aspects of the pharynx has been overcome.[5,8–10]

Direct pharyngolaryngoscopy is a commonly performed and easily accomplished office procedure (Fig. 7–4). The more patent nasal fossa is usually used, and often no anesthetic or decongestant is necessary. However, for patient comfort and reassurance, most physicians spray the nose with a small amount of Neosynephrine and a topical anesthetic such as xylocaine.

After waiting a few moments, the flexible scope can be passed. Examination of the nasal fossa can be accomplished while passing it through the nose, and the nasopharynx can be visualized for obstructive lesions or adenoid hypertrophy. The scope can then be passed down to just above the epiglottis where the larynx and hypopharynx can be seen. Vocal fold mobility, mucosal abnormalities, and mass lesions can easily be identified. To visualize the vocal folds or subglottic area more closely, passing the scope right up to the vocal folds may be easily accomplished after the onset of phonation.

The larynx itself can be well anesthetized by applying a topical anesthetic directly on the epiglottis and vocal folds with a curved laryngeal topical applicator or syringe. With such anesthesia, close and more prolonged visualization is possible, and the subglottic area can be evaluated.[11] For the professional vocalist, the author does not inject the superior laryngeal nerves with anesthesia in the office, but this may play a role in the surgical setting.

The entire procedure of nasopharyngolaryngoscopy generally takes less than a few minutes. The flexible laryngoscope can be attached to a camera and videostroboscope for videorecording (Fig. 7–4) and for stroboscopic assessment in the patient difficult to visualize with rigid laryngoscopy. The examiner may visualize the larynx by looking directly through the eyepiece of the scope (Fig. 7–4A) or by viewing the procedure from the videomonitor (Fig. 7–4B). Some authors have reported the simultaneous use of a rigid oral laryngoscope and nasopharyngoscope in the nasopharynx to assess simultaneous movement of the larynx and palate.[12] There is a potential to be able to utilize naso-pharyngolaryngoscopy in vocal pedagogic training,[5] but such investigation is still in its early stages. Some investigators have noted differences in vocal tract gestures between countertenor, baritone, and bass–baritone voices when viewed with a fiberscope.[13] The flexible scope is also valuable in assessing velopharyngeal competence and closure.[5,12]

RIGID ENDOSCOPY

Rigid 70 degree and 90 degree telescopes are now being used commonly in the office to evaluate the larynx. This generally provides a magnified view of the larynx and allows for videorecording for documentation and treatment response assessment.[14] These instruments are used in association with a stroboscope to evaluate vocal fold mobility (see Chapter 10). The rigid telescopes can also be used to perform office-based laryngeal procedures under topical anesthesia and can even be used for cancer staging in the office setting.[14]

ANCILLARY TESTING

Rhinomanometry is now commonly used for an assessment of nasal patency, nasal resistance and airflow.[15–17] The value of this study may be dependent on nasal pathology. In

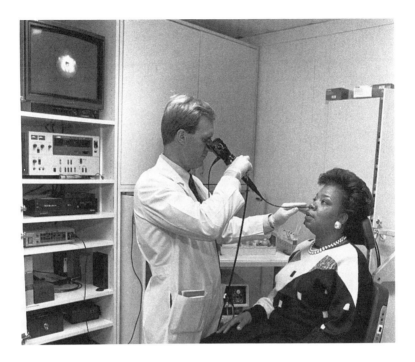

A

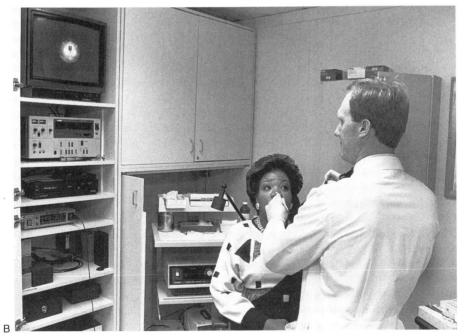

B

Figure 7–4.   Office flexible pharyngolaryngoscopy with videotape documentation. **A**, Examination with direct visualization; **B**, Visualization from the videomonitor.

particular, rhinomanometry is valuable for pre- and postoperative assessment of a patient undergoing nasal surgery such as septoplasty or turbinate reduction. Some people notice significant problems with nasal obstruction without obvious anatomic or physiologic causes and rhinomanometry can help to verify the degree of their obstruction.[17] Nasometry has also been shown to be of value in the assessment of nasal patency and airflow.[18] In addition, this will give valuable information regarding the nasal quality of voice production.

Pulmonary function tests can be performed to evaluate lung function. Quantification of air volumes and the rate of movement of air to and from the lungs are used to assess ventilatory function.[19] Two measurements are commonly used to assess lung volumes: total lung capacity (TLC), or the volume of gas contained in the lungs following maximal inspiration, and residual volume (RV), which is the volume of gas remaining after maximal expiration. Tidal volume (TV) is the amount of gas exhaled in quiet breathing, and vital capacity (VC) measures the volume of gas exhaled from the lungs (TLC − RV). Three measurements are usually obtained to evaluate airflow: forced expiratory volume in 1 second (FEV_1) measured in the first second of forced expiration; forced vital capacity (FVC); and forced expiratory flow rate from 25 to 75 percent of vital capacity ($FEF_{25-75\%}$), which is a measure of the average flow rate.[19]

Assessment of volume and flow rates gives valuable information regarding ventilatory function and helps to categorize abnormal ventilatory function into two major patterns: restrictive and obstructive (see Chapter 14). In patients with bronchoconstrictive disorders such as asthma, pre- and post-treatment responses can be evaluated to determine if bronchodilatation will improve pulmonary function.

Assessment of velopharyngeal competence often requires objective testing. As noted previously, flexible and direct nasopharyngoscopy can assess the palatal movement and velopharyngeal closure.[5,12] Lateral plane x-rays and lateral cephalograms can help to evaluate the nasopharynx and are particularly valuable for assessing nasal masses and adenoid hypertrophy.[20] Lateral x-rays and cephalograms are static and do not give an assessment of palatal movement and velopharyngeal competence. Videofluorography does allow the dynamic visualization of velopharyngeal closure[21] and is commonly performed jointly by the radiologist and speech–language pathologist. Nasometry can be helpful in evaluating the hypo- or hypernasal voice and is discussed in more detail in Chapter 10 on objective voice analysis.

Radiologic evaluation of the larynx is usually not necessary in the performing vocalist. Direct visualization of the larynx and appropriate evaluation of voice production through the voice laboratory will almost always give sufficient information for diagnosis and management. Although plane x-rays of the larynx have been utilized in the past to assess the larynx and even to study laryngeal function in singers,[22] these are no longer commonly performed. High resolution computed tomography does have a role in evaluation of certain pathologic conditions of the larynx, particularly fractures and neoplasms,[23] and magnetic resonance imaging will likely have applicability for such disorders. These studies, however, are expensive and time intensive and usually will add little to the evaluation and treatment of the performing voice.

Many ancillary studies that might be performed would be directed at specific medical problems. An in-depth analysis of these procedures is beyond the context of this chapter. A more thorough discussion of medical disorders in the performer is given in Chapter 14.

If a study is planned within a short time before a performance, care must be taken if topical anesthetics need to be used. Topical anesthetics can interfere with the normal proprioception and sensation necessary for appropriate voice production and prevention of injury. Similarly, long-acting nasal decongestants that might be utilized for flexible direct laryngoscopy or rhinoscopy can result in changes in sensation for the performer with respect to resonation. Since these procedures can frequently be accomplished without the use of topical agents, such examinations may be performed within a short time of performing, if necessary. Care, however, must be made to perform any study atraumatically.

SUMMARY OF THE MEDICAL EXAMINATION

In summary, the medical examination relies on an appropriate and thorough history. Close attention to the myriad of medical problems that can affect the voice will guide the clinician to examine the relevant organ systems adequately. Close observation of the larynx can be achieved through indirect, mirror laryngoscopy or flexible or rigid laryngoscopy. A thorough physical examination in concert with the voice assessment and objective vocal laboratory tests will provide an appropriate framework for the treatment of disorders in the performing vocalist.

REFERENCES

1. Pirsig W: History of rhinology: Nasal specula around the turn of the 19th–20th century. *Rhinology* 28:113–122, 1990.
2. Stammberger H: Endoscopic endonasal surgery—Concepts in treatment of recurring rhinosinusitis. Part I. Anatomic and pathophysiologic considerations. *Otolaryngol Head Neck Surg* 94:143–147, 1986.
3. Benninger M, Mickelson SA, Yaremchuk K: Functional endoscopic sinus surgery: Morbidity and early results. *Henry Ford Hosp Med J* 38:5–8, 1990.
4. Levine HL: The office diagnosis of nasal and sinus disorders using nasal endoscopy. *Otolaryngol Head Neck Surg* 102:370–373, 1990.
5. Benninger MS, Carwell MA, Finnegan EM, et al: Flexible direct nasopharyngolaryngoscopy in association with vocal pedagogy. *Med Probl Perf Art* 4:163–167, 1989.
6. Abelson TI, Tucker HM: Laryngeal findings in superior laryngeal nerve paralysis: a controversy. *Otolaryngol Head Neck Surg* 89:463–470, 1981.
7. Sataloff RT: Physical examination, in Sataloff RT (ed): *Professional Voice: The Science and Art of Clinical Care*. New York, Raven Press, pp 91–100.
8. Selner JC: Visualization techniques in the nasal airway: Their role in the diagnosis of upper airway disease and measurement of therapeutic response. *J Allergy Clin Immunol* 82:909–916, 1988.
9. Rosevear WH, Hamlet SL: Flexible fiberoptic laryngoscopy used to assess swallowing function. *Ear Nose Throat* 70:498–500, 1991.
10. Yanagisana E, Estill J, Mambrino L, Talkin D: Supraglottic contributions to pitch raising: Videoendoscopic study with spectroanalysis. *Ann Otol Rhinol Laryngol* 100:19–30, 1991.
11. Bastian RW, Collins SL, Kaniff T, Matz GJ: Indirect videolaryngoscopy versus direct endoscopy for larynx and pharynx cancer staging. Toward elimination of preliminary direct laryngoscopy. *Ann Otol Rhinol Laryngol* 98:693–698, 1989.
12. Yanagisana E, Kmucha ST, Estill J: Role of the soft palate in laryngeal functions and selected voice qualities simultaneous velolaryngeal videoendoscopy. *Ann Otol Rhinol Laryngol* 90:18–27, 1990.
13. Lindestad P-A, Sodersten M: Laryngeal and pharyngeal behavior in countertenor and baritone singing—A videofiberscopic study. *J Voice* 2:132–139, 1988.
14. Bastian RW: Laryngeal videostroboscopy and photography for the diagnosis and management of voice disorders. *Insights Otolaryngol* 2:1–8, 1987.
15. McLean JA: Nasal rhinomanometry and experimental nasal challenges. *Am J Rhinol* 1:73–82, 1987.
16. Pallanch JF, McCaffrey TV, Kern EB: Normal nasal resistance. *Otolaryngol Head Neck Surg* 93:778–785, 1985.
17. Jones AS, Willatt DJ, Durham A: Nasal airflow resistance and sensation. *J Laryngol Otol* 103:909–911, 1989.

18. Parker AJ, Clarke PM, Dawes PJD, Maw AR: A comparison of active anterior rhinomanometry and nasometry in the objective assessment of nasal obstruction. *Rhinology* 28:47–53, 1990.

19. Weinberger SE, Drazen JM: Disturbances of respiratory function, in Wilson JD, Braunvald E, Isselbacher KJ, et al (eds): *Harrison's Principles of Internal Medicine*, 12th ed. New York, McGraw-Hill, 1991, pp 1033–1040.

20. Weimert TA: Evaluation of the upper airway in children. *Ear Nose Throat* 66:17–24, 1987.

21. Neime S, Bell Berti F, Harris KS: Dynamic aspects of velopharyngeal closure. *Folia Phoniatr* 34:246–257, 1982.

22. Kovacs A: Roentgenologic study of the laryngeal function in singers. *Acta Radiol (Diagn)* 6:548–560, 1967.

23. Suartz JD, Lansman A, Marlowe FI, et al: High resolution computed tomography: Part 3, the larynx and hypopharynx. *Head Neck Surg* 7:231–242, 1985.

8

Clinical Voice Assessment

ALEX F. JOHNSON, PhD

Clinical voice assessment includes those activities carried out by the speech–language pathologist in the evaluation of the phonatory system. These activities, which can be specified as a series of tasks and decisions, are used to systematically determine the type, severity, and characteristics of a patient's vocal disturbance. Most important, these activities lead to the interpretation (diagnosis) of the behavioral symptoms and also to the recommendations and activities of treatment. Typically, this assessment is conducted as a complementary activity to the otolaryngologic examination and voice laboratory studies. The clinical voice evaluation in assessment of professional voice users (singers, actors, broadcasters, and so forth) is a variation of the general voice evaluation protocol recommended in many voice pathology texts.[1-3] The information presented in this chapter therefore will be a protocol for the general voice examination, with special attention to necessary adaptations that need to be made by the examining clinician for professional voice users.

STANDARD ASSESSMENT PROTOCOLS: A REVIEW

A variety of clinical approaches to voice assessment are found in the literature and are summarized here. Numerous authors and investigators have discussed basic clinical tasks, standardized assessment techniques, instrumental approaches, decision frameworks, interviewing techniques, and so forth for use in clinical voice diagnosis. While only a few authors have explored the special adaptations and techniques for professional voice users, the work to date is significant and represents contributions from a variety of disciplines and perspectives.

In general, the clinical voice evaluation can be divided into a number of components (Table 8–1), including identification of the chief complaint, general medical and social history, voice use history, examination of the perceptual and physiologic aspects of phonation, oral motor examination, hearing screening, formulation of diagnosis (interpretation), and recommendations. Each of these components presents the clinician with important decisions and relates to the various other parts of the assessment. In general, each component is represented in both the general voice examination *and* in the examination of the professional voice user.

Table 8–1 Components of the Assessment Process

	SOURCE OF INFORMATION	SPECIAL CONSIDERATION FOR THE PROFESSIONAL VOICE USER
Identification of the chief complaint	Patient report, history form	Information from voice or acting instructor, audience feedback
Medical/social history	Referring otolaryngologist, medical records, history form	N/A
Voice use history	History form, patient report	Detailed questionnaire
Examination of the perceptual and physiologic aspects of phonation	Tests and observations in the speech examination	Observation of professional voice use
Oral motor examination and hearing screening	Examination by speech–language pathologist/otolaryngologist/ audiologist	N/A
Formulation of diagnosis (interpretation)	Medical diagnosis: otolaryngologist Speech diagnosis: speech–language pathologist	Input from voice teacher, acting coach
Recommendations	Medical/surgical: otolaryngologist Behavioral: speech–language pathologist	Professional use: voice or acting instructor

The Context for Assessment

Professional Context

Before proceeding with discussion of the various individual components of clinical assessment, it is important to emphasize the context in which voice assessment for the professional voice user typically occurs. Regardless of the setting itself (clinic, hospital, private practice), the context in which the speech–language pathologist operates when evaluating the professional voice user is always *multidisciplinary*. Thus, whether the patient is seen simultaneously with other professionals present or with only the speech–language pathologist present at the examination, the nature of the information utilized in decision making is always collected from a variety of professional sources. While numerous texts discuss the significance of the relationship between the otolaryngologist and the speech–language pathologist in diagnosis of voice disorders, Stemple[4] (p 91) succinctly states:

Management of patients with voice disorders is increasingly being accomplished through the teamwork of the speech pathologist and the otolaryngologist. The otolaryngologist is trained to examine the laryngeal mechanism for pathology and to determine the need for surgical or medical intervention. The speech pathologist is trained to identify the causes of voice disorders and to establish improved vocal functioning through various therapeutic approaches.

While from the point of view of achieving a thorough and efficient examination the otolaryngologist and the speech–language pathologist should be viewed as partners, it is essential to note that every patient seen by the speech–language pathologist with a complaint related to voice production must be examined by an otolaryngologist. This examination should be completed either before or immediately after the speech–language examination session. In no case should voice treatment be initiated prior to a thorough examination of the head and neck by the otolaryngologist. Given the multitude of medical problems, some very serious, that induce phonatory change as the first sign of illness, every patient with any vocal difficulty is entitled to appropriate medical intervention and diagnosis before any focus on behavioral modification or vocal hygiene instruction is initiated. Also, given the cost of health care, it is very important that all treatment— medical, surgical, and behavioral—be provided in the most timely and cost-efficient manner. Clearly a factor that increases the efficacy in both cost and quality of a treatment is a precise understanding of the cause and nature of the presenting difficulty. This precision can only be accomplished through the discipline-specific contributions of each of the professionals involved in voice assessment and diagnosis and begins with the information provided by the otolaryngologist regarding the patient's physical characteristics and condition.

The second relationship that must be emphasized in the discussion of the assessment of the professional vocalist is the role of the voice teacher. Numerous chapters in this text are authored by professionals from the field of vocal instruction. Each of these contributions demonstrates the unique input provided by professionals involved in the teaching, coaching, and rehabilitation of the professional with voice problems.

Thus the professional context in which voice assessment occurs is one that emphasizes the unique and essential contributions of the otolaryngologist, the voice teacher, and the speech–language pathologist in providing care for the vocalist. The specific expertise provided by each discipline allows for the collection of a complete set of data for decision making throughout the diagnostic process.

Physical Context

The specific clinical setting where vocal assessment occurs is subordinate in importance to the issue of the professional contributions described above. The exact physical specifications of the clinical environment will be dictated by the nature of the practice.

For a multidisciplinary clinical setting the physical requirements include rooms for individual patient examinations by the various disciplines represented on the team, special instrumentation set-ups for the otolaryngologist, a voice laboratory, and a room equipped with a piano or electronic keyboard for assessment by the vocal instructor. While this arrangement may seem elaborate, it is ideal for the operation of a multispecialty voice clinic that operates on a regular basis and accommodates many professional voice users.

While the setting described in the previous paragraph is ideal, the speech–language pathologist who operates in a hospital or private practice setting is typically conducting examinations in a standard speech and language clinic environment. The minimum requirements for completion of a voice assessment are a private and quiet room for testing, good tape recording equipment (preferably audio and video), and access to the services of a comprehensive voice laboratory. Although there has been apparent rapid growth in the number of voice laboratories in various settings around the country, the establishment of these labs is costly due to the specialized equipment required, the employment of a qualified clinician for direction and operation of the laboratory, and the amount of dedicated space needed. It would appear that the ideal arrangement would be for voice laboratories associated with various institutions to make their services available to speech–language pathologists and otolaryngologists from around the community. This would allow improved utilization of difficult to obtain resources while providing state of the art care for patients with voice disturbances. Complete descriptions of the various instruments in use in most voice laboratories are available in numerous texts and articles and are beyond the scope of this chapter. Chapter 10 deals specifically with the role of objective voice assessment in overall patient management.

In summary, the professional context for the clinical assessment of the professional voice user is multidisciplinary in nature, with essential sources of input being the otolaryngologist, speech–language pathologist, and the voice instructor. While the professional context for assessment does not vary, clinical services may be delivered in a variety of settings—clinic, physician's office, private practice, hospital, and so forth.

Assessment Components

The Patient Interview

There are two major aspects to the patient interview process. These include identification of the patient's chief complaint and securing the patient's medical, social, and vocal histories. **Identification of the Chief Complaint.**   While the elicitation of the patient's reason for coming to the assessment appointment sounds obvious at the outset, clinical experience indicates that patients pursue evaluation of their vocal problems for a variety of reasons. Occasionally, naive clinicians assume that their understanding of the patient's complaint and reasons for coming to the appointment are clear without asking the patient. This can lead to faulty decision making and poor patient management. Even when the patient's reason for coming seems perfectly clear (e.g., very hoarse voice) it is essential that the clinician ask the patients to clarify their motivation in coming and to describe their problem. The patient who states "I think I have to change the way I talk and sing. I'm really concerned about the way my voice is impacting on my career. . . . I've been overlooked for key roles in two musicals and my agent tells me it is because my voice is just not strong enough for the part" is demonstrating different insight and motivation than the patient who presents with "I'm not exactly sure why I came to see you today, but my doctor just wanted me to do it."

Obtaining the patients' primary complaint as well as their understanding of their vocal difficulties is essential to assessing their potential for behavioral change. The patients' statement of what is wrong reflects their own understanding of the problem. If the patient's perception of the problem or its causes is significantly different from the clinician's understanding, then intervention in the form of behavioral treatment will be quite difficult despite the clinician's best attempts until they can find common ground. Aronson[1] provides a comprehensive review of the importance of the patient–clinician relationship in the voice evaluation. He states that: "The speech pathologist who is most likely to succeed in providing psychologic support of the patient with a voice disorder is one who has a high degree of acceptance of self and others, is understanding, is skillful in asking questions, knows how to listen, is sympathetic and trustworthy, and is persistent."

In addition to providing the focus for the establishment of the clinician's relationship with the patient, the patient's description of the problem is one key to the overall assessment of the complaint. Colton and Casper[2] have identified eight major categories of vocal symptoms: hoarseness, vocal fatigue, breathiness, reduced range of phonation, aphonia, pitch breaks or inappropriately high pitch, strain/struggle voice, and tremor. The patient's statement of the problem can serve to cue the clinician toward these key symptoms. This cueing from the patient is one of the fundamental keys to diagnosing the voice disorder. While examination of the physical characteristics of the larynx and procurement of clinical data in behavioral testing or the voice laboratory are the fundamental approaches to voice assessment, it is frequently only from a carefully elicited description of the problem that the clinician can come to understand the daily fluctuations in vocal performance that the patient perceives throughout the day and the associated sensory symptoms for which objective measures are not available.

In the case of the vocal professional, complaints of vocal fatigue, irritation, or soreness after a performance can be most useful in the identification of the pattern of vocalization that may be producing the problem. The importance of utilizing this type of information in making the assessment and planning treatment is underscored in the case of the patient with a normal sounding speaking voice or a normal appearing laryngeal mechanism. It may be that these early sensory complaints can lead to appropriate preventive treatments so as to minimize long-term effects of vocal misuse/abuse and allow for the patient to maintain his or her rehearsal or performance schedule. Thus in a professional voice user these complaints might be thought of as "pre-clinical," indicating the need for a careful preventive approach.

Obtaining the History.   Data gathering through history taking serves two important functions. First, most voice disorders can be understood best in the context of the patient's history—medical, socioemotional, vocational, and so forth. Vital data that contribute to the clinician's understanding of the nature and causes of the voice problem are revealed in this process. A general form for collecting basic history information from patients is found in Appendix A. Other examples have been published by Colton and Casper,[2] Bastian,[5] and Sataloff.[6]

A second purpose, that of establishing and shaping the relationship between the patient and the speech–language pathologist, is also a key factor in the process. In addition to the medical and social history, a detailed history of voice use is essential to understanding the problem of the professional or avocational singer, actor, broadcaster, teacher, or preacher. In most cases related to vocal overuse or misuse, it is the carefully and precisely elicited history of vocal use that provides necessary information for planning intervention for the patient. Even in patients with documented vocal nodules and polyps, it is important to remember that it is the behavior that is producing the lesion that is contributing to the hoarseness.

It is essential, then, that the daily vocal habits of the patient be carefully explored. In our own clinic, a form is used to elicit information about daily use of the voice in both professional and social interactions. Actually completing a schedule of daily vocal use such as the one found in the history form in the Appendix serves as a tool for providing valuable information to the clinician, but also demonstrates for the patient the extent to which he or she is using (or abusing) his or her voice.

For the professional voice user, a number of other questions are important in clarifying the issue of behavioral contributions to the voice difficulty. Table 8–2 presents a list of topics that must be considered. The factors listed assist the clinician in understanding the type, frequency, and loudness of daily vocal use. It has been made evident from clinical experience with professional singers and actors that precise clarification of these issues is both time consuming and tedious; however, it provides a backdrop for virtually all of the behavioral treatment decisions that need to be made. In addition, as this information is

**Table 8–2   Questions and Topics for Professionals
Regarding Daily Vocal Use**

Practice schedule	Social talking (outside of practice)
No. of hours per day	a. On telephone
No. of days of practice	b. With friends
Conditions for practice	c. With children
Position for practice	Travel
Type of accompaniment or background music	Type (mode)
Performance schedule	Frequency
Performance conditions	Home situation
Typical audience size	Noise level
Frequency and length of performances	Number of family members
Type and effectiveness of amplification	Other activities
Typical posture/position during performance and practice	Musical instrument
Type of accompaniment or background music	Physical exercise
	Teaching activities

gathered it is important to understand that the interactions among and within the categories outlined in Table 8–2 are important to understand. For example, it is not unusual to meet patients who teach music classes during the day to large groups of young children (usually in a poor acoustic environment), perform two to three times per week, and work with a voice teacher. Understanding the exact number of hours per day of demanding vocal use is important to acknowledge if the goal is going to be to change this pattern. In general, the interactions between type of phonation (singing, speaking), length of time, frequency, and acoustic characteristics of the environment are of greatest interest to the voice clinician.

In referring to Table 8–2, the rationale for the inclusion of information regarding practice, performance, and social schedules is obvious to those who work in the area of voice disorders. Three categories, however, need explanation. These are travel schedule and type of travel, the home situation, and the "other activities" of the patients.

Travel

Many singers and actors are involved in extensive travel. In addition to the stress and fatigue associated with frequent travel, there are other potential hazards for the professional voice user. In general, airplane cabins are thought to be quite dry and the quality of the air is frequently reported to be unsatisfactory. In addition, the level of ambient noise within the cabin is quite high. If the patient is prone to extensive interaction with fellow passengers, there may be some temporary effect on phonatory quality. For most people this causes only slight inconvenience. For the singer or actor, however, the results can be devastating.

Home Situation

The concern is with the general noise level in the home, as well as the number of family members and their ages. Most important, the type of communication that occurs at home is of greatest interest. If there is a large family and the communication style of the patient is one of verbosity, the potential for overuse of voice is increased.

Other Activities

Many performing artists simultaneously work to develop skills in a number of areas—dancing, singing, acting, playing a musical instrument. Also, because of the emphasis from potential employers on physical appearance, many are involved in extensive exercise programs. When patients present with vocal difficulties it is worthwhile to explore the effects of these activities on the process of effective phonation. On occasion, an individual whose primary activity is vocal music presents for evaluation with the understanding that she must be doing something wrong when singing. After extensive questioning, it is not unusual to find that this person also engages in other vocally demanding activities. In such cases, it may not be the singing process that is causing the difficulty: it may well be that the patient's nonmusical demands are the source of the problem.

Summary

In summary, a detailed history is essential to the assessment and subsequent care of the professional voice user by the speech–language pathologist. All aspects of the history—social, educational, vocational, medical—are important in understanding the patient's voice disorder. A detailed and precise description of the patient's daily vocal use in various social, vocational, and performance contexts is crucial to the assessment process and patient management.

EXAMINATION OF THE PERCEPTUAL AND PHYSIOLOGIC ASPECTS OF PHONATION

The remainder of this chapter deals with the activities of clinical assessment used by the speech–language pathologist in voice assessment. It is the patient's history of voice use and misuse that provides the backdrop for these activities and allows the clinician to formulate hypotheses about potential causes of the problem and possible treatments that might be most efficacious. In the assessment process the clinician tests hypotheses regarding causation and remediation using tasks that sample speech processes.

It should be noted that instrumental approaches to assessment are treated in Chapter 10 of this text and are not dealt with here. It is safe to say that, as technology has developed in recent years, clinicians are relying quite heavily on the instrumentation of the voice laboratory for information for both assessment and treatment. The technology of the voice laboratory apparently has changed the practice of voice diagnosis and rehabilitation forever. Clinicians can now analyze the acoustic and aerodynamic aspects of speech production with considerable accuracy in a relatively short period of time. Through videostroboscopy, images of the laryngeal structures can be obtained with great clarity. In addition, the simulated slow motion pictures of the stroboscope allow for observation of the movements of the vocal folds, providing the clinician (and the patient) with direct feedback as to the effectiveness of any treatment program.

While these objective measures of voice production are essential components of the process of management of voice disorders, they are only one piece of the puzzle. The core of voice assessment lies in the systematic observation of the voice user. Given that the majority of voice disorders affecting professional voice users are disorders of function, it is important that observations of vocal behavior in a variety of contexts be made.

These careful observations need to be juxtaposed against the findings from the physical examination performed by the otolaryngologist and those findings from the speech production laboratory. The clinician who attempts to modify vocal behavior without data from all of these sources is placing himself and the patient at a disadvantage. It is valuable to the patient, rewarding to the clinician, and efficacious for treatment when the relationships between the patient's history and vocal practices are consistent with the physician's findings and the results of objective testing in the laboratory. The identification of these consistencies and inconsistencies in clinical findings allow for the development of patient management hypotheses that can be tested in treatment and modified based on the response of the patient (and the vocal mechanism) to the approach being used.

Recording and Documenting Clinical Assessment Results

Audio and Video Recording

All aspects of the examination should be recorded (with documented patient permission). There are a range of acceptable recording systems that are currently in use in speech clinics. In addition to standard audio recording practices, many clinicians are beginning to use video recording as a primary source of documentation in the voice clinic. In addition to providing a high quality of vocal output, other aspects of communication that impact on the voice can be identified with the visual image. Clinical experience indicates that many patients identify aberrant speaking behaviors themselves, once they see the video recording that has been made.

In the case of the vocal performer, it is very important to allow the patient to have as much information about the voice problem and potential causes as possible. Especially when causes are "behavioral," patients frequently need "proof" that their own practices in breathing, vocal initiation, articulation, loudness, or muscular tension might be contributing factors. Demonstration of these practices via video recording provides feedback that is objective, direct, and immediate. Once the performer can identify the particular behavioral factors that may be contributory to their problem (e.g., excessive vocal strain, hard glottal attack, poor breath support) then it is much more likely that a sincere attempt at change in pattern can occur. If the recommendations from the speech–language pathologist seem inappropriate, illogical, or inconsistent with the patient's own observations and perceptions, it is far less likely that compliance will occur, especially around issues of professional voice use.

All clinicians involved in the treatment of performing artists should remember that when asking these special patients to make adjustments in their behavior, they are also frequently asking that the patients make a shift in the way that they carry out their professional activities. It is imperative that all of the changes clinicians request have clear logical explanations. Patients will then feel justified in making the adjustments, which may present some risk from a performance standpoint. Careful recording—audio and/or video—helps in making clinical recommendations about voice use both clear and logical.

Written Documentation

In addition to audio and video recording, written documentation of the clinical evaluation is important for communication with other professionals, measurement of progress over time, and for medicolegal purposes. For the speech–language pathologist, the written documentation of the evaluation appointment usually consists of a narrative report that summarizes the reason for referral: significant history (medical, social, and vocal); perceptual observations of the patient's pitch, loudness, quality, resonance, prosody, articulation, and fluency; results of the hearing screening and oral mechanism examination; and clinical impressions and recommendations. In some clinics, where the clinical assessment and the voice laboratory procedures are performed by the same clinician or as part of a specialty clinic, then the results of the speech production analysis (voice laboratory) are included in the clinical report. In other situations, results of objective aerodynamic, videostrobic, electroglottographic, and acoustic analyses are maintained on a separate form. An example of the former type of report is included in the Appendix to this chapter.

The Speech Sample

A sample of the patient's conversational speech is very important in every evaluation of communication. In the typical voice evaluation appointment, the speech–language pathologist will have collected much valuable information about conversational speech patterns during the course of the initial history taking activity with the patient. The skilled clinician begins listening to the patient's vocal output in the waiting room, noting changes that occur throughout the evaluation.

Although it is frequently difficult to replicate the various situations in which voice is used, attempts should be made in the evaluation to have the patient demonstrate the various aspects of communication, including singing, in which he or she participates on a regular basis. It is not unusual to identify exceptionally abusive patterns in one mode of communication, while finding essentially normal speaking behaviors in another. Every attempt should be made to elicit speaking samples under a variety of conditions so as to identify such discrepancies among the various communicative contexts.

In addition to sampling connected speech in conversation, it is helpful to use some standard passages such as The Rainbow Passage[7] to elicit a sample of speech for comparison with other patient and normal voices and also for comparison before, during, and after treatment. The clinician may also find it beneficial to observe a performance by the patient or to observe a lesson conducted by the patient's voice teacher. If this is impossible, it can be very helpful to watch a videotaped performance.

Speech Testing and Perceptual Analysis

In addition to making observations about the patient's use of voice in various communication situations and contexts, it is also usually necessary to elicit more limited samples of speech and voice production in order to address questions regarding the modal use of the system, the limits of the patient's speech production capabilities, the flexibility of the patient in making speech modifications, and, most important, to isolate the speech symptoms by speech production subsystem. This analysis is typically completed quickly and efficiently given a cooperative and motivated patient and a talented clinician with refined perceptual skills. This type of analysis cannot be accurately performed by clinicians who have not developed expertise in perceptual analysis or have not demonstrated reliability (agreement) with other experts. Unfortunately, this tends to be a somewhat "underrated" aspect of training in speech–language pathology. The inexperienced clinician with an interest in the area of voice disorders quickly discovers that in the area of perceptual speech production analysis the act of collecting the data is far more easy than the act of making the perceptual judgments as to degree of deviation from a reference population, clinical significance of the observed production, degree of difference from other productions by the same speaker, and so forth. Clinicians from any of the disciplines interested in care of the professional voice patient should spend considerable time and effort in acquiring the skills for reliable perceptual analysis. Procedures for developing reliability are given in numerous tests[8-10] and articles.[11-13]

Speech Tasks: Basic Measures in the Voice Evaluation

There are numerous protocols for sampling specific vocal behaviors, which are described in the basic texts cited earlier in this chapter.[1-3] In Table 8–3, typical tasks used by the clinician in the standard voice assessment are summarized. These tasks serve a variety of important clinical purposes:

1. Measurement of the ranges of strength, flexibility, and movement within the vocal system: tasks 1, 2, 3, 4, 6, 9, 10
2. Identification of areas of relative normalcy and those of relative inefficiency and/or deviation from normal: tasks 1 through 10
3. Physiologic "localization" of the problem (laryngeal, respiratory, articulatory, or neurologic subsystems): tasks 1 through 10
4. Identification of abusive vocal patterns: tasks 3, 4, 5, 6, 7, 9
5. Identification of ability to improve voice: tasks 3, 6, 7, 9, 10
6. Identification of potential facilitating behaviors for therapy: tasks 3, 6, 9, 10

From this part of the assessment the clinician gathers essential information to balance with observations of other examiners and with data obtained in the laboratory or the medical examination. If the patient is a voice therapy candidate, the information obtained in this component of the examination can be most useful in planning behavioral treatment and in measuring progress.

The importance of knowing normal ranges for the various measurements summarized in Table 8–3 cannot be overstated. Basically normative value in nonlaboratory voice measurement is established in three ways, depending on the type of task under consideration. These three approaches include comparison with published normative values, comparison with "local" norms, and judgment of normalcy against a perceptual reference.

Comparison of a patient with published ranges provides the illusion of safety for the clinician. It needs to be noted that there are few, if any, complete studies across the life span for most of the tasks in widespread use in voice assessment. A thorough review of various normative studies was done by Baken[14] for a number of parameters of production including maximum phonation time, s/z ratio, and pitch range. While most of the literature reviewed in the cited text are significant contributions and provide a framework for further study, all clinical interpretations made against these "norms" should be quite conservative. While they serve as good descriptions of "what some normal voice users do on a task," the values presented rarely are representative of a true normative sample. Because so many genetic factors (age, sex, ethnicity, dialect), medical factors (health history, medications, psychological factors), and experiential factors (daily voice use, profession, voice training,

Table 8–3   **Clinical Tasks Involved in the Voice Evaluation**

	TASK	SUBSYSTEM FOCUS	DESCRIPTION OF PROCEDURE
1.	Maximum phonation time	Respiration, motor control, glottal efficiency	Patient is asked to take a deep breath and sustain the vowel /a/ for as long as possible. Usually done at comfort level, high pitch, and low pitch
2.	s/z Ratio	Respiratory/phonatory efficiency	Patient is asked to take a deep breath and sustain /s/ for as long as possible; then asked to do the same for /z/. The time recorded for /s/ is divided by the time for /z/
3.	Pitch range	Laryngeal	Patient is asked to sing a scale as high and low as possible
4.	Endurance testing	Motor strength	Patient is asked to count vigorously to at least 100
5.	Musculoskeletal tension tests	Laryngeal musculature	The external laryngeal musculature is palpated by the clinician with the patient identifying points of pain. Resistance to shifting of position of the hyoid bone and larynx is noted
6.	Loudness testing	Respiratory, phonatory	Patient is asked to count with gradual increase in loudness
7.	Testing for hard glottal attack	Glottal closure	Patient is asked to count from 80 to 90, stopping between each number
8.	Coughing	Glottal closure	Patient is asked to cough forcefully
9.	Production of reflexive sounds	Phonation in reflexive activity (quality)	Patient is asked to cough, say "uh-huh," laugh, and clear the throat
10.	Changing voice focus	Change in voice quality	Patient is asked to "chant" sentences with high proportions of nasal sounds

daily practice schedule) impact on voice production, it is important to know the demographic characteristics of the sample normative population prior to comparison with the patients. This is probably especially true for the professional speaker and/or singer. The less representative the sample population is with regard to the specific patient's demographic and historical factors, the less useful the normative values can be.

Some investigators and clinicians have attempted to develop normative data for specific groups of patients by testing a small group of individuals who can be contrasted with a target patient population under study. For example, Jacobson et al[15] examined a group of university level vocal students at various experience levels in order to establish "local" norms for purposes of comparing various aspects of phonatory function with clinical populations who attend the professional voice clinic. Again, this approach adds some validity to the use of the normative data because the groups under comparison have "more" in common. However, this approach also requires extensive interpretive caution. While the comparison group may reflect particular variables of interest (ie, professional vocal experience), other key variables (age, sex) may not have been included in the local normative sample. In addition, local normative studies rarely reflect a sample size to be considered statistically viable. Use of such data, which can be supportive and clinically helpful, requires interpretive conservatism and is rarely definitive.

A third approach to establishing "normalcy" is to use perceptual scaling methods. In this case, an experienced clinical listener rates some aspect of production against a scale. In some cases the scale is numeric and in others it is descriptive.[16] In these scaling procedures a perceptual judgment is made by the examiner, usually with regard to degree of deviance from a perceptually normal voice. In addition to the importance of availability of an established scale that is valid for use in voice assessment, the issue of obtaining reliability among clinical users, already discussed, is essential. Because the major benefit of the utilization of such scales is that they provide a comparative reference, it is necessary that users of the scale exert considerable energy in comparing their judgments with others who are also using it. Once a range of reliability is obtained for the scale, the skilled examiner literally becomes an "objective" measurement tool.

Thus, while none of the three approaches for comparing clinical patients to normal persons are perfect, careful, conservative, and precise use of each method should be encouraged and should become standard practice in the voice clinic. Until such time as fully acceptable standard behavioral measurements are established these approaches assure quality and accuracy.

SUMMARY

Assessment of the professional speaker and/or singer is a unique and exciting opportunity for the voice clinician. Experience in careful observation and listening, clinical management, and an appreciation for the physiologic and psychological effects for professional voice use are the prerequisites for the practicing professional. In this chapter an attempt has been made to present a view of the concepts and practices used by the speech–language pathologist in voice assessment with a focus on care of the professional.

REFERENCES

1. Aronson A: *Clinical Voice Disorders*, 3rd ed. New York, Thieme, 1990.
2. Colton RH, Casper JK: *Understanding Voice Problems: A Physiological Perspective for Diagnosis and Treatment*. Baltimore, Williams & Wilkins, 1990.
3. Stemple JC: *Clinical Voice Pathology: Theory and Management*. Columbus, OH, Charles E. Merrill, 1984.
4. Stemple JC: *Clinical Voice Pathology: Theory and Management*. Columbus, OH, Charles E. Merrill, 1984.
5. Bastian RW: Factors leading to successful evaluation and management of patients with voice disorders. *Ear Nose Throat* 67:211–220, 1988.
6. Sataloff RT: Clinical evaluation of the professional singer. *Ear Nose Throat* 66:267–277, 1987.
7. Fairbanks G: *Voice and Articulation Drillbook, 2nd ed.* New York, Harper & Row, 1960.
8. Ventry IM, Schiavetti N: *Evaluating Research in Speech Pathology and Audiology: A Guide for Clinicians and Students*. Reading, MA: Addison and Wesley, 1980.
9. Hedge MN: *Clinical Research in Communicative Disorders*. Boston, Little, Brown, and Co, 1987.
10. Silverman FH: *Research Design in Speech Pathol and Audiology*, Englewood Cliffs, NJ, Prentice Hall, 1977.
11. Kreiman J, Gerratt BR, Precoda K: Listener experience and perception of voice quality. *J Speech Hear Res* 33:103–115, 1990.
12. Murry T, Singh S, Sargent M: Multidimensional classification of abnormal voice qualities. *J Acoust Soc Am* 64:81–87, 1977.
13. Kempster GB, Kisteler DJ, Hillenbrand J: Multidimensional scaling analysis of dysphonia in two groups. *J Speech Hear Res* 34:534–543, 1991.
14. Baken RJ: *Clinical Measurement of Speech and Voice*. College Hill Press, 1987.
15. Jacobson BH, Johnson AF, Benninger M, Jacobson B, Johnson A: Normative Data on Professional Voice Students. Paper presented at the American Speech–Language–Hearing Association Annual Meeting, Washington DC, 1990.
16. Silverman FH: *Research Design in Speech Pathol and Audiology*, Englewood Cliffs, NJ: Prentice Hall, 1977.

Appendix

PROFESSIONAL VOICE CLINIC

Reason for Evaluation: This 43-year-old female was referred by her otolaryngologist for assessment of voice. On 2/4/92, the doctor reported bilateral nodules.

Medical History: Information was obtained from an interview with the patient and from her medical record. She has a history of childhood kidney problems, tuberculosis that was identified at age 16, bronchitis, leg and wrist fractures, and hernia. She has had a tonsillectomy and adenoidectomy. She has no known allergies other than to fish. She is currently taking iron and ascorbic acid supplements.

Social History: The patient lives with her young adult children. She works in a hospital laboratory and is a professional singer. Her present singing activities include taking courses, performing at the local repertory theater, singing in church choir, teaching youth groups (which requires additional singing), and working on personal projects such as singing for television and radio commercials. She talks approximately 8 hours per day and sings 10 hours per week. She has no history of vocal training. The patient sings in the contralto range from middle C to G above middle C. She warms up prior to rehearsals with singing scales. She does not perform any cool-down exercises.

The patient reported onset of voice problem 5 years ago, following bronchitis. She "lost her voice." Since then, she frequently loses her voice after illnesses, in air-conditioned rooms, on airplanes, and when she is tired. She reported that in December 1991 she had lost her voice following influenza. She complained of excessive saliva in her larynx. She reported that she drinks approximately three glasses of water, one cup of caffeinated coffee, and one to two cups of decaffeinated coffee per day. She does not regularly drink alcoholic beverages. She has never smoked. The patient reported that after working at the hospital from 4 AM to 1 PM she frequently takes a nap within 1 to 2 hours following lunch.

CLINICAL FINDINGS

General Observations: The patient was pleasant and cooperative throughout the evaluation.

Hearing: She passed the hearing screening test at 1,000, 2,000, and 4,000 Hz bilaterally.

Oral Peripheral Examination: Oral structures and functioning were within normal limits for voice production. Mild laryngeal tension was noted during digital manipulation, and excessive neck muscle tension was visible as she spoke.

Perceptual Voice Analysis: On 2/6/92, the patient's speaking voice was character-ized by a moderately hoarse quality with more breathiness than harshness, periods of

109

aphonia, and low pitch. She tended to use a thoracic breathing pattern during conversation and while singing. Frequent throat clearing, hard glottal attacks, and loud laughing were observed throughout the evaluation. She was able to sustain phonation of /a/ for 22 seconds and /i/ for 13 seconds (normal mean = 18 to 20 seconds); /s/ for 25 seconds; and /z/ for 14 seconds. The latter resulted in an s/z ratio of 1.7, which perceptually suggests abnormal vocal fold vibration (mean for normal quality = 1.4 or less). Pitch range was approximately 10 to 12 notes. Breathiness, aphonia, and strained quality appeared to increase with increased pitch while singing.

On 2/14/92, following 1 week of strict vocal rest, the patient continued to demonstrate moderately hoarse quality, periods of aphonia, and low pitch. Each characteristic was slightly improved since 2/6/92. No other perceptual changes were noted since 2/6/92.

Videostroboscopy: On 2/6/92, the patient demonstrated increased redness and vascularization of the lateral portion of the right vocal fold (suggesting possible hemorrhage). Bilateral nodules were noted at the one-third to one-half anterior portion of the vocal folds (right larger than left). Mild swelling in the arytenoid area and increased saliva in the laryngeal area were observed. Glottic closure with a posterior glottic chink was noted. Excessive compression of the ventricular folds was noted during phonation. Other than the bilateral nodules, the vocal fold edges appeared to be smooth. Amplitude of vibration for both vocal folds were moderately decreased. Mucosal wave of the right vocal fold was moderately decreased and that of the left vocal fold was slightly decreased. Phase closure was characterized by regular symmetry and a predominating open phase.

On 2/14/92, the patient exhibited resolving nodules and redness/vascularization. Bilateral nodules at the one-third to one-half anterior portion of vocal folds were mildly decreased when compared with their condition on 2/6/92. A small streak of redness was observed from the lateral middle portion to the medial posterior portion of the right vocal fold. Swelling in the arytenoid area and the amount of saliva in the laryngeal area were slightly reduced since 2/6/92. Amplitude of vibration for both vocal folds was slightly reduced (considered to be improved since 2/6/92). The mucosal waves of each vocal fold were within normal limits (WNL). These changes appeared to be related to the resolving hemorrhagic-like vascularization and reduced size of nodules, which are most likely a result of vocal rest. No other dimensions of vocal fold functioning had changed since 2/6/92.

Acoustic Analysis: Data were taken on 2/14/92. The patient's fundamental frequency during sustained vowel phonation at habitual pitch was 160 Hz, which is considered to be at the low end of normal for sex and age (mean = 180 to 250 Hz). Her frequency ranged from 108 to 447 Hz (24.56 semitones), which is considered to be reduced for sex and age. Jitter (frequency perturbation), shimmer (intensity perturbation), and signal to noise ratio (SNR) were WNL at all pitch levels. SNR was significantly increased during high pitch, which corroborated with excessive strain noted perceptually. These findings suggest low habitual frequency of phonation, which corroborates with her perceptually low pitch.

Aerodynamic Analysis: Airflow volume during phonation at habitual, high, and low pitches ranged from 2,460 to 2,990 ml, which is considered to be generally WNL for sex and age (normal mean = 2,000 to 3,000 ml). Mean phonation times were WNL at all pitch levels but were at the low end of normal during high pitch (normal mean = 18 to 20 seconds). Airflow rates were WNL (mean = 80–200 ml/s), highest during high pitch (139 ml/s), and lowest during habitual pitch (109 ml/s). These findings suggest efficient laryngeal valving. However, the increased rate during high pitch corresponded to the increased breathiness and aphonia noted perceptually, while the lower rate during habitual pitch corresponded to the increased laryngeal tension noted perceptually and on video-stroboscopy.

Impression: The patient demonstrated moderate dysphonia characterized by moderate hoarseness, low pitch, and periods of aphonia and strain. Although acoustic and aero-dynamic analyses revealed normal parameters, hyperfunctional use of muscles for voice production was observed perceptually and videostroboscopically. Although etiology for the hemorrhagic-like observations on 2/6/92 were unclear, it appeared to be related to abusive behaviors, as it resolved with strict vocal rest. The existence of bilateral nodules appears to be related to abusive speaking and singing behaviors. The presence of swelling in the arytenoid area may be a result of gastric reflux. Functional communication is good to excellent. Prognosis for improvement with voice therapy is considered to be good based on the patient's dissatisfaction of current vocal characteristics and appropriate motivation.

Recommendations: Following a discussion with the otolaryngologist on 2/6/92, it was recommended to the patient that she observe strict vocal rest for 1 week and avoid participating in singing and performing activities for several weeks. It was also recom-mended that she consider hiring a voice teacher prior to continuing her professional sing-ing and performance career. Based on the fact that the hemorrhagic-like characteristics resolved and that the nodules were reduced on 2/14/92 and appeared to be related to abusive vocal behaviors, it was recommended that the patient receive therapy on a weekly basis for 6 to 8 weeks, goals to include (1) education about and improvement in vocal hygiene; (2) increased pitch and changed vocal focus; (3) decreased laryngeal tension; (4) improved diaphragmatic breathing during phonation; and (5) counsel as needed.

The patient appeared to understand these findings, impressions, and recommen-dations.

9

Assessment of the Singing Voice

JOHN-PAUL WHITE
EDITH DIGGORY, DMus

This chapter is for an audience not necessarily fluent in the language of the voice studio in an attempt to give a better understanding of the role of the voice teacher in the overall management and care of the professional voice. The assessment process is described in detail using a sample vocal evaluation form, followed by a description of basic vocal technique in order to give the reader a better understanding of the principles on which an evaluation is based.

Though a thorough and methodical assessment would seem to be a given when beginning vocal study, one would likely be surprised at the infrequency of such an evaluation in the typical vocal studio. An introductory audition is relatively common, but that may range from merely singing part of a song to a much more complete process of scales and vocal testing. There is no doubt that better and more detailed assessment would improve the overall quality of studio voice instruction and better serve the needs of the voice student. The voice teacher who is interested in being part of a treatment team must certainly take the same care as the other members of the team.

The assessment of the singing voice by the voice teacher presents difficulties, however, because it is an almost entirely subjective process and there are a great many opinions as to what is "technically correct" singing. There exists no real standard, even among the various vocal styles, let alone between them. It is important to note that at this time very few voice teachers rely on the sophisticated instruments found in voice laboratories for the evaluation of a singer's technique. Perhaps this will change in the future, but for now it is safe to assume that most evaluation is done visually and aurally, without the aid of instruments. The main tool of the voice teacher, the ear, is subjective by nature, and therefore there will likely never be a consensus of opinion among all vocalists or teachers.

EVALUATION

The evaluation begins with taking a history, not dissimilar to that used by a laryngologist or speech pathologist, though somewhat less detailed. If in fact the voice teacher has access to a history from one of the other team members, this step can be greatly shortened. The history should include information based on the following sample form (Figs. 9–1, 9–2).

112

SAMPLE VOCAL EVALUATION FORM

HISTORY:

NAME: _____   DATE: _____

AGE: _____ SEX: _____   OCCUPATION: _____

TYPE OF USE: _____   FREQUENCY OF USE: _____

STUDENT'S ASSESSMENT OF VOICE TYPE: _____ RANGE: _____ to _____

PREVIOUS VOICE TEACHERS: DURATION OF STUDY:

_____   _____

_____   _____

_____   _____

_____   _____

LAST TEACHER: _____   FOR HOW LONG: ____ LAST LESSON: _____

MUSICAL PROFICIENCY: _____

PRACTICE FREQUENCY: _____ DURATION: _____ DESCRIBE: _____
_____

WARM-UP: ____ COOL-DOWN: ____ DESCRIBE: _____
_____

TOTAL TIME SINGING DAILY: _____

AVERAGE HOURS OF SLEEP PER NIGHT: _____ SMOKER: ____ HOW LONG: _____

DRUGS OR PRESCRIPTION MEDICATIONS: _____
_____

OTHER RELEVANT PHYSICAL CONDITIONS (ALLERGIES, TMJ, REFLUX, ETC.): _____
_____

PROBLEMS OR DIFFICULTIES WITH VOICE: _____
_____

OTOLARYNGOLOGIST: _____

SPEECH-LANGUAGE PATHOLOGIST: _____

MEDICAL DIAGNOSIS: _____
_____

Figure 9–1.

AURAL EVALUATION:

(+) = effective
(o) = adequate
(-) = problematic

SPEAKING VOICE: _____

SCALES USED: _____
_____

SONG(S) PERFORMED: _____

POSTURE / ALIGNMENT:

FEET AND LEGS _____
HIPS _____
RIB CAGE / CHEST_____
SHOULDERS _____
ARMS / HANDS_____
HEAD / NECK _____

INHALATION:

LOW ABDOMINAL _____
RIB CAGE / CHEST _____
BACK _____
DURATION _____
AUDIBILITY _____
TENSION _____

SUPPORT:

ATTACK _____
SUSTAIN _____
RELEASE _____
LOW ABDOMINAL _____
RIB CAGE EXPANSION _____

HEAD / NECK:

LARYNGEAL POSITION _____
NECK MUSCLES _____
JAW _____
TONGUE _____
SOFT PALATE _____
FACE (lips, forehead, etc.) _____

TONE QUALITY:

FREEDOM _____
CLARITY _____
FOCUS _____
PHARYNGEAL RESONANCE:
    NASO - _____
    ORO - _____
    LARYNGO - _____
VIBRATO _____

OTHER:

RANGE _____
REGISTRATION _____
VOWEL PRODUCTION _____
DYNAMIC CONTROL _____
INTONATION _____
FLEXIBILITY _____

CONSISTENCY OF PRODUCTION FROM SPEAKING TO SINGING SCALES: _____
FROM SCALES TO SONGS: _____ FROM STYLE TO STYLE: _____

TEACHERS ASSESSMENT OF:

VOICE TYPE: _____ RANGE: _____ to _____
INHERENT BEAUTY: _____
POTENTIAL TO FULFILL GOALS: _____
_____

PERSONALITY EVALUATION:
LEARNING TYPE: _____
STRESS FACTORS: _____

Figure 9–2.

Aural Evaluation

Speaking Voice

The aural evaluation should begin by paying careful attention to the speaking voice. While most voice teachers have had no formal training in speech–language pathology and should be careful not to venture beyond their expertise in giving advice, the obvious connection between the speaking and singing voice should not be overlooked. Those elements of vocal quality in speech that we listen for in determining the condition of the singing voice include

> pitch—too high, too low; naturalness; correlation with the singing voice
> range—excessively wide, narrow; voice skips from one range to another; change of quality as the voice modulates up and down
> timbre—dark and heavily weighted, or bright and light; nasal, strident, pinched, full, resonant
> clarity—clear, breathy, hoarse, poorly focused
> placement—forward nasal resonance; nasal twang; throaty; trapped in the mouth
> attacks and releases—glottal, aspirated, coordinated
> breathing—audible, tense, shallow inhalation; consistent, sustained exhalation; abrupt, inefficient exhalation; breath holding

While there may appear to be a great deal of contrast when those factors come to bear in singing, one should be concerned if the speaking and singing voices are vastly different in production. In fact, many teachers approach the training of the singing voice based on the speaking voice in an attempt to attain freedom and naturalness, and, assuming that the speaking voice is produced correctly, this can be a valid method. This does not mean that a good singer will necessarily produce the speaking voice correctly, but if they do not, it is likely that they sing well in spite of that fact, not because of it. In any case, the teacher who is already sensitive to the qualities that yield healthy tone in singing should be listening for them in the speaking voice as well. Many clues to the solution of a singer's problems can be found at this stage, before ever hearing a note of music.

Singing Voice

A healthy, well-produced voice will have an easy, clear sound, with forward placement, good breath support, and be even from top to bottom with no audible variation of tone production. A healthy well-trained voice will have a range of two and a half to three octaves, an untrained voice may have only an octave and a half, and an unhealthy voice may have as little as an octave or less.

When the sound is not clear and free, the teacher must discern whether this is due to improper technique or possible pathology. For instance, a very airy sound can be caused by improper breath support, incorrect sound placement, or pathology of the vocal folds themselves. Through various exercises the teacher will try to get the singer to produce a clearer sound. If some improvement of the sound occurs relatively quickly, the teacher will suspect faulty technique. If it is impossible for the singer to produce a clear sound at all, the teacher may suspect some damage to the vocal folds. Sometimes this distinction is very easy to make. When it is less clear, the teacher might relate the singing voice to the speaking voice. If the speaking voice is clear and the singing voice is not, poor technique is more likely the problem. However, if both the speaking and singing voices are very breathy or husky, it is reasonable to suspect physiologic problems. Whenever there is any doubt about the condition of the vocal folds, the teacher should recommend a consultation with a laryngologist and possibly a speech pathologist.

The teacher will use a variety of vocal exercises to examine all aspects of the singer's technique. When evaluating the singing voice, the singer should be warmed up. A beginning student will likely not have thought of it, but the more advanced singer may have. In any case, it can be telling to ask the singer to demonstrate his or her own way of warming up. An insufficient or too demanding warm-up may be revealed, and either extreme will need alteration.

The next step should include several simple scales to determine the singer's actual range. Depending on the type of singer and the level of experience, this may or may not correspond to the range revealed in the history. One of the biggest problems clinicians see is singers who are pushing beyond their currently usable range. This is especially true of, though not limited to, pop singers. In addition, indicators of potential problems may show up here.

A noticeably audible breath is a sign of tension in the throat and probably also indicates that the singer is not breathing deeply enough. Difficulties in negotiation of a smooth transition among the various registers of the voice, pushing through the passaggio (transition), lack of flexibility or agility, improper vowel production, poor placement or focus, poor intonation, inappropriate and uncontrollable dynamic (volume) level, an artificially produced and encumbering timbre (color), and glottal or overly aspirated attacks and releases are all potential if not immediate problems.

Vibrato is a good indicator of the overall health of the voice. Within a range of frequencies considered to be normal (the average is six to seven times per second) what is desirable is a matter of esthetics. The absence of any perceptible vibrato, a too slow and wide vibrato or a too fast and narrow vibrato, may well indicate problems in production, usually with their origins either in tension or in the breath support system.

The performance of one or two songs is helpful in determining other problems that may arise as the singer confronts the added burden of adding words, rhythm, and varying intervals. The possibility of imitating another singer, something that can have both positive and negative effects, and other factors may come into play at this point because the singer is now "performing." Interestingly, some singers sing much more technically correct when they are involved in performing a song; others seem to forget everything technical and concentrate solely on "selling" the song, sacrificing all else.

Voice Classification

Voice classification is determined by several factors, including the singer's range, timbre (quality of tone), and comfortable tessitura—that range in which the voice performs best in terms of quality and ease of production. It is this last quality that many singers ignore in determining appropriate repertoire. Singing in an inappropriate tessitura can be as harmful to the voice as singing beyond one's usable range. Most voices will fit into one category or another, but some defy a specific label or seem to fit in the overlapping areas of two or more categories. It is not so important that a voice have a label, but a singer trying to recover from vocal misuse or abuse know his or her current range limitations and comfortable tessitura and stay well within those bounds. Most healthy voices with no technical problems should possess at least two octaves of range and *may* fit conveniently into one of these general categories:

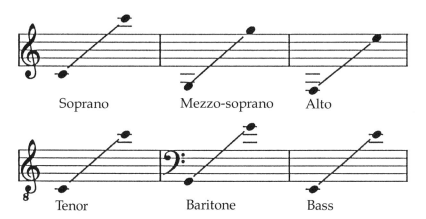

Soprano   Mezzo-soprano   Alto

Tenor   Baritone   Bass

Visual Evaluation

In addition to the aural observation, the voice teacher must also be concerned with what may be observed visually, beginning with overall posture, and specifically with the proper alignment of the throat in relation to the head and chest. A neutral "studio posture" is discussed in detail later, but singers are often called upon and should be able to sing with their bodies in any number of nontraditional postures. This is especially true when acting or dancing is required, which is why correct alignment is emphasized here as the crucial point. Such signs as rounded shoulders, swayback, uneven distribution of body weight, a collapsed ribcage, the jaw jutting forward, craning the head upward, or tilting it downward, habitually turning the head to one side while singing, singing out of the side of one's mouth, while they may stem from other problems, all demonstrate improper alignment, indicating the use of those muscles involved (incorrectly so) in the production of sound. Any physical abnormalities that would affect alignment should be noted at this point. Not that these are necessarily problematic, but such conditions as unequal leg length, rounded shoulders, scoliosis, or remarkable asymmetry of any kind can create problems and should be taken into consideration in the evaluation.

Tension, which for our purposes is any unnecessary use of the musculature that interferes with the production of tone, is probably the biggest single obstacle to correct singing. Tension can often be observed visually before it is heard in the sound. Upper body tension is indicated by the elevation of one shoulder or the other, hence shortening one side of the neck, or by the shoulders raising simultaneously. Such signs as excessive or exaggerated jaw usage, a wobbling jaw, trembling lips or lips that appear rigid, any excessive tongue movement such as a fluttering tongue or a groove or dip in the tongue indicate tension. In addition, contraction of the mylohyoid and geniohyoid muscles and tightness and protrusion of the musculature of the neck in general and specifically around the larynx causing too wide a fluctuation in the position of the larynx are relatively easy to spot, yet all too often go unnoticed by the singer.

Abdominal tension is particularly troublesome because of its inhibiting effect on inhalation from which other problems are certain to follow and because of the possibility of the singer confusing it with the desirable use of abdominal support. It is more difficult to observe visually, but palpation may reveal quivering or shaking of the abdomen or chest during phonation, especially in the upper range. Also, if inhalation appears shallow and of short duration, abdominal tension (as opposed to support) may be present.

Personality Evaluation

Because the voice teacher must deal with the whole person, elements other than the purely physiologic must also be evaluated. The sensitive observer will learn a great deal in the preliminary evaluation about those personality traits that will directly or indirectly affect the use of the voice. Short of using some type of personality assessment testing such as the Myers-Briggs Type Indicator (which may prove very helpful in understanding how best to work with different learning styles), this may begin by trying to determine the singers' levels of motivation and their attitudes toward learning. An enthusiastic, "over-achiever" type may tend to approach vocal technique in a too aggressive manner and may need to be tempered with some restraint, whereas the "laid back," lethargic personality may lack the dynamic energy needed to support the voice properly. Either extreme will affect the voice negatively, but both can be used positively with the proper instruction.

As discussed earlier, the elimination of unwanted tension is a major factor in good production of sound, and since stress can be directly related to muscular tension, the voice teacher must be aware if there are factors from outside the vocal studio that contribute to the problem. This is often difficult to do without seeming to pry into the singer's private life. However, the stress produced by divorce, death of a loved one, unemployment, overwork, or problems with children, for instance, will inevitably affect vocal production and needs to be acknowledged. Does the tension observed in the jaw, for example, stem only from poor breath support and improper vowel production, or is it also there at the end of a stressful day and carried over into the voice lesson?

Certainly most voice teachers are not trained counselors, and the professional boundaries that separate the two must be acknowledged and respected, but we cannot escape the fact that the voice is a complex instrument that involves the mind and personality as much as the diaphragm and soft palate. Ultimately, all must work together in singing.

RECOMMENDATIONS

One of the most difficult questions for the voice teacher to answer is in regard to the career aspirations of the singer and whether or not those goals are realistic and consistent with the instrument, the production, and the personality. A teacher would certainly be ill advised to make a judgment too hastily, and some choose to avoid the subject altogether, but if the singer is pushing the voice to be something that it is not in order to fulfill some unrealistic career goal, then that should be addressed sooner rather than later. The inherent or natural beauty of the voice, and its suitability and marketability for the desired medium must be considered, as well as the size of the voice. Technical considerations include range, timbre (the "color" of the voice), and the natural tessitura (the pitch range in which the voice feels most comfortable). Temperament, motivation, and discipline are a few of the personal factors that must be taken into account. This can be difficult to do, but it is incumbent on the voice teacher to give this advice, especially if vocal damage may occur as a result of not doing so.

The voice teacher should seek to establish a rapport with an otolaryngologist and speech-language pathologist who have an interest in the special needs and problems of singers. If the slightest doubt exists about the health of the voice, it is recommended that the student be seen as soon as possible, certainly before beginning continuous study.

Other recommendations may include learning relaxation techniques such as the Alexander technique to help lessen body tension, changing the warm-up/cool-down or other practice habits, reducing or increasing the amount of time spent singing and speaking each day, changing vocal hygiene habits, and changing vocal technique. Professional counseling may be indicated for severe performance anxiety or for other reasons that would undermine a singer's ability to successfully cope with the stresses of a performing career.

In most instances, continued vocal study will be the major prescription. Performing places such incredible demands on the voice and the singer's concentration that even singers with a seemingly flawless technique may unwittingly develop poor habits that need to be addressed immediately.

VOCAL TECHNIQUE

To evaluate the voice, there must be some standard against which vocal production can be measured. While not espousing any one technique or method, we describe here the basic tenets of healthy voice production on which we base an evaluation.

There are those who would argue that the use of vocal technique varies with the vocal style, and that may be true. It is also true that some singing has become legitimized as a "vocal style" because of the success of a given performer and the subsequent imitation that follows that success. Never mind that it was produced with poor, or no vocal technique to begin with. The "rasp" is a fairly recent example of what has become an accepted, and even sought after, sound, which is dangerous to any voice and fatal to many. The voice is a wonderfully flexible instrument capable of making an incredible array of sounds, but there are several principles that must be followed, whatever the style, to maintain vocal health.

The singing voice, like every other musical instrument, involves three elements in its production. There must be *initiation*, *vibration*, and *resonation*. To use a violin as an analogy: drawing the bow across the string initiates the vibration. The tone is amplified by the body of the instrument, which provides the space for resonation. Likewise, the initiator of the voice is the breath, the vocal folds vibrate, and resonation occurs in the naso-, oro-, and laryngopharynx and sympathetically in the chest. This seemingly oversimplified statement is the essence of correctly produced tone, and any discussion of vocal technique must begin and end with the function and coordination of these three things.

Posture

For the system to operate efficiently, energetically, and free from unwanted tension, we begin with a discussion of correct standing posture for singing. As mentioned earlier, alignment of the instrument is the chief concern, and this can be achieved in a variety of positions, from standing to lying down, but the rib cage, neck, and head must remain aligned and unrestricted. The head should feel as though it is suspended by the crown from above, almost marionette fashion, with the chin neither jutting upward nor pulled down and back, but able to move freely within a range of up to approximately 30 degrees. The chest and rib cage will be held in a comfortably high position, but not so high as to compromise a feeling of expansion in the back at the same time. The spine should feel a small upward stretch, as though the vertebrae were separating while the shoulders and arms feel somewhat weighted, supported by the trunk. One way of creating this is to raise the arms over the head like a diver, inhaling deeply, then, without exhaling, lower the arms slowly to the sides. The abdominal muscles should be relaxed, but not flaccid, and the pelvis should be rolled under in a position that will minimize the curve of the lower spine. The knees should be flexible, not locked. The feet may be perpendicular to each other or one slightly ahead of the other, and should be a comfortable distance apart with the weight directed forward toward the balls of the feet. The sensations achieved with this posture should be that of relaxed poise, balance, confidence, and strength. The same basic posture can be achieved from the hips up while seated.

Breathing and Breath Support

Correct breath support is perhaps the most crucial component of singing. Without it, nothing about the sound production will be truly correct. Much of the extraneous tension in singing can be attributed to various muscle groups compensating for the absence of a good air supply.

There are three basic categories of breathing: clavicular, intercostal, and abdominal. Clavicular breathing is the equivalent of panting—very shallow breaths inhaled and exhaled quickly. This type of breathing does not create enough breath pressure to produce a full, clear vocal sound, nor does it provide adequate amounts of air to sustain long musical phrases. Hence it is not practical for singing.

Intercostal breathing is characterized by the expansion and contraction of the ribs. While this type of inspiration brings in substantially more air than clavicular breathing, exhaling with the intercostal muscles is inappropriate for singing. The air tends to come out in one rapid gush, which is insufficient for sustaining long phrases. Also, compression of the rib cage causes the throat to contract as well, which makes it difficult, if not impossible, for the larynx to vibrate freely.

Abdominal breathing utilizes the relaxation and contraction of the muscles in the lower third of the abdominal wall, those between the hip bones. Used in proper conjunction with the intercostal muscles, the abdominal muscles will provide the strongest and most efficient means of breath support for singing.

Inhalation

With the rib cage already in the partially expanded position described above, the breath should be taken so that the rib cage in front, back, and sides will expand completely with inhalation. At the same time, the abdominal muscles relax and expand out and slightly downward, and one should attempt to feel expansion as low as possible in the pelvic area. For some, the analogy of water filling a glass the way it does from the bottom up is useful in achieving this sensation. Others may find it easier to achieve at first by lying down, probably because they allow their muscles to relax more than when standing. Inspiration should be considered the relaxation phase of respiration for singers. Any signs of muscular tension such as an overly distended abdomen indicate that this feeling of passive relaxation has not been achieved.

Breathing through the nose warms, filters, and humidifies the air and requires that the breath be taken slowly and deliberately, which for most singers results in a deeper, fuller breath. Breathing through the mouth allows the singer to establish the open position of the vocal tract in anticipation of phonation. A combination of the two is probably most effective. It is at this point that the singer is preparing the throat for phonation by consciously relaxing the larynx down with the breath in preparing for the attack (onset of sound). A useful tool in achieving this is recreating the very beginning sensations of a yawn. A noisy, gasping breath is a sure sign of constriction in the throat and should be avoided.

Support

As the initiator and sustainer of sound, support may be simply defined as the coordination of those muscle groups (dominated by the abdominals, intercostals, and diaphragm) which at the same time compress and pressurize the breath and propel it upward to the vocal folds, supplying the main energy to set them in motion. *Support* is a much used but often misunderstood term. Most singers know that they are supposed to do it, and yet ineffective support is one of the most common problems seen.

The Italian word for support, *appoggiare*, which means, "to lean upon" or "rest upon," is perhaps more descriptive of how support should feel. Though mostly a conceptual difference, a sensation of the voice "resting" upon a pressurized airstream is less likely to force the voice than the feeling of "driving" the voice with the breath.

It is important that support be initiated as soon as inhalation is completed, without holding the breath for any length of time and simultaneously with the attack. This will occur most effectively when one thinks of support immediately preceding the attack. Support will be generated by gently engaging the rectus abdominus muscle as low as possible, in the same area where inhalation was conceived, and mentally initiating the attack from there. If expansion of the rib cage is maintained at the same time, the epigastrium will protrude slightly (or greatly, depending on proficiency of coordination and the vigor with which the attack is commenced). It is helpful to think of the rib cage expanding further as a result of the low abdominal contraction rather than as a separate function. This interaction will result in the compression of air necessary to set the vocal folds in motion and begins the process of support that must be continued in varying degrees throughout the vocal line. Support must always be present. It should be increased and intensified when ascending in pitch and lessened but always continued when descending. It should also be increased or relied upon more when either greatly increasing or decreasing the amplitude of sound.

Configuration

Unlike other musicians, singers need to recreate the shape of their instrument with each use, with each breath. We are referring here to the resonating cavities over which the singer has a large degree of control, primarily the mouth and throat. The correct shape will allow maximum efficiency, ease of production, and resonance. This can only be accomplished with heightened sensory awareness and well-developed muscle memory.

The Pharynx

The sound of the voice is greatly dependent on the configuration of the three primary resonators of the head and neck: the nasopharynx, the oropharynx, and the laryngopharynx. Each voice is unique, and the right proportions of resonance must be fine tuned by a discriminating ear, but the overall goal is to maintain proper alignment and relaxation and to enlarge each of the cavities to maximize their role in amplifying and enhancing the tone.

Since the nasopharynx is fixed, there is little control to be exercised except for determining a desirable amount of nasality. Hypernasality, or nasal twang, is generally considered esthetically unpleasant, but a certain amount of nasal resonance can enrich tone quality. In most singers the elevation of the soft palate will correct any excessive nasality, and the use of some nasal resonance, especially with beginning singers, may increase the likelihood of developing a forward vocal placement, which is highly desirable.

The elevation of the soft palate is also prerequisite in enlarging and enhancing resonance in the oropharynx. In addition, the base of the tongue should be slightly lower than normal, without depressing the larynx, so that the back wall of the pharynx is fully visible when the mouth is open. The very beginning of a yawn is quite similar in the way it enlarges the pharyngeal walls, and using it as an example can be helpful in establishing the sensation.

To open and enlarge the laryngopharynx, the most desirable position is achieved when the larynx is slightly lower than its normal position when at rest. It should remain relatively unchanged on the attack and throughout the duration of the vocal line. If it rises dramatically with either increased amplitude or ascending pitch, the resulting tone will sound strained and tight. Here, too, the yawn sensation can help in establishing the proper position for the larynx and help stabilize it while singing. It should be emphasized again that only the very *beginning* of a yawn is the desirable sensation, as too much of it can cause tension. The shaping of the resonators can vary depending on several things, including interpretation and vocal style. The one exception to this is the relaxed, unraised position of the larynx, which is implicit in healthy singing.

The Tongue

The position of the tongue on all vowel sounds should be such that the tip rests against the lower front teeth. A slight forward arching of the tongue will occur on [i], and a gradual flattening and lowering as one proceeds through the tongue vowels to [a], remaining basically in that position through all other vowels. The tip of the tongue should not retract or curl, nor should the base of the tongue either rise or form a large groove, especially if this is associated with change in pitch. If the tongue appears grooved, scooped, or narrows significantly, there is evidence of tension. Some singers have used these means (likely unconsciously) to color the tone, sometimes with an esthetically pleasing effect, but the tension that results can cause unnecessary vocal strain and should be avoided. As mentioned earlier, a fluttering tongue is also a sign of tension, which often will have a negative effect on the vibrato. The source of tension may be the tongue or any number of the muscles connected to it. Any protrusion under the chin should be checked by palpation of the area. The mylohyoid should remain relatively soft and pliant while singing.

The Jaw and Lips

The jaw should be totally uninvolved in producing any vowel sound. It should remain relaxed throughout the vocal line, never quivering or shaking. The jaw should relax downward from its hinge without jutting forward or pressing into the neck. Moderation should be the guide in determining the appropriate opening. Too little space traps the sound; overextension creates tension.

In order for the jaw to remain relaxed when changing pitch and especially when moving into the upper range, it is recommended that the necessary opening be attained in anticipation and in advance of the note, rather than on it. Likewise the lips should remain relaxed and pliant, used only in a supplementary manner to help shape the lip vowels and articulate consonants. Quivering, trembling, or stiffness are results of overusing the lips.

As noted previously, proper configuration depends on the head and neck being aligned with the spine, the jaw parallel to the floor. Singers who sing with a microphone or use music when they practice or perform should take special care to position the microphone and the music so that the head can remain level.

Placement and Focus

When it comes to the issue of placement, the teacher and singer move from the realm of the purely physical to the conceptual. In doing so, the vocabulary changes from simple commands for specific physical manipulation to metaphors and imagery. This is not to suggest that the goals are any less real or significant to a well-produced tone, but that the vocabulary is not as precise. This is due to two factors. First, the teacher is describing a sensation, which is very subjective. Second, the teacher is no longer describing a physical action, but a mental one.

Vocal teachers run the gamut from those who dismiss the concept of placement altogether as unscientific to those who base their teaching solely on the imagery of placement. The truth probably lies somewhere in between. To one who views singing solely from a physiologic perspective, the idea is of little use, but that would be to ignore the creative element in singing that calls on the imagination to do its part in the process. There may be ways of making the same adjustments to the sound by using purely physical means, but a combined approach that also uses the imagination, first to realize the sensation, and then sensory memory to recreate it, while not scientific, has consistently proven itself to be an effective pedagogic tool.

One can certainly feel vibration in the areas of the nose, hard palate, front teeth, cheek bones, and sinus cavities when one sings; that much is not imagined. Placement is the concept of using the imagination or will power to direct the voice to one or more of those areas before the sound ever begins and to continue to use it as an imaginary focal point throughout the vocal line. There is debate as to whether this forward placement adds to that desirable quality of singing known as "ring." There is also debate as to just how effective the sinus cavities are as resonators. What is of great effect is that focusing on a point relatively far away from the throat often leads unconsciously to the relaxation of those muscles that interfere substantially with the process of phonation when engaged. This, if for no other reason, makes the concept of placement a valid one.

Focus, a term that is sometimes used interchangeably with *placement*, is actually more descriptive of what is accomplished when a sound is both supported and well placed. That is to say, one can achieve the forward placement described above without sufficient support, and the resulting tone will sound like what a picture out of focus looks like: unclear, fuzzy, and lacking definition.

Coordination

After the three basic elements of tone production are studied and developed separately, the next and probably most difficult step is the coordination of the three working together as one.

Vowel Production

When most singers think of good diction, they think of emphasizing the consonants. However, it is with the vowel that good diction in singing begins. It is the vowel that carries and projects the sound. The singer's objective therefore is to ensure that all the vowels are placed correctly and are well focused. This is achieved by maintaining the size and configuration of the vocal tract as consistently as possible while still allowing for discrete and distinct vowels. Specifically, this means minimizing the movement of the mouth, tongue, and lips. Ironically, many singers try to exaggerate these motions, believing that this will lead to clear diction. However, it leads to different timbres for each vowel and inconsistent placement of the sound, which results in diminished resonance on some, if not all, of the vowels. The effect is like a melody played one note at a time on a succession of different instruments of varying quality.

Consonant articulation must also be scrutinized to check for any interference with sound production. When singing, the consonants must be crisp, clear, and, in general, short. If the consonants are prolonged to the point where they inhibit the airflow, the sound will stop and the diction will become unintelligible.

Adapting diction to the spatial requirements of the singing voice is frequently a difficult task. In many instances a singer can perform vocal exercises easily and then have difficulty transferring this into a song. This is most often due to singers trying to make the shape of their instruments conform to their speech patterns instead of expanding their diction to accommodate the size and shape of their instrument.

Registration

As the singer sings up and down a scale, there are physiologic changes that take place in the length and thickness of the vocal folds that are controlled by the intrinsic muscles of the larynx. To achieve an even, seamless sound from top to bottom of the range, the singer must learn not to interfere with this process.

Most untrained singers do not possess the muscular coordination to allow this process to occur and therefore exhibit some kind of timbre or quality change at some point(s) in the range, commonly referred to as a *register break*. This is usually caused by the swallowing muscles interfering with the coordination of the intrinsic muscles of the larynx. The singer must learn to relax these swallowing muscles to eliminate this tension.

To accomplish this, the singer will try to follow the same process of sound production on each tone, concentrating on breath support, making an optimum resonating chamber, and placing the sound to achieve maximum focus. Problems occur when the singer has a different physical and mental approach for various pitches.

If muscular interference is the main inhibitor to healthy singing, understanding and using a "legato" approach to vocal production may be the best aid. *Legato*, the Italian word for *bind* or *connect* as a musical directive, is one of many different effects or styles that can be used by the singer interpretively; but as an approach to singing technique, its definition of "smooth, connected transition" becomes vitally important. First, the supported breath must feel connected to the placement of the tone, without interference along the way; second, smooth and connected intervalic transition with pitch changes occurring gently, without altering the position of the larynx; third, smooth and connected transition between vowels in order to maintain an even vocal line; and fourth, the smooth and even connection of the so-called registers of the voice, by successfully achieving the connection and coordination of the first three.

Practice and Exercises

The importance of establishing good practice habits, both mental and physical, cannot be overemphasized. Through practice, the singer programs the muscles and the brain to respond in specific ways to specific commands, even under the stress of performance. Mindless repetition of a song from start to finish in the hope that it will improve with time is not likely to modify behavior patterns efficiently. Practicing should be careful and methodical, with a lot of attention to detail.

A typical practice session should consist of warming up the voice slowly and carefully, then exercising the voice with vocalises (musical scales on various sounds) that address the singer's particular needs. Only then should repertoire be practiced, followed by cooling down the voice on vocalises to end the session.

This process may take from 10 minutes to an hour and a half, depending on the expertise and stamina of the singer. The less advanced the student, the shorter the practice sessions should be. This is especially true for damaged voices. Frequent repetition of 10 minute practice intervals will actually allow singers to train their muscles and their concentration more quickly and more effectively.

Generally speaking, the warm-up should begin in the lower middle part of the singers' range at an effortless dynamic level, working the voice in half steps, first downward, then upward into the upper middle part of the range, and then descending again in whole steps. The time involved will vary with the individual and the time of day, but ventures into the upper extremes of the range should occur only after the voice is thoroughly warmed up. The cool down is simply the same process in reverse.

The single most important element of successful practicing is concentration. An acute sensory awareness of the physical manifestations of each element of the technique must be developed. It is through reproduction of these physical sensations that the singer acquires a consistent approach to singing. Then the separate components of the technique must all be coordinated. Finally, the singer must integrate the technical aspects of singing with the musical and expressive elements.

Scientific Fact Versus Functional Fiction

It is important that the members of the treatment team understand the vocabulary used by each other and are able to communicate effectively. To the reader who is well versed in anatomy and physiology but unacquainted with vocal technique and teaching methods, we have discussed several things that may appear confusing and even misleading. While a scientifically based knowledge of the structure and function of the voice is absolutely necessary to the voice teacher, so too is a creative imagination that can aid the student in stretching beyond the purely physical. The imagination can play a very important role in stimulating muscular responses that allow the singing mechanism to work in its most natural, uninhibited way. Directives of this sort may appear to contradict scientific fact.

For example, to take in the deepest breath possible and to utilize the abdominal muscles more effectively in support, a student might be instructed to "inhale deeply, all the way to the pelvic area." One assumes that no one would believe that achieving that feeing would result in the air actually going below the lungs, yet imagining that sensation may aid the singer with deeper inhalation and improved breath support. As another example, we describe inhalation as the passive part of breathing and exhalation as active. In breathing for singing, it is functionally more effective to associate relaxation with inhalation, and the active engagement of the breathing muscles during exhalation in order to support the sound.

We speak of relaxing the muscles of the throat during phonation, when obviously the muscles must be engaged and working efficiently to produce tone. The truth is that it would be counterproductive for a singer to be concerned with the intricate workings of each muscle group in the throat while singing, and it is more beneficial simply to conceive of the entire throat as being open and relaxed.

The concept of placement and the imagery used to achieve it falls into this category as well. Although it may not be measurable, its validity is proven in practical application. One must bear in mind that these and other such "functional fiction" are only tools that the voice teacher may use to help the student achieve proper vocal production, not the underlying truths.

EXERCISES

The following exercises are presented as a suggested regimen for developing and coordinating the basic elements of vocal technique. All of the musically notated exercises should be executed at various pitch levels throughout the singer's range, starting in the lower middle, ascending by semitones, descending by whole tones. Any vowel may be substituted for the one indicated in the exercise.

Posture

1.   To feel the proper alignment of the head and torso, stand against a wall with the head and spinal column as flat as possible. To accomplish this, one may have to move the feet several inches away from the wall. Note that the pelvis will be tilted forward.
2.   The same alignment can be achieved while lying on the floor with the knees bent and feet flat on the floor. In this position, most singers will feel much more relaxation of the abdominal muscles. This is especially recommended for dancers, weight lifters, and persons who are very conscious of their figures, who frequently maintain more tension in the abdominal area than is desirable for singing.

3.   In a standing position, bend forward from the waist until the head, neck, shoulders, and arms are hanging freely, without any tension. Gradually, "unfold" one vertebra at a time, keeping the neck and shoulders rounded for as long as possible, until a well-aligned, relaxed stance is achieved. Maintain the center of gravity over the instep and balls of the feet. This exercise will relax the stance that is too rigid, with the chest held too high, and the shoulder blades pressed together.

4.   This exercise, which we refer to as the *diver's stance*, focuses on breathing as well as posture. In a standing position, with body weight centered over the balls of the feet, raise the arms and clasp the hands over the head. Let the abdominal muscles relax, and breathe deeply. The singer will feel the rib cage lift and expand. Repeat this several times. In this position, it will be difficult for the singer to breathe by raising the shoulders. Repeat once more, and while holding the breath, slowly let the arms relax to the sides. This will leave the rib cage in the expanded position that should be maintained while singing. Now inhale and exhale several times with the rib cage in this position.

Breath Control and Support

1.   Sit in a chair, resting the elbows on the knees with the head in the palms of the hands, and breathe in and out normally. In this position, the expansion of the lower back and relaxation of the abdominal muscles will be emphasized. Return to a standing position and try to duplicate the same feeling of relaxation upon inhalation. This is especially useful for singers who feel tension while inhaling.

2.   Breathe in for a slow count of five, feeling the back ribs expand and the abdominal muscles *relax* outward. Hold for a slow count of five to develop the expansion and strength of the intercostal muscles. Then gently release the air on [s] by contracting the lowest abdominal muscles while holding the ribs in this expanded position. Keep the sound steady and even for as long as possible. Time the exhalation.

      a.   Repeat the entire exercise substituting a very soft, sung [o] for the [s]. Use a medium pitch range, c¹, d¹, e¹, f¹, one note at a time.

      b.   The exhalation times for the [s] and [o] should be approximately the same. A dramatic difference between the two times indicates inefficient usage of the air. A reasonable goal is a duration of 30 seconds.

3.   Pulsation of a sustained sound will help the singer become aware of and develop proper abdominal support. After initiating a sound, either spoken or sung, the singer should contract the lowest abdominal muscles with short, energetic pulses, relaxing them completely after each pulse. The sound should remain uninterrupted, but the pitch may vary due to increased breath pressure.

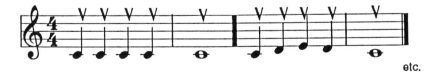

etc.

4.   Staccato articulation will also develop abdominal support. The singer must take care to leave the throat open between each note.

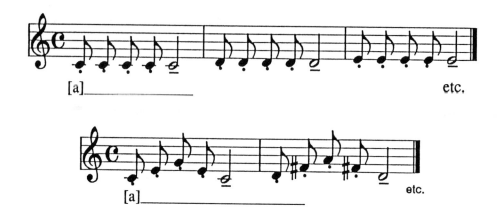

5.   Alternation of staccato and legato will ensure correct support not only on an attack, but throughout a phrase.

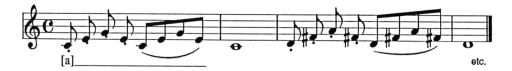

6.   Exhale completely while contracting the lowest abdominal muscles. Then let the muscles quickly release downward and outward to feel the "passive" intake of air. This exercise will counteract a tendency to push the abdominal muscles out while inhaling, which creates tension.

7.   Using a short, sharp contraction of the lower abdominal muscles, alternate [s] and [a]. Let the abdominal muscles relax completely between each sound. This strengthens the abdominal muscles and helps the singer achieve a coordinated attack.

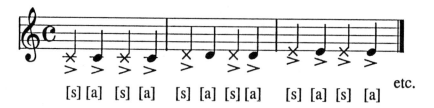

8.   With the mouth open, breathe in slowly and deeply until full. Then holding the throat in the same expanded position, exhale very gentle on [a] on any comfortable pitch. Repeat exercise substituting several short puffs of air for the long, slow breath. This will train the throat not to close between inhaling and exhaling.

Relaxation and Creating Space

1.   With the mouth closed, try to create the sensation of stifling a yawn. Notice the relative positions of the soft palate, tongue, walls of the throat, and larynx. The soft palate will

stretch upward and backward. The tongue should lie along the bottom jaw with the tip touching the lower front teeth. The throat will feel expanded and the larynx somewhat low, but not artificially depressed. This position expands and relaxes the pharynx and creates optimal resonation space.

2. Place index fingers on the hinges of the jaw and drop the jaw open. Feel the motion of the jaw as it swings from this hinge. It should neither jut forward nor press in toward the throat.

3. To gain control over raising and lowering the soft palate, sustain one pitch while alternating [ŋ] and [a]. When the [ŋ] is sounding, the soft palate and tongue are touching. In moving to [a], the soft palate will pull up and the tongue will relax downward.

   a. Sing a triad letting the jaw swing freely from the hinge on each note, using the syllable [ja]. This will help to loosen a tense jaw.

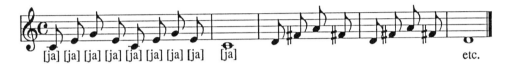

   b. To separate the motion of the tongue from that of the jaw, sing the triad again on the syllable [ja]; however, this time let the jaw hang motionless so that only the tongue articulates the syllable. Any motion of the jaw will indicate that the singer is trying to use the jaw to generate the sound.

4. To allow the larynx to remain in a low, relaxed position, gently slide on one vowel. The key is to use the air to achieve the legato; the throat will remain relaxed.

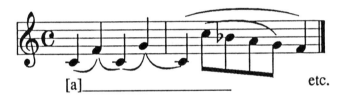

5. Simulate the beginning of a yawn. While maintaining this sensation, initiate a descending scale as if sighing. This will result in an easy, coordinated attack.

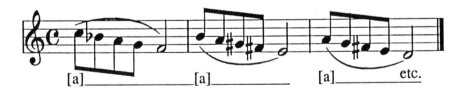

Placement and Focus

1. Humming is a relatively easy way for a singer to experience the high, forward placement that helps give a tone "ring." Any one of the nasal consonants can be used, [n], [m], or [ŋ]. The singer should experiment with all three and select the consonant that is the most resonant.

2.   Having experienced this "buzzing" sensation in the sinus cavities on a consonant, singers should then practice beginning each vowel sound with their most resonant consonant, trying to keep the placement of the vowel the same as the consonant. Although the sensation will not be identical, the placement of the sound should remain the same.

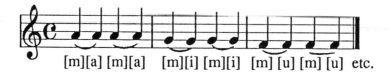

[m][a] [m][a]   [m][i] [m][i]   [m] [u] [m] [u] etc.

3.   Initiate a pitch using a very nasal quality. Gradually raise the soft palate while maintaining the forward "nasal" placement. The tone should become clear, losing the unpleasant nasal "twang." Be careful not to create a false nasal sound by closing the throat.

4.   Using the hand to close the nostrils, begin a pitch by trying to breathe out through the nose. While this will not be possible, one should feel a very forward placement of the sound. Release the nose and keep the same placement. As in the previous exercise, the nasal quality of the tone should disappear, while the nasal resonance should remain strong.

5.   Trilling an [r] will also affect the desired placement of a tone. In addition, it positions the tongue forward in the mouth and requires a constant flow of air to be sustained. If the breath support is not consistent, the trill will stop.

Coordination and Agility

To execute the following exercises successfully, the singer must concentrate on all components of sound: or; support, relaxation of the throat, and placement of the tone. These exercises should be performed in a variety of tempi and on all vowels.

1.   Legato fifths and octaves.

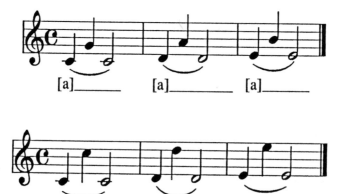

[a]_____   [a]_____   [a]_____

[a]_____   [a]_____ [a]_____ etc.

2.   Legato scales ascending to the fifth, ninth, and eleventh degrees of the scale should be broken into sections to fit the singers' expertise. Only the most advanced singers should attempt to sing the entire pattern on one breath. If they have difficulty articulating the

pitches at faster speeds, they should alternate the syllables [hwi] and [u] on successive pitches until the feeling of legato on separate pitches is achieved.

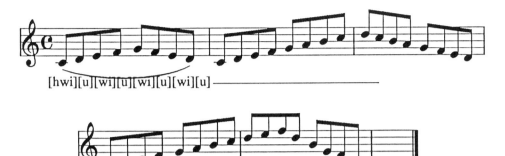

3. Arpeggios should be practiced with both staccato and legato articulations at different tempi.

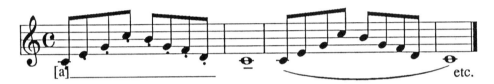

4. Advanced singers should also include extended arpeggios.

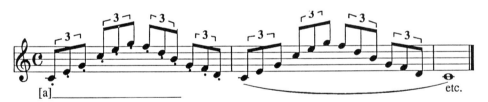

5. Alternating staccato and legato attacks will aid in developing the flexibility of the support mechanism.

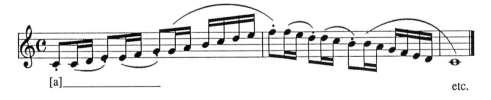

6. To minimize timbre changes between vowel sounds, slide on one pitch from [i] to [e] to [a], moving the tongue, lips, and jaw as little as possible. Repeat substituting [u], [o], and [a]. When this has been mastered, insert these vowel progressions into various scales and chords.

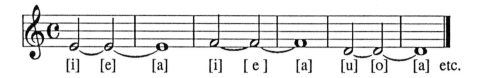

[i]   [e]   [a]   [i]   [e]   [a]   [u]   [o]   [a] etc.

7.   Chanting a text on one note will help the singer to achieve a legato approach to diction. The duration of the vowels should be emphasized. Consonants will be short and will form clusters at word junctures, except where this would obscure the meaning. Voiced consonants should be sung on pitch.

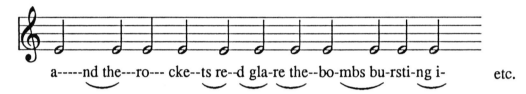

a-----nd the---ro--- cke--ts re--d gla-re the--bo-mbs bu-rsti-ng i-   etc.

8.   The "messa di voce" is one of the oldest and most effective vocal exercises.

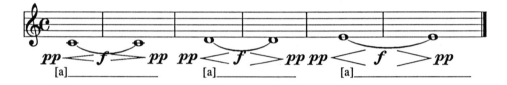

pp ‹ f › pp   pp ‹ f › pp   pp ‹ f › pp
[a]_____   [a]_____   [a]_____

Range Extension

1.   Do–do, ti do re do, etc.

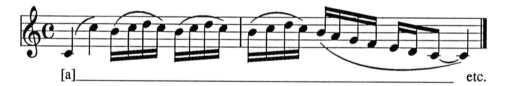

[a]_____ etc.

2.   Do–re with messa di voce on re

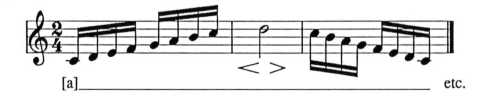

[a]_____ etc.

3.   Do–re, alternate do and re, then down

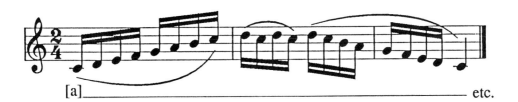

RECOMMENDATIONS FOR THE INJURED VOICE

"Mend your voice a little, lest you mar your fortune."
William Shakespeare

In dealing with a voice that has been diagnosed as having sustained injury, it is recommended that the voice teacher work closely with the student's physician. A singer with nodules, for example, should be seen frequently for assessment of progress, and together the Ear Nose Throat specialist and voice teacher should determine how much time should be spent in daily vocalises and other voice use. The voice teacher should also be involved in devising a regimen of good vocal hygiene consistent with the doctor's advice.

The first recommendation given to a singer with vocal pathology or one recovering from any kind of throat surgery should be to begin singing as soon as their doctor approves, but not to perform for 6 weeks to 6 months. The actual length of time involved will vary from one individual to the next and will depend on the severity of the damage to the vocal folds, the technical problems, and the determination of the singer to modify the vocal behavior. Chances are that if the problem was due to technique, it will reoccur in the pressure-filled atmosphere of a performance, where the singer will do "whatever it takes to get the job done." The right way is to exercise the voice in a controlled environment, with no fear of taking the time and risks to undo bad habits and learn new ones. This is difficult for most singers to accept, especially if their income is dependent on performing, but it will greatly shorten the recovery time and greatly lengthen their singing careers.

We would also recommend that singers suspend work on their current repertoire for a time. This will allow them to concentrate fully on the mechanics of voice production without being distracted by musical or interpretive considerations. It is also easier to adopt new vocal habits in new repertoire than it is to rework old material in which undesirable vocal habits are ingrained.

Exercises

Through the information furnished in the history, the evaluation process, and from consultation with the physician, the teacher will try to determine the cause of the problem and design exercises to suit the individual voice. Vocal exercises for the injured voice will not differ substantially from those for the healthy voice, with two major exceptions. Exercises specifically designed to extend the pitch or dynamic range should probably be avoided until the voice has fully healed and the singer has become comfortable with a new technique in the upper range of voice. These kinds of exercises require the most muscular strength and coordination and are the ones most likely to add strain to the singing process when done incorrectly. In general, most singing should be done in a medium pitch range and at a medium to soft dynamic level.

Practice

It is especially important for singers with vocal pathology or those recovering from voice surgery to be working with an experienced teacher who can guide them through their practice and exercise sessions and help them develop a sensitivity to healthy tone production. The teacher's primary function should be to teach the singer how to practice, for it will be in the practice sessions that real progress will be made.

Practice sessions should be short, perhaps 5 to 10 minutes, and repeated frequently throughout the day. The same procedures involving warming up and cooling down the voice, mentioned earlier, apply to these practice sessions as well. Should there be any indication of fatigue or strain, however, the singing should be immediately terminated.

CONCLUSION

The innately subjective nature of vocal instruction can be made more objective through a thorough and systematic assessment process. The assessment should take into account the singer's history, vocal health (including the speaking voice), personality, and aspirations.

Vocal technique has been the subject of much disagreement over the years, mostly among voice teachers themselves. This may be confusing and even frightening to the voice student choosing a teacher, as well as to a physician or speech–language pathologist seeking to refer a patient for good vocal instruction. Since there is no licensing or regulatory body for voice teachers, they are free to teach as they wish. Caveat emptor! No one teaching method may suit every student, and there is room for differences of opinion on the fine points of technique, but every aspect of vocal technique can be evaluated by its relevance to the three basic elements of tone production: initiation, vibration, and resonation. Technique that is not based on the development and coordination of these three things is questionable.

10

Objective Voice Analysis: The Clinical Voice Laboratory

BARBARA H. JACOBSON, PhD

In the past 10 years, there has been an explosion in the amount of technology available for voice analysis. In many cases, development of instrumentation is far ahead of scientific and clinical knowledge regarding phonatory behavior. In particular, we do not yet know how useful this instrumentation will become to the practicing otolaryngologist or speech–language pathologist specializing in voice. Currently, there is little standardization of protocols for various measures of voice and a great deal of variability in equipment and the way phonatory data are analyzed.

During a discussion in laboratory instrumentation and measures at the annual Voice Foundation Symposium on the Professional Voice in 1991, panel participants were asked to name one piece of equipment that they found to be indispensable in their clinical voice laboratories. Many responded with "the ear." Many of us feel, when pressed, that the ear remains the most secure, most reliable way to measure parameters of voice. However, Kreiman et al[1] found that perceptual ear judgments were sensitive and reliable for "normal" voices but that judges differed widely when rating "pathologic" voices. The appeal of objective voice analysis to describe and quantify phonatory behavior remains strong in the face of many uncertainties regarding its reliability and reproducibility and ultimately its usefulness in the clinical setting.

For the professional voice user, the clinical voice laboratory can serve several functions. "Well voice" assessment can provide the singer or speaker with a baseline regarding voice production when healthy. Particular pieces of equipment are useful in monitoring efficient voice production over the extent of a singer's range. Of course, instrumentation in the voice laboratory is important in the diagnosis of acute and chronic voice disorders and frequently is used during treatment. In this chapter, we discuss the types of voice production analysis possible, specific equipment configurations and needs, establishment of norms, and meaningfulness of voice analysis measures.

VOICE ANALYSIS

In this section, we discuss the various types of analysis available and generally used in the clinical voice laboratory. For reference, it is important to remember that there are many customized systems in use in addition to the commercially available equipment. Many people who operate clinical voice laboratories—that is, laboratories whose main emphasis is providing clinical care to persons with voice disorders—rely on commercially marketed equipment. Consequently, our survey of available equipment will concentrate on a sample of those items that are commercially available.

Videostroboscopy

Techniques for visualization of the larynx have been available since Garcia adapted a dental mirror for indirect laryngoscopy in 1854. The next advance came with the application of high speed photography for the demonstration of slow motion of the vocal folds and the development of fiberoptics for full laryngeal view. However, no one technique alone or combination of techniques was adequate or convenient enough to provide simultaneous examination of laryngeal appearance and vibratory motion of the vocal folds. For many years, high speed photography was the only method for viewing vocal fold motion; however, the cost of equipment and film was prohibitive for routine use. With the merging of the techniques of stroboscopy and laryngeal visualization (using flexible and rigid endoscopes) has come the field of videostroboscopy.

Stroboscopy is a technique used to observe motion in cases in which the movement is so quick that the human visual system cannot capture and process the image. The human eye can only "see" five vibrations per second. Using stroboscopy, a light is flashed on the target object either in synchrony with the motion or slightly out of phase. When the light flashes are synchronous with the movement, the image appears to be motionless. When the light flashes are slightly out of synchrony (approximately three to four cycles per second for phonation), then the image appears to be moving in slow motion. The stroboscope lights one segment of the movement as it flashes, and the visual system puts these successive images together to reproduce motion. Examples of the use of stroboscopy are timing lights used in engine mechanics and strobe lights used at dance clubs. The important concept to remember when viewing an image filmed under stroboscopy is that the motion is *simulated* slow motion and that you may miss some detail that would be present in a film made using high speed photography.

When a stroboscope is connected to a lens and videocamera that is joined to an endoscope of some kind, then it is possible to record the stroboscopic image. This is what is now commercially available today as a videostroboscopic unit used to visualize the larynx. Other attachments may include a sound microphone, a stethoscope-type microphone that allows the stroboscope to track the vibration of the vocal folds, a videotape recorder, and a videomonitor.

Endoscopes in general use today include 70 degree and 90 degree rigid endoscopes and flexible fiberoptic scopes. Each type of scope has its own advantages and uses. Rigid scopes generally provide detailed views of the vocal folds, with excellent visualization of vibratory characteristics. However, the patient is only able to produce the sound "ee" (/i/). Flexible scopes provide a better view of the entire larynx, and it is possible for the patient to perform speech and nonspeech movements with little interference from the instrument. However, flexible scopes require a very strong light source to reproduce enough laryngeal detail.

Regardless of the type of scope, it is important that the user remember that the image is distorted by the optics of the scope. This means that the image on the videomonitor cannot be used directly to measure the length of the vocal folds or the size of any mass or lesion. Peppard and Bless[2] have described a method whereby it is possible to get an approximate comparison of the relative size of the glottic opening or laryngeal mass by using a transparency overlay on the monitor screen and tracing the image. This is used to compare the image with a prior one. Figures 10–1, 10–2, and 10–3 show examples of videostroboscopic units.

A basic protocol for recording vocal fold appearance and motion includes: (1) production of the vowel /i/ at comfortable or habitual pitch and loudness; (2) phonation at sustained high pitch; (3) phonation at sustained low pitch; (4) loud phonation; (5) soft phonation; (6) ascending and descending glissando or vowel glide; (7) fast repetition of "ee" (/i/–/i/–/i/–/i/); (8) fast repetition of "hee" (/hi/–/hi/–/hi/–/hi/); (9) quiet breathing; (10) forced inhalation/exhalation; (11) throat clearing. In other words, the examiner wants to capture a sampling of the possible variations in phonatory and nonphonatory movements of the vocal folds. For the singer, there are several maneuvers that should be added. These include phonation at the passagio or register break, phonation at extremes of the range, and phonation at "problem areas" of the singing range. Often, vocal fold movement during singing can best be observed using the flexible fiberoptic scope. Since the optimal singing voice is produced not only by vocal fold vibration but also by proper configuration of the structures *above* the vocal folds, the flexible scope often can reveal what the supraglottic structures may be doing to enhance or inhibit good voice production.

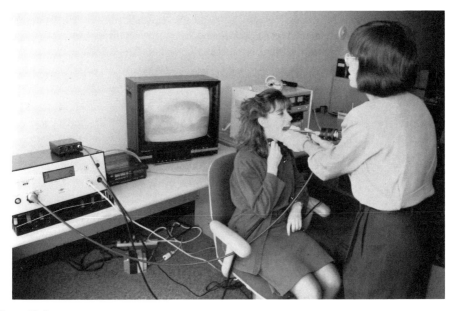

Figure 10–1.

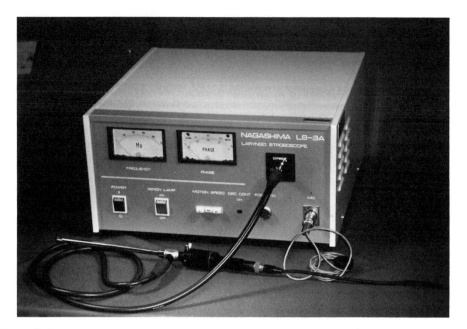

Figure 10–2.

Once the image has been recorded, there are several specific parameters or characteristics of appearance and movement that may be rated for "normalcy." Typically, judgments and ratings are based on samples obtained during comfort or habitual pitch phonations. Glottic appearance and vibratory motion are the two major categories into which visual observations are organized.

Glottic Appearance

The glottic appearance category describes various vocal fold characteristics that are visualized best under full light. Ratings and judgments made with these parameters correspond to those made using indirect laryngeal examination with a mirror.

Glottic Configuration.   The glottic configuration is the position of the vocal folds during phonation. Typical patterns include *complete* closure, where the vocal folds come together or adduct along their entire length. A *posterior* closure pattern, with a small "chink" or opening at the posterior commissure at the arytenoid cartilages, is seen commonly in women (approximately 80%). "Hourglass" configurations are seen when vocal nodules are present.

Supraglottic Activity.   The term *supraglottic activity* is generally used to describe excessive ventricular fold movement or "assist" during phonation. In addition, one should always mention whether there was an "anterior to posterior press." This is indicative of vocal hyperfunction and often is evident by an outpouching of the epiglottis at its base.

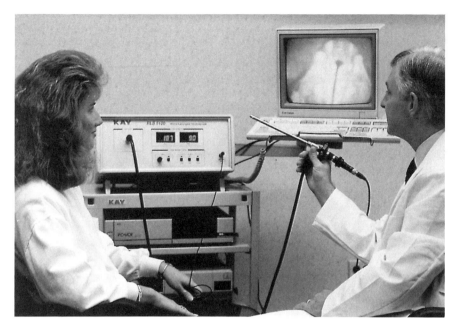

Figure 10–3.

Vertical Level Approximation.   The vocal folds should be parallel on the vertical plane. While this can be difficult to see on a two-dimensional representation, occasionally it is possible to see a shift in the level. This has implications for vocal fold weakness (paresis) or paralysis.

Appearance.   When rating this parameter, the examiner describes color and shape of each vocal fold. One might observe redness (erythema) or obvious blood vessels on the surface of the vocal folds.

Vocal Fold Edge.   Vocal fold edge is the integrity of the vocal fold mucosa. If the edge of the vocal fold is smooth and straight, then it is rated as normal. If there is scarring or a mass lesion along the edge, then the rating is a degree of abnormality.

Vibratory Motion

In the vibratory motion category, parameters of movement are judged and rated. These characteristics relate most closely to the clarity of the tone produced by the vocal folds. While an examination of vibratory motion is helpful in determining the effect of a mass on vocal fold movement, it is crucial to understanding dysphonia in the face of an absence of any vocal fold lesion.

Mucosal Wave.   As discussed in Chapter 3, the integrity of the mucous membrane is central to the quality of the tone generated by the vocal folds. One of the great advantages of videostroboscopy is the ability to determine the presence or absence of the mucosal wave and its viability. The mucosal wave will be reduced in vocal fold paralysis or with scarring. If a vocal nodule is particularly chronic, then there is reduced mucosal wave.

Amplitude.   Amplitude is the maximum excursion of the vocal folds during phonation. The overall stiffness of the phonatory system is reflected in the magnitude of vibration. Vibratory amplitude decreases at high pitch. It will increase more than normal when vocal fold paralysis is present and the vocal fold has reduced muscle tone.

Phase Symmetry.   Phase symmetry is the extent to which each vocal fold's movement "mirrors" the other. Potential causes of irregular symmetry include recent excision of a nodule or polyp, vocal fold edema, muscle imbalance, or vocal fold weakness.

Duration of Open Versus Closed Phase.   Ideally, the vocal folds should remain open and closed for relatively equivalent periods during a typical vibratory cycle, although electroglottography indicates that the vocal folds are in contact for a slightly shorter period than they are apart. This parameter reflects the degree of hypo- or hyperfunction of the vocal folds. When the open phase of vibration predominates, then generally the voice produced is somewhat more breathy. A closed phase of vibration corresponds to a more tight, strained voice.

Nonvibrating Portion.   The nonvibrating portion relates to the stiffness of each vocal fold and has implications for the degree of infiltration of a lesion on the vocal fold. It also tells us something about the degree of scarring, if present, in an individual who has had phonosurgery.

Periodicity.   The vocal folds should exhibit enough regularity of motion to enable the stroboscope to show simulated slow motion. A "flutter" motion of the vocal folds during stroboscopy indicates aperiodicity. Voices that are extremely hoarse or that are characterized by some aphonia are often difficult to represent stroboscopically because the stroboscope cannot track the vocal fold vibration accurately. To register some vocal fold vibration, it may be necessary for the examiner to place the stethoscope microphone against his or her own neck to produce some slow motion.

There are many uses for videostroboscopy that extend beyond diagnosis. Much of this value is gained in looking at changes not only in the appearance of the vocal folds but also in the quality of the vibration after surgery, voice therapy, or medical intervention. For the speech–language pathologist, videostroboscopy can serve as feedback for use with the patient during specific therapy tasks. In addition, the clinician can use videostroboscopy as a "treatment probe" to assist in determining whether certain treatment tasks have the potential to change phonatory behavior and voice production.

Training and Reliability

Finally, the issues of training and reliability must be addressed. For most clinicians, the relatively static image as obtained by indirect laryngeal examination is familiar and customary. However, videostroboscopy reveals an entirely new aspect of laryngeal function. Some time is needed in specific training to learn to interpret videostroboscopic images. It has been estimated that it takes approximately 20 hours of training to learn to distinguish normal from abnormal phonatory behavior as shown by videostroboscopy. Merely being able to perform the examination does not ensure that interpretations of motion will be correct. At this time, videostroboscopy is performed by otolaryngologists and speech–language pathologists. It is our opinion that those speech–language pathologists using videostroboscopy should be specially trained in vocal fold physiology and function and perform the examination under institutional approval and with appropriate precautions. Speech–language pathologists do not make medical diagnoses. However, with specific training, they are qualified to make descriptive statements about the quality of vocal fold movement and its relation to voice production. It is also important that reliability in judgment of parameters of vocal fold motion be obtained among users and that persons within a program demonstrate intra- and inter-judge reliability.

Acoustic Analysis

Acoustic analysis is the measurement of the sound signal as produced by the vocal folds. Acoustic analysis enables one to objectify elements heard in the voice: pitch, loudness, hoarseness, and so forth. Acoustic analysis has always been an important measure obtained in clinical voice laboratories. However, there has been little standardization in measurement across laboratories. Some centers have developed their own equipment configurations for extracting acoustic information from a voice signal. Even when using the same equipment, centers often differ in the way in which a portion of the voice signal is selected for analysis. Titze et al,[3] Karnell,[4] and Karnell et al[5] have described this phenomenon, and the reader is referred to their articles for clear discussions of the issues and some potential solutions. Examples of acoustic analysis systems are shown in Figures 10–4 and 10–5.

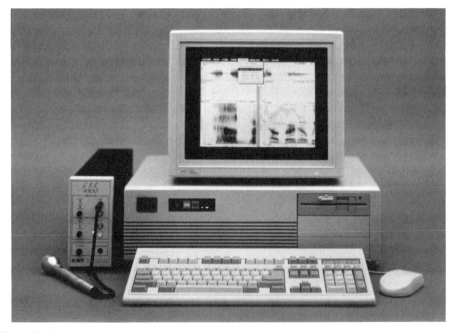

Figure 10–4.

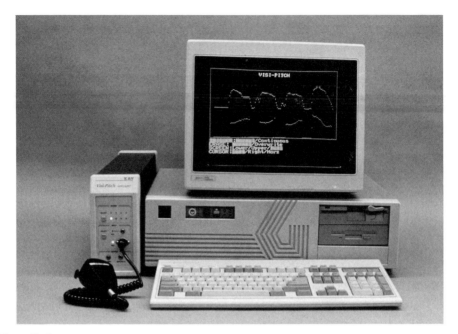

Figure 10–5.

The rationale for performing acoustic analysis is that it provides objective data relative to a set of normal values. Although at times it appears that there is little direct relationship to impressions gained through perceptual analysis, acoustic analysis does provide concrete information for comparison in different points in time. While there can be a wide degree of variability among individuals performing the same vocal task—for different age, sex, smoking history, voice use—the value of acoustic analysis lies in the comparison of voice production for the same individual at different points in time.

Regardless of the methodologic issues, there are several basic acoustic measures that are part of a standard acoustic analysis. In the following paragraphs we will describe them.

Fundamental Frequency

Simply stated, fundamental frequency (F_0) is the number of vibrations per second produced by the vocal folds. The measurement generally is expressed in hertz (Hz). Pitch is considered to be the perceptual correlate to fundamental frequency. The faster the vocal folds vibrate, the greater the fundamental frequency and the higher the pitch appears to the ear. The most direct method of measuring F_0 is by asking a person to sustain a vowel sound. Of course, in speech F_0 fluctuates constantly. This presents a difficulty in measuring F_0 reliably for a rapidly changing conversational signal. There is a long history of acoustic studies investigating F_0 for a number of populations. The reader is referred to Baken[6] for an excellent review of those studies and a summary of normative values for various groups of speakers.

Jitter

An electronic signal generator can produce a tone of a given F_0 with virtually no variation. Over time, the number of cycles per second may change only minimally. However, there is less consistency in human voice production. *Jitter* is the term given to frequency perturbation or the variability in F_0 from vibratory cycle to vibratory cycle. In other words, jitter is a measurement of the short-term variability in the voice production system. As an illustration, the vocal folds may be vibrating at 134 Hz for the first cycle, then at 137 Hz for the next cycle, then at 132 Hz for the next cycle, and so on. The examiner might calculate the percentage difference in F_0 across the entire sample or might average the difference in fundamental frequency. Regardless of the method chosen, the resulting value is regarded as jitter.

It is important to remember that there are a number of methods to calculate jitter. Terms in the literature or clinical evaluation reports include *jitter factor*, *jitter ratio*, and *relative average perturbation*. These are expressed in various units (milliseconds, percentages). It is vital that the reader understand the method by which a particular analysis extracts this measure so that a valid assumption can be made about the results. This is especially true if the analysis was done in an unfamiliar laboratory or if one wants to incorporate specific jitter values from a journal article into one's own laboratory.

Frequency Range (Maximum Phonational Range)

Another important measure of vocal function is the highest and lowest frequencies produced by an individual's voice. Frequency range or maximum phonational range often is related to the health of the vocal folds. In persons with dysphonic voices, frequency range is often reduced. For singers, this is often the first symptom of vocal dysfunction. Frequency range, as measured in the voice laboratory, should be distinguished from singing range. In assessing frequency range, the quality of the vocal tone is not essential; rather, it is the ability to produce the highest and lowest note possible, generally elicited via a vowel glide. As F_0 is measured on a logarithmic scale, frequency range is not quantified in hertz. It is measured in *semitones*—calculated from the difference from the highest to lowest note.

Intensity

Intensity is the acoustic correlate to loudness. It is measured in decibels (dB). Intensity reflects the amplitude of the vocal signal. It is important to remember that the measure of intensity is directly related to the distance of the microphone to the lips. If the microphone is further away from the lips, then the intensity measure will be reduced. For example, if the microphone is placed at 5 cm for one patient and records 75 dB, then the patient whose voice is recorded at 10 cm could provide the same intensity level but be measured at 72 dB (or 69 dB if recording sound pressure). Consequently, it is important to maintain a constant microphone-to-mouth distance in the clinical laboratory. One simple way to do this is to use a microphone mounted in a headpiece and measure the distance from lips to microphone for each patient.

Shimmer

Shimmer or intensity perturbation is a measure of the fluctuation in the amplitude of a sound signal from vibratory cycle to vibratory cycle. Shimmer is another component of what is perceived as hoarseness. Shimmer is measured best during sustained phonation of a vowel. It can be expressed as a percentage or in decibels.

Dynamic Range

Dynamic range is the range of intensity capable of being produced by an individual. In the laboratory it is measured by asking the patient to produce the softest sound possible and to produce a shout. While there is a great deal of variability in this measure from person to person, it is useful in measuring change in an individual with a particular voice disorder such as vocal fold paralysis. As with measuring habitual intensity, it is important to maintain a consistent microphone-to-mouth distance.

Signal-to-Noise Ratio/Harmonic-to-Noise Ratio

The signal-to-noise ratio (SNR) contrasts the periodic or regular signal produced by the vocal folds with the "noise" or aperiodic signal from the vocal folds and vocal tract. This is usually expressed in decibels. The more hoarse or "noisy" a voice is, the lower the SNR. A high SNR indicates a relatively clear voice. Algorithms for computing SNR are included in several commercially available computerized acoustic analysis systems.

Spectrography

Spectrography is a method for measuring the acoustics of speech. The output of a spectrograph is the signal produced at the vocal folds and the alterations of that signal imposed upon it by the vocal tract (Fig. 10–6). A spectrogram shows the fundamental

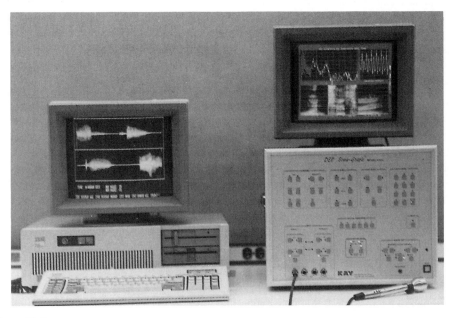

Figure 10–6.

frequency of a given complex sound signal (speech) as well as the other frequency components that make up that sound and that are produced by the changing configurations of supraglottic structures. Spectrograms accurately reflect the influences of resonance and articulation upon the voice signal generated at the vocal folds. Rather than relying on sustained vowels for acoustic analysis, spectrography allows the examiner to measure acoustic information within the context of speech. Acoustic analysis via spectrography was formerly a tedious task. However, with the advent of digital signal analysis and computerization, convenience has been improved (for an in-depth review of the principles of physics and acoustics involved in sound spectrography, see Baken[7]).

Aerodynamic Analysis

One of the crucial components of voice production is that of adequate airflow from the lungs. In aerodynamic analysis, instrumentation is used to measure the patient's ability to use the respiratory system and vocal fold valving appropriately for voice production. Various measures give some idea of the amount of air available for voice production (tidal volume, vital capacity), the amount of air used during phonation (flow volume/phonation volume), the ability of the vocal folds to maintain adequate closure against the flow of air from the lungs (pressure), and the amount of airflow through the adducted vocal folds (airflow rate). In some clinical voice laboratories, complete pulmonary function tests are performed routinely. Sataloff et al[8] present a case for collecting information on pulmonary function for singers. They have found that, for some singers who present with suspected technical singing problems, in fact the cause of the difficulty is previously undiagnosed asthma.

Flow Volume/Phonation Volume

Flow volume is the amount of air used for voice production. It is measured in liters. While a relatively small percentage of vital capacity is used for speech, flow volume typically is measured after a maximum inhalation. Consequently, flow volume values should be close to vital capacity values.

Airflow Rate

The airflow rate is the amount of air expelled during voice production over a given period of time. For a sustained vowel production, it is the flow volume (milliliters) divided by the maximum phonation time (seconds). Among patients and conditions (varying pitch and loudness) there is a great deal of variation.[9]

Subglottic Pressure

While technically not an aerodynamic measure, subglottic pressure is included in this discussion because of the interdependency of phonation volume, flow and pressure. Direct measurements of subglottic pressure are invasive and involve placing a pressure transducer directly beneath the vocal folds via a puncture into the trachea. This is not acceptable for routine clinical use. Indirect measures include the insertion of a catheter with a pressure transducer into the esophagus and inferring subglottic pressures from the changes in pressure against the esophagus from the trachea. Unfortunately, this can be an unreliable measure because of individual differences. More commonly, clinical voice laboratories are measuring an extrapolation of actual subglottic pressure by measuring intraoral pressure through a specific task. The patient is asked to repeat the sound "pa" (/pa/) or "pee" (/pi/) rapidly at a constant pitch and loudness. Pressure peaks produced by this method are considered to be an estimate of subglottic pressure. There are currently several pieces of equipment that allow for the collection and analysis of this measure (Phonatory Function Analyzer [Nagashima]; Aerophone II [Kay Elemetrics]) (Figs. 10–7, 10–8).

Electroglottography

Electroglottography (EGG) is a method by which the contact area of the vocal folds is measured via surface electrodes applied to both sides of the thyroid cartilage. The basic principle behind the design of EGG instrumentation is that human tissue conducts electrical current variably, depending on its density. When there is an opening or space in the structure, the resistance to the current is increased. In the larynx, when the vocal folds are open, there is decreased conductance of electrical current. When the vocal folds are closed, there is increased conductance of electrical current. This is represented graphically by upward and downward slopes of a tracing. This graphic representation can be used to

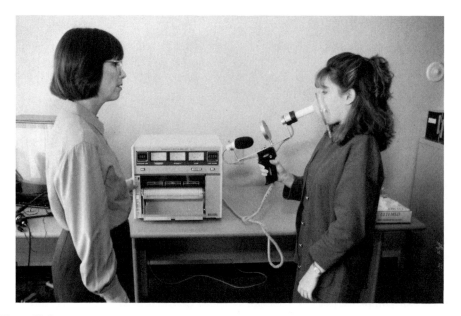

Figure 10–7.

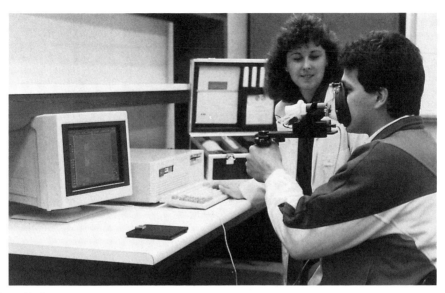

Figure 10–8.

estimate the time spent by the vocal folds in opening, open, closing, and closed phases of vibration.

While a version of the device most commonly used today was first described in 1971 by Fourcin and Abberton[10] and the principle is well understood, its usefulness in the clinical laboratory continues to be debated (Fig. 10–9). As Colton and Conture[11] describe, there are several drawbacks to this type of analysis ranging from equipment constraints to patient variability that limit the ability of researchers and clinicians to interpret and apply its data. Much of the existing research on the EGG is descriptive rather than quantitative. Its current promise appears to be in the ability to record electroglottographic data simultaneously with other types of analysis such as videostroboscopy or inverse filtering. Measures that may be obtained through EGG include F_0, qualitative descriptions of the shape of the glottal waveform as measured by EGG, and quantitative measures such as open quotient (open phase/time).

Resonance

To the singer or speaker, the production of the appropriate balance of oral and nasal resonance is crucial. Listeners may find the presence of hypo- or hypernasality extremely distracting. For the singer, the overall quality of the singing tone is disturbed when there is poor resonance functionally or anatomically. When surgery is considered in the hypopharynx or nasopharynx in the adult (e.g., tonsillectomy and/or adenoidectomy), the clinician must consider the possible effects on resonance postoperatively.

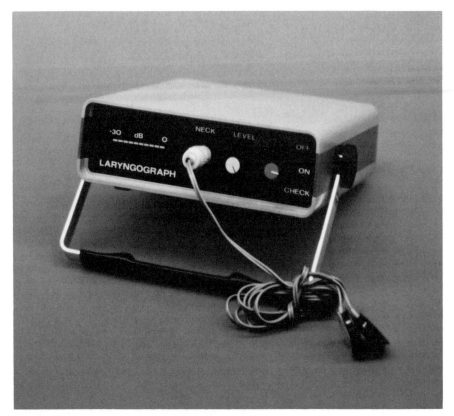

Figure 10–9.

There are several methods available for measuring resonance. In almost every case, the techniques compare values obtained orally and nasally. One can measure oral versus nasal air pressure, oral versus nasal airflow, oral versus nasal resistance, and oral versus nasal accelerometer values. The sound spectrograph also demonstrates spectral changes when excessive or inadequate nasality is present (Fig. 10–10). The Nasometer (Kay Elemetrics) is a commercially available piece of equipment that compares oral and nasal sound pressure, and results are expressed in the percentage of "nasalance" present. Stimuli used for measuring resonance include sustained vowels, nasal and nonnasal sentences, and standardized paragraphs, such as the Rainbow Passage.

Other Measures

Inverse Filtering

Inverse filtering is a method by which the factors contributing to the acoustic signal *above* the larynx are filtered. This results in a signal that is considered to be equivalent to the

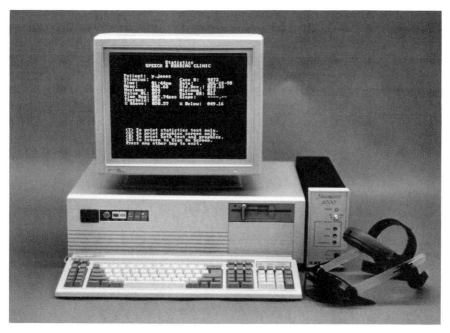

Figure 10–10.

signal generated by the larynx alone. One may also use the airflow waveform that has been filtered to extract the signal at the larynx using a specially designed mask. As mentioned above, this signal is teamed with the EGG signal to provide more information about the vibratory characteristics of the vocal folds. A special piece of equipment called a *Rothenberg mask* is used to measure the airflow waveform for inverse filtering.

Electromyography

All of the measures noted above give information about how the various systems that contribute to voice production are functioning. However, none of these techniques can tell directly about the function of the muscles that produce voice. Electromyography is a technique whereby electrodes are inserted directly into the muscle and the activity of muscle fibers is recorded. In laryngeal electromyography, electrodes record activity from the thyroarytenoid, cricothyroid, and posterior cricoarytenoid muscles most commonly. The measurement of laryngeal muscle fiber activity is by no means routine in the clinical voice laboratory; however, it can help provide information that is helpful for the differential diagnosis of vocal fold weakness and paralysis versus arytenoid fixation. It can also be used to guide injection of botulinum toxin for treatment of spasmodic dysphonia. Special training is required to place the electrodes and interpret the muscle activity, both visually and auditorially. Specialists who perform this procedure are neurologists, neurophysiologists, otolaryngologists, and, in some cases, speech–language pathologists.

GUIDELINES FOR EQUIPMENT SELECTION

A detailed description of the equipment needed to perform the above analyses is beyond the scope of this chapter. However, there are several principles to keep in mind when selecting equipment for the laboratory.

1.   Keep clinical and research needs in mind when purchasing equipment. Many "pre-packaged" analysis systems come with many more "bells and whistles" than may be needed, and these can boost the cost significantly.

2.   Read the research and clinical literature to determine which systems appear to produce the most reliable, reproducible data.

3.   Purchase the best system that is the most affordable. This is especially true for videostroboscopic components.

4.   Check for availability of "loaner" equipment when a system requires service. In a busy clinical laboratory, dysfunctional equipment results in lost revenue.

5.   Visit several clinical voice laboratories to learn applications for equipment and "real world" experience.

Table 10–1 lists some of the commercially available equipment for each type of analysis discussed above. This list is not meant to be exhaustive, as there are certainly many other types of equipment available. (The reader is referred to Read et al[12,13] for reviews of speech analysis systems.)

ESTABLISHMENT OF NORMATIVE VALUES

The driving question for the clinician when inspecting data obtained from the clinical voice laboratory is what distinguishes normal vocal behavior from abnormal behavior. Unfor-

Table 10–1   Commercially Available Equipment for Voice Function Analysis

ANALYSIS	EQUIPMENT	MANUFACTURER
Videostroboscopy	Rhino-Laryngeal Stroboscope	Kay Elemetrics
	Laryngostroboscope (model LS3-A)	Nagashima
Acoustic	Computerized Speech Lab (CSL)	Kay Elemetrics
	CSpeech	Paul Milenkovic (Univ. of Wisconsin)
	DSP Sono-graph	Kay Elemetrics
	Sound level meter	Bruel & Kjaer (other manufacturers)
Aerodynamic	Aerophone II	Kay Elemetrics
	Phonatory Function Analyzer	Nagashima
	Pneumotachograph	OEM, Inc. (other manufacturers)
Electroglottography	Laryngograph	Kay Elemetrics

tunately, the range of "normal" can be quite large. While there are several available studies that report normal values for laryngeal function measures for various groups (e.g., by sex, age, smoking history, profession), these measures are often referenced to a particular equipment configuration or data collection protocol. Practicing clinicians must always interpret such data cautiously when applying values to their own laboratories.

A solution for this dilemma is for clinicians to produce normative values for their own individual laboratories. While this activity can be cumbersome and time consuming, it provides a reference for the comparison of subsequent pathologic and normal patients. By incorporating this information into a database, the clinician can discuss a patient's laryngeal function descriptively, in terms of statistical measures of means and standard deviations. A clinician can also follow the progress of treatment using established laboratory measures. This is particularly helpful for documentation of progress for third party payers.

The accumulation of normative measures of laryngeal function should be a cumulative process. Initially, a normal subject group of 20 should be sufficient to begin a database. However, a clinician should always be aware of opportunities to collect more data—from patients' spouses, co-workers, friends and acquaintances. Careful collection of such data will help to corroborate the reliability of laryngeal function measures.

THE RELATIONSHIP OF OBJECTIVE VOICE ANALYSIS TO DIAGNOSIS AND TREATMENT

As with any measurement of behavior, whether it is perceptual or objective in nature, the interpretation of results cannot be made in a vacuum. No one measure provides a definitive diagnosis. Even perceptually, clinicians incorporate several distinct components of voice production into their final assessment of dysphonia and its possible etiology. Through experience with laryngeal function measures for various disorders of voice production, a clinician can assemble a montage of typical laboratory values that correspond to a particular diagnosis. For example, low airflow rates, elevated shimmer values, a restricted frequency range, and anterior to posterior supraglottic "press" with reduced amplitude of vibration most likely indicates a hyperfunctional pattern of voice production.

While objective voice analysis may help to answer the diagnostic question for a particular patient, one of the benefits of laboratory assessment is for the determination of appropriate treatment directions for a patient. In the example above, instrumentation can be useful to "probe" the efficacy of certain treatment techniques for the alteration of this hyperfunctional pattern. Do changes in pitch or loudness result in more normal-appearing airflow rates or acoustic measures? Does reduction of extrinsic muscle tension produce less supraglottic activity on videostroboscopy? For most patients with voice disorders, the element of feedback of functional measures is extremely reinforcing. With the population of professional voice users, this effect is magnified.

Initially, the accumulation of information obtained in the voice laboratory may appear overwhelming. Frequently, in attempting to explain results, a clinician may become lost in a flurry of percentages, milliseconds, and semitones. However, in conjunction with perceptual measures and patient history, measures of laryngeal function provide crucial information about laryngeal physiology and, more importantly, about changes in laryngeal physiology as voice behavior is manipulated by the patient and the clinician.

SUMMARY

The evolution of objective voice analysis for clinical use has come about in the last 10 years. In many cases, the sophistication of basic science and instrumentation in this field has exceeded knowledge of how to use these measures in the voice clinic. To develop and operate clinical voice laboratory adequately, one must have a solid core knowledge of vocal pathology, laryngeal and speech physiology, acoustics, and respiratory dynamics. Thus a clinician is prepared to interpret the information obtained through videostroboscopy, acoustic analysis, aerodynamic analysis, EGG, and resonance analysis. Ultimately, the value of objective voice analysis emerges from the ability of the clinician to integrate the results from these components into a cohesive impression of laryngeal function as a whole.

REFERENCES

1. Kreiman J, Gerratt BR, Precoda K, Berke GS: Individual differences in voice quality perception. *J Speech Hearing Res* 35:512–520, 1992.
2. Peppard RC, Bless DM: A method for improving measurement reliability in laryngeal videostroboscopy. *J Voice* 4:280–285, 1990.
3. Titze IR, Horii Y, Scherer R: Some technical considerations in voice perturbation measurements. *J Speech Hear Res* 30:252–260, 1987.
4. Karnell MP: Laryngeal perturbation analysis: Minimum length of analysis window. *J Speech Hear Res* 34:544–548, 1991.
5. Karnell MP, Scherer RS, Fischer LB: Comparison of acoustic voice perturbation measures among three independent voice laboratories. *J Speech Hear Res* 34:781–790, 1991.
6. Baken RJ: *Clinical Measurement of Speech and Voice.* Boston, College Hill Press, 1987, pp 125–196.
7. Baken RJ: *Clinical Measurement of Speech and Voice.* Boston, College Hill Press, 1987, pp 315–392.
8. Sataloff RT, Spiegel JR, Carroll LM, et al: Objective measures of voice function. *Ear, Nose Throat J* 66:307–312, 1987.
9. Hirano M: *Clinical Examination of Voice.* Wien, Springer-Verlag, 1981, pp 27–29.
10. Fourcin AJ, Abberton E: First applications of a new laryngograph. *Med Biol Illus* 21:172–182, 1971.
11. Colton RH, Conture EG: Problems and pitfalls of electroglottography. *J Voice* 4:10–24, 1990.
12. Read C, Buder EH, Kent RD: Speech analysis systems: A survey. *J Speech Hear Res* 33:363–374, 1990.
13. Read C, Buder EH, Kent RD: Speech analysis systems: an evaluation. *J Speech Hear Res* 35:314–332, 1992.

Disorders of Speaking in the Professional Voice User

ALEX F. JOHNSON, PhD

The purpose of this chapter is to present the various disorders of speech production typically seen in persons with voice disorders. Specifically, those aspects of speech that contribute to the types of disorders frequently seen in professional voice users are addressed, and behavioral/perceptual perspectives of voice disorders rather than an anatomic classification are emphasized.

ASPECTS OF NORMAL SPEECH PRODUCTION

In 1977, Nation and Aram[1] introduced the Speech and Language Processing Model as a way of categorizing the various processes that underlie speech and/or language and relating these processes to their outputs. The outputs (or products) for speech are, of course, the acoustic realization of these underlying processes. In the case of speech production, the underlying processes are understood as being physiologic subsystems that allow for the occurrence of speech.

Speech production is accomplished through interactions of the respiratory, articulatory, phonatory, and prosodic subsystems. It is these subsystems that account for the speech products of voice, phonetic structure (articulation), resonance, and prosody. *Voice* refers to that aspect of speech production that is driven by the respiratory cycle and is generated by the vibration of the vocal folds. The listener attends to the various perceptual characteristics of voice, with loudness, pitch, and quality being the most prominent. *Phonetic structure* is the result of the articulatory processes that result in the production of the recognizable segments of speech, the consonant and vowel sounds. Each sound has certain features—voicing, place of articulation, manner of articulation—that distinguish it from other sounds. Articulation is accomplished via movements of the tongue, lips, jaws, palate, and larynx.

Resonance refers to the modifications made in the sound generated at the level of the larynx by the various supralaryngeal tissues and cavities. For example, in normal speech production there is a perceptually acceptable balance of nasal and non-nasal resonance that is accomplished through the valving mechanics of the soft palate. The vocal tone that

153

we perceive when we listen to a speaker is actually the acoustic realization of the vibratory characteristics of the voice, modified by the resonating characteristics of the vocal tract.

Prosody can be defined as the nonsegmental aspects of rate, fluency, intonation, and stress. The parameters involved in the prosodic system allow for the smooth flow of connected speech. Variations in prosody, which are used in a most effective way by excellent professional speakers and singers, are accomplished through a very delicate balance of respiratory dynamics with the vocal and articulatory functions. These dynamics allow for very rapid (yet predictable, organized, and consistent) adjustments in the loudness, rate of speech, and pitch level that enhance the communicative intent of an utterance.

Table 11–1 presents examples of the function of voice production in the various characteristics of each speech production parameter. While each process of speech production has unique anatomic, physiologic, and acoustic features, the essential role of voice is obvious. When phonation is severely impaired, the effects on all aspects of speech production can be devastating to communication and intelligibility. Conversely, impairment of resonance, articulation, breathing for speech, or prosody can contribute to a voice that is perceptually deviant.

PATHOLOGIES OF SPEECH PRODUCTION IN PROFESSIONALS

Professional voice users are susceptible to the same etiologies as the general population for factors that produce various speech disturbances. General categories of causation of speech disturbance include etiologies that are developmental, neurogenic, structural, psychogenic, environmental, or functional. It is the selective impairment of voice production in the professional singer and speaker resulting from disordered use of the mechanism that is the focus of this chapter. The general causes for these disturbances are functional (misuse, abuse), environmental (e.g., exposure to smoke), or psychogenic (e.g., musculoskeletal tension). It is not unusual to have interactions between functional and psychological factors that cause the development and maintenance of a voice disturbance.

Professional singers and speakers represent a specific subgroup of high-risk patients for a set of environmental and functional causative factors. In the same manner that athletes are susceptible to a unique set of injuries that can limit their efficient performance, the professional voice user is at greater risk than the normal speaker for disorders caused by

**Table 11–1   Role of Voice Production
With Other Levels of Speech Production**

LEVEL OF SPEECH PRODUCTION	ROLE OF PHONATION
Articulation	Provides a differentiating feature for various phonemes (e.g., /t/ vs /d/)
Resonance	Generates tone that is modified by the resonating characteristics of the tissues and cavities of the head and neck
Prosody	Rapid adjustments in loudness and pitch signal inflectional changes and syllabic stress

overuse or by inefficient use of the speech production system. In the context of performing, preaching, public speaking, or broadcasting, minor variations in vocal efficiency may become prominently notable. What might be a "little hoarseness" to the nonprofessional speaker may have devastating effects on the performance of the professional singer or speaker. Even minor variations in vocal quality, range, or flexibility may prove quite disabling to the performer, preacher, or broadcaster. The remainder of this chapter is devoted to the issues that place the professional at risk and to particular symptoms and causes that clarify the nature of voice disturbances.

High-risk factors that contribute to voice disturbance in the singer can be divided into three sets: misuse, exposure to irritants, and psychogenic causes. Table 11–2 summarizes factors believed by many voice specialists to contribute to disordered vocal function.

Misuse

Vocal misuse is believed to be a common cause of dysfunction. While the precise mechanisms for vocal problems secondary to misuse of the phonatory mechanism are not well understood, practicing voice clinicians give much attention to these factors in clinical practice. Specific behaviors that are often cited as causal can be divided into activities that occur while speaking (eg, loud talking, hard glottal attack) and those that occur as nonspeech vocal behaviors (grunting, throat clearing, loud and hard laughing).

Problematic Speaking Behaviors

The normal human voice has a broad range of physiologic capabilities, allowing for broad variance in the production of loudness, pitch, and quality characteristics. For some speakers, it appears that, when there is a habitual pattern of voice use at the extremes of these ranges, both esthetic and pathologic changes may occur. The typical acoustic changes seen in persons with deviant speaking patterns are hoarseness, harshness, and breathiness. In addition, singers and professional speakers often experience reduced vocal range for loudness and/or pitch. Vocal fatigue is another common complaint in singers who are using inappropriate patterns.

Loud Talking, Yelling, and Screaming. Some variations that involve the use of extremes of loudness and pitch in conversational or vocational situations are demanding

Table 11–2 Factors Believed to Contribute to Voice Disturbance

Misuse	Exposure
Loud talking, yelling, screaming	Alcohol consumption
Hard glottal attack	Medications
Singing or speaking outside acceptable physiologic range	Caffeine
Speaking in a noisy environment	Recreational drugs
Excessive coughing and throat clearing	Smoke
Grunting (as in exercising and lifting)	Reflux of stomach contents
Excessive talking	Psychogenic causes
Loud, hard, abusive laughing	Musculoskeletal tension
Producing voice when laryngeal tissues are inflamed	

for the normal speaker, but are of special concern to the vocal professional. Chronic patterns of excessive loudness are found in certain personality types and certain vocational situations (ie, coaching, classroom teaching). Because many very serious singers and speakers are unable to survive on the income derived from performing they frequently can be found in other professional situations, for at least part of the day. It is not unusual to come across a patient who teaches elementary school music classes during the day, studies and practices in the evenings, and performs on the weekend.

According to Colton and Casper[2] (p. 82):

the mechanism for increased loudness requires the creation of increased resistance of the laryngeal valve until an appropriate level of air pressure is produced and released. The vocal folds must be adducted strongly to create the increased medial compression. . . . The laryngeal mucosa, especially along the glottal edge, may become irritated, inflamed, and swollen.

This behavioral pattern can result in localized inflammation and swelling and ultimately in development of a lesion at the point of maximum contact of the vocal folds.

Alterations in vibration secondary to swelling or formation of nodules are likely to result in hoarseness, and the inability of the glottis to achieve maximum closure due to obstruction by nodules will increase the turbulent sound that is perceived as breathiness. Again, for the nonprofessional patient these variations may be small problems. However, for the professional these patterns result in vocal fatigue, inability to make fine vocal adjustments during performances, and ultimately significant changes in the perceived quality of the performer.

To date there has been no systematic investigation of the vocal habits (in speaking) of trained professional voice users. A number of studies have demonstrated that persistent misuse/overuse of the vocal mechanism can lead to vocal difficulties. Groups studied have included female army instructors and recruits,[3] professional welders,[4] and cheerleaders.[5,6]
Hard Glottal Attack.   The abrupt, almost explosive, onset of vowel-initiated words and phrases by some "harsh" speakers has been labeled as *hard glottal attack*. This type of attack on vowels is perceived as a popping sound that accompanies the actual production of the target phoneme. Colton and Casper[2] describe the movement patterns that allow this phenomenon to occur as being either medial compression associated with the onset of phonation or prephonatory constriction of the larynx and supralaryngeal structures with a springing open of the larynx at phonatory onset.

Observation of many individuals indicates that hard glottal attack frequently occurs in persons who are normal speakers. In addition, it is also observed, at least occasionally, in most speakers. It is likely when the predominant manner of vowel onset is with the hard onset, or when the patient is talking loudly all day, using this type of talking, that there is a problem. Most likely, the hard glottal attack is one of many possible vocal symptoms of either poor speaking style or underlying musculoskeletal tension.
Singing or Speaking Outside Acceptable Physiologic Pitch Range.   Each voice has distinctive characteristics and capabilities. While normal ranges for pitch, volume, range, and so forth are published and used clinically, the performer is in the unique position of being called upon to use his or her voice at the limits of the range. It is clear that well-trained singers and performers can increase their range and can use the limits of the range without considerable difficulty. Those individuals who do not study with an expert teacher are at some risk. The classic picture is, of course, one of the person who works in a verbally demanding position during the day and then performs in a theater, church choir, or night-

club in the evening. These persons are at considerable vocal risk and are common patients in the voice clinic setting.

Lack of Vocal Training.   One of the greatest risk factors for singers (and even professional speakers) is lack of professional vocal training. It is possible for a professional to develop a vocal output that is quite pleasing to an audience while using poor vocal technique. Professionals should be cautious, however, in assuming that experience in singing or speaking guarantees long-term success in maintaining vocal health. In a most interesting study, Teachey et al[7] studied a group of 30 singers with less than 2 years of vocal training. Using instrumental (voice laboratory) assessment and perceptual judgments they demonstrated (1) deficits in technique, (2) that those singers with "some" vocal training outperformed those without such experience, and (3) that vocal nodules were present in 60% of the singers. The authors suggested (p. 55) that training "should include career counseling, education in vocal hygiene, rigorous development of good vocal technique, and accurate descriptions of voice mechanics."

Problematic Nonspeech Vocal Behaviors

The patient's use of the vocal mechanism in nonspeech activities is also a concern for the clinician assessing the professional voice user. Personality type and lifestyle, as well as development of vocal habits, can all contribute to a healthy or nonhealthy phonatory pattern.

Excessive Coughing and Throat Clearing.   Many persons with vocal difficulties develop a pattern of frequent throat clearing and coughing. Again, the abrasion produced by this type of vocal behavior is believed to contribute to swelling of the vocal folds.

Our clinical experience suggests that this pattern develops as a behavioral symptom. There is no evidence upon fiberoptic or videostroboscopic examination to support a need for constant throat clearing activity. Patients often report that they cough and throat clear "to make it feel better" or "because I feel like something is caught there." It may be that the patient is responding to the sensation of the added mass of vocal swelling or a nodule rather than to any loose material in the proximity of the vocal folds. While the recurrent harsh coughing or strong throat clearing may provide a temporary reduction in the sensation that is uncomfortable, this behavior has potential for being quite aggravating for the lesion, if present.

Grunting.   In exercise and heavy lifting, the vocal folds are brought tightly together to increase upper body strength. While this activity, performed in moderation, probably has many beneficial effects for most persons, it can be detrimental for the singer. During this activity there is tight compression of the vocal folds. Persons who engage in this activity repeatedly may experience some vocal swelling. Singers who participate in heavy weight-lifting as a form of exercise may find some voice changes following completion of such a session.

Loud, Hard, Abusive Laughing.   With the loud, hard, driving laughter that is frequently found in outgoing or aggressive personality types, it is not unusual for development of vocal problems to occur. During hard laughter there is rapid forced expulsion of air from the lungs, usually with the elastic vocal folds snapping open and closed. Again, this type of behavior may produce localized edema if it occurs repeatedly. In addition, long-term abusive laughing, along with other inappropriate vocal activities, may be quite damaging to the professional, limiting vocal range and efficiency.

Playing Wind Instruments.   Playing a wind instrument is not a common cause of vocal disturbance. However, there is preliminary evidence to suggest that some individuals who do play such instruments may be at risk for the development of voice problems. Ocker et al[8] studied vocal output in 63 wind instrumentalists. After 1 hour of playing (flute, reed, brass), 19 exhibited a perceptually worse voice. These authors suggest that the greatest risk is for individuals with existing voice disorders who persist in playing their instrument.

Exposure

Exposure to a variety of substances can have adverse effects on the vocal mechanism and its efficiency. These effects may be seen in the way that structure or movement are impaired. In some cases of exposure, both movement within the vocal tract and structure can be affected.

Exposure to Smoke

Smoke can be inhaled, for example, from cigarettes, from the air (secondary smoking), or from marijuana. The extreme effect of smoking is laryngeal cancer. Precancerous conditions such as leukoplakia and hyperkeratosis are also associated with smoke inhalation. While these more obvious effects of extended exposure to smoking are well known to clinicians who work in the field of voice disorders, it is also important to recognize the effects of these substances on phonatory production. Laryngoscopic examination will reveal redness and irritation of the vocal mucosa,[2] and there is a tendency toward dryness in the vocal tract. It is likely that the singer will find that it is difficult to maintain vocal stamina for a performance if these effects along with those affecting respiration are experienced.

Sataloff[9] reports that singers who perform in smoky rooms may suffer similar effects to those who smoke. This is of special concern to the nightclub singer who may have relatively constant exposure to a smoky environment.

Alcohol Consumption

Abuse of alcohol can be another cause of faulty performance ability for either the professional speaker or singer. Intake of large amounts of alcohol results in generalized incoordination of muscular activity. This type of incoordination has been associated with slurring of speech production at the articulatory level. There is also a predictable loss of ability to control fine neuromuscular adjustments in the larynx, thereby producing loss of volume or pitch control.

In smaller quantities, according to Sataloff,[9] alcohol consumption is a concern for singers or speakers with food allergies to wine or beer. These can cause nasal congestion or rhinorrhea.

Drugs

Medicines and recreational drugs all have potential for limiting vocal efficiency. This may be either through increased dryness or from impaired movement of the vocal cords and/or the articulators. The observed variations are similar to those seen in exposure to smoke or alcohol, as noted above.

One of the significant effects of many of the agents described—smoke, drugs, alcohol—is their dehydrating effect. Many voice clinicians (see Stone, this text) have expressed considerable concern about the effect of dryness on vocal production. The vocal quality of the person with a very "dry" hoarseness is well known to the experienced voice clinician. For some patients, almost immediate improvement in vocal output is obtained with improved hydration.

Gastric Reflux

A common problem among singers and other performers is reflux laryngitis. According to Sataloff,[9] the typical symptoms in reflux are prolonged warm-up time before singing, hoarseness, halitosis, a feeling of "lump in the throat," frequent throat clearing, chronic irritative cough, and frequent tracheitis or tracheobronchitis. Reflux is increasingly recognized as a source of voice disturbance and should be addressed in the management of the professional voice user.

Psychogenic Factors

Psychological factors play a part in many aspects of human behavior as it relates to vocal performance. The major psychological factor that contributes to problems for the performing vocalist is increased musculoskeletal tension. Aronson[10] [(p. 121)] states:

> The extrinsic and intrinsic laryngeal muscles are exquisitely sensitive to emotional stress, and their hypercontraction is the common denominator behind the dysphonia and aphonia in virtually all psychogenic voice disorders. . . . In general, however, the extent of visible pathology is incongruously minor or absent in comparison with the severity of abnormal voice.

The professional singer and/or performer is frequently involved in a stress-producing lifestyle. Travel, competition, inconsistent income, problems with maintaining a consistent diet, and irregular eating times all can contribute to excessive tension, which can be reflected in a high-positioned larynx. Manual manipulation of the muscles of the neck in the area of the larynx and hyoid bone will produce pain or discomfort.

The vocal effect of excessive musculoskeletal tension may be hoarseness, reduction of pitch range, or poor vocal focus due to tight laryngeal/pharyngeal constriction, tongue retraction, or limited mandibular excursion. While these factors may produce voices that are tolerable in general speakers (if not attractive), it is likely to produce unacceptable voices for singing or public speaking. When excessive musculoskeletal tension is present in the professional speaker or singer it must be addressed and treated.

Finally, when professional voice users have concerns about their voice, their habitual speaking pattern should be studied very carefully. It is not infrequent to find the patient who has learned relaxed, appropriate vocal movements for the professional situation, but exhibits the tight, strained, restricted vocalization associated with excessive musculoskeletal tension during spontaneous conversation.

CHARACTERISTICS OF VOICE DISTURBANCE

Colton and Casper[2] have identified eight "primary symptoms" of voice disturbance. These symptoms, which are frequently the presenting complaints for many patients, are hoarseness, vocal fatigue, breathiness, reduced phonational range, aphonia, pitch breaks or inappropriately high pitch, strain/struggle voice, and tremor. For the voice clinician, laryngologist, and voice teacher these symptoms provide the window into the patient's difficulties and often contribute to the formulation of the diagnosis of the problem.

While the patient's presenting complaint may be a combination of any of these symptoms, it should be noted that tremor is typically seen only in neurogenic disorders and is rarely the single presenting complaint of the professional singer or speaker. Aphonia (complete loss of voice) may be experienced after a significant vocal trauma (ie, hemorrhage) or as a conversion (hysterical) symptom. Aphonia is not a typical presentation among professional voice users. The other vocal symptoms are reported to varying degrees by professionals and are discussed below.

Hoarseness

A hoarse quality is the classic presentation of vocal disturbance. Hoarseness can be the result of the increased mass that results from a vocal nodule or polyp or localized edema, or it can be observed in the absence of a mass lesion of any sort. This perceived quality disturbance does not differentiate among causal factors.

Hoarseness is perceived as a rough, sometimes harsh, breathy quality and may vary in severity from patient to patient. The various components of hoarseness have been attributed to "irregular" laryngeal behaviors, that is, behaviors that alter the glottal cycle in such a way that it is unpredictable and/or considerably different than the cycles adjacent to it. Hoarseness has also been referred to as *aperiodic noise*.[11] When the duration of each cycle is irregularly variant, perturbations in pitch (jitter) are most notable. Conversely, when the intensity of the signal varies considerably, perturbations in loudness (shimmer) are present.[12]

Vocal Fatigue

A fatigued voice is a common complaint, heard from many patients with voice disorders, who report that their laryngeal musculature "feels tired" at the end of a performance or rehearsal. It is not unusual for a patient to be able to go into great detail to describe the type of fatigue, how long it lasts, when it occurs, and so forth. Soreness in the throat muscles, as well as an intermittent weakness and/or hoarseness, may also accompany the vocal fatigue.

Reduced Range of Phonation

For both the professional speaker and singer, phonatory range is crucial to vocal effectiveness. This symptom of voice disorder is sometimes an early sign of a more serious disturbance. It is most apparent in the singer who is quick to observe that a note at the extreme end of the scale cannot be produced as well as in previous performances. This may develop without any change in overall vocal quality, and even without notable fatigue. Whenever a singer begins to notice a loss of notes at the extreme end of the scale, a work-up should be initiated to determine the cause. If no organic cause is present then voice therapy should be initiated immediately.

In the professional speaker, reduced range of phonation may present as difficulty with elevation of the pitch during speaking activities for purposes of emphasis and inflection. Thus a speaker may come across as being quite stilted and monopitched in situations that call for increased animation. When this speaker attempts to move into the desired range he may experience a variety of vocal symptoms and therefore compensates by reducing pitch variability in speaking parts.

Breathiness

Breathy voice quality occurs as the result of inefficient closure of the vocal folds, a process known as *hypolaryngeal valving*.[13] In breathiness, what is usually most notable is a significant amount of air turbulence that accompanies a weak vocal tone. In this speech pattern, phrases are shorter than normal.

Breathy voice quality may signify neurologic pathology (ie, vocal fold paralysis), the presence of added mass to the vocal folds (ie, edema) that causes irregular variations between the two folds in opening and closing activity, thereby allowing an irregular release of air, or it may be produced by nodules along the edge of the vocal folds that prevent normal closure and allow some air escape. In the professional speaker or singer, breathiness may also represent a learned speaking pattern.

Strain/Struggle Voice

In strain/struggle voice, there is a strident, harsh, vocal quality. This pattern is associated with "hyperlaryngeal valving"[14] and is a most unpleasant voice from an aesthetic perspective. This type of voice pattern is most readily associated with the phonatory pattern seen frequently in patients with musculoskeletal tension disorders. The patient usually complains of discomfort when speaking, and, in addition to a "strained" perceptual quality, obvious physical strain is apparent when watching the patient communicate verbally.

The "tightness" in strain/struggle phonation is accomplished through tension in the larynx, as well as in the supralaryngeal vocal tract. Thus the perceived vocal quality is best understood as a combined disorder involving both voice and resonance.

REFERENCES

1. Nation JE, Aram D: *Diagnosis of Speech and Language Disorders*. St. Louis: CV Mosby, 1973.
2. Colton RH, Casper JK: *Understanding Voice Problems: A Physiological Perspective for Diagnosis and Treatment*. Baltimore: Williams & Wilkins, 1990.
3. Sapir S, Atias J, Shahar A: Symptoms of vocal attrition in women army instructors and new recruits: results from a survey. *Laryngoscope* 100:991–994, 1990.
4. Ohlsson AC, Jarvholm B, Lofquist A, et al: Vocal behaviour in welders—a preliminary study. *Folia Phoniatr* 39:98–103, 1987.
5. Andrews M, Shank K: Some observations concerning the cheering behavior of school girl cheerleaders. *Language, Speech, Hear Serv Schools* 14:150–156, 1983.
6. Campbell SL, Reich AR, Klockars AJ, McHenry MA: Factors associated with dysphonia in high school cheerleaders. *J Speech Hear Disord* 53:178–185, 1988.
7. Teachey JC, Kahane JC, Beckford NS: Vocal mechanisms in untrained professional singers. *J Voice* 5:51–56, 1991.

8. Ocker C, Pasher W, Rohrs M, Katny W: Voice disorders among players of wind instruments. *Folia Phoniatr* 42:24–30, 1990.
9. Sataloff RT: Common diagnoses and treatments in professional singers. *Ear Nose Throat J* 66:278–288, 1987.
10. Aronson AE: *Clinical Voice Disorders*, 3rd ed. New York, Thieme, 1990.
11. Morris HL, Spriestersbach DC: Appraisal of respiration and phonation, in Darley F, Spriestersbach DC (eds): *Diagnostic Methods in Speech Pathology*. New York, Harper and Row, 1978.
12. Perkins WH, Kent RD: *Functional Anatomy of Speech, Language, Hearing*. San Diego, College Hill Press, 1986.
13. Moncur JP, Brackett IP: *Modifying Vocal Behavior*. New York, Harper and Row, 1974.

Disorders of Singing

HOWARD L. LEVINE, MD

The professional singer may suffer from all of the disorders of the nonsinger; however, when they do it is often anxiety provoking, performance impeding, or even career devastating. The problem is further complicated by the countless individuals—singing colleagues, accompanists, directors, producers, followers—who depend on the singer's performance. Even the most minor disorder may be a major illness or injury to the professional singer. Voice disorders can affect a singer of any style to the same extent. While some vocal instrumentalists with greater training have more reserve to fall back on, others with less may attempt to sing through illness, only causing greater damage to the voice.

When dealing with the professional singer with a voice disorder, history often becomes a critical portion of the evaluation, while physical examination usually confirms the diagnosis suspected by history. In addition to the usual questions about an illness, history must include past and present training, type of singing, performance length and frequency, type of material performed, environment of practice, rehearsals, and performance such as acoustics, temperature, humidity, noise level, pollutants, speaking activities, conducting activities, and musical instrument playing.

UPPER RESPIRATORY TRACT INFECTION

Upper respiratory tract infections typically create mucosal congestion, increased nasal secretions that are often purulent, and nasal obstruction. The secretions may bathe the pharynx and cause pharyngitis. Fever that may accompany the infection may produce mild to moderate dehydration. If the infection has caused lower respiratory tract involvement, a productive or nonproductive cough may be present.

The professional singer will often self-medicate with over-the-counter "cold remedies" in the hopes of rapid recovery. The singer must be knowledgeable about these medications and understand that they typically contain a combination of several different agents. They must realize that probably nothing will shorten the infection, but that some of these medications may give symptomatic relief. Antihistamines are usually to be avoided, since they typically dry and thicken secretions, often making performing even more difficult. They may be used in the early stages of infection, in which secretions may be thin and watery. While many antihistamines are sedating, terfenadine and astemizole provide long-acting relief with minimal, if any, sedation.

Most often mucolytic agents and decongestants give the greatest symptomatic relief. The singer should know that most decongestants are sympathomimetic and can cause some degree of sleeplessness and anxiety. Non-narcotic cough suppressants are usually effective for cough associated with most upper respiratory infections. Since vascular engorgement usually accompanies most episodes of moderate inflammation, it is best to avoid aspirin or aspirin-containing products because of the possibility of vocal cord hemorrhage with coughing.

Fluid intake should be increased, using fluids that do not increase mucus and secretions. Nasal irrigations of commercially available agents or home preparation of a saline solution often helps to reduce the volume of the infectious inoculum and thin the secretions. For those singers with purulent secretions, antibiotics should be considered.

The singer may perform if there is no vocal cord vascular engorgement and if the singer feels that the quality of voice is acceptable. Any throat clearing should be done with minimal vocalization.

LARYNGITIS

With any upper respiratory tract infection, laryngitis may occur due to mucosal edema of the vocal folds. These singers are treated like individuals with upper respiratory tract infections. Voice rest should be considered. If an individual is able to practice, it should be done for only short periods of time during the day, with a few brief sessions rather than a single long session. Any singing should be within a narrow pitch range, avoiding the extremes. Vocalization during other daily activities should be minimized and preferably avoided. While many professional voice users believe that they can whisper or whistle their parts while rehearsing with an upper respiratory tract infection or laryngitis, this usually is ineffective. Whispering puts as much or more strain on the vocal mechanism as singing or talking and therefore is an ineffective and sometimes harmful way to rest the voice. Likewise, whistling to rehearse creates vocal strain and should be avoided.[1] When laryngeal inflammation is accompanied by vocal hemorrhage, voice rest is mandatory and practice and performance should be curtailed.

While many singers believe that gargling is effective for laryngitis, it does little and probably no good. Steam inhalation is soothing for the inflammation and to reduce the tenacity of the secretions. Ultrasonic treatments, if available, are ideal. It should be emphasized that, with any method of humidification, it is important to keep the humidifier clean and free of mold and mildew since the spread of spores can perpetuate the upper respiratory tract infection.

If it is important to perform during an episode of laryngitis, an attempt should be made to alter the material performed to one with limited pitch range and volume. During the rehearsals, practice, and performance, the vocal teacher ideally should be available to coach during this stressful period. Prolonged "laryngitis" necessitates examination by a trained laryngologist.

VOCAL CORD HEMORRHAGE

Vocal cord hemorrhage (see Appendix B, Fig. A–13) can occur with an upper respiratory tract infection, laryngitis, or coughing. It is also seen as part of vocal abuse, especially with single shouting episodes. A few women may be predisposed to vocal cord hemorrhage at the onset of the menstrual period. In all individuals it is important to maintain strict vocal rest, since additional trauma can cause organization of the hematoma and the creation of fibrous tissue within the vocal fold. This is one disorder that necessitates cancellation of performance.

A few patients will experience frequent episodes of hemorrhage because of prominent blood vessels on the surface of the vocal folds. The use of the laser to photocoagulate the vessels is helpful in resolving the problem.

TONSILLITIS

The treatment of acute tonsillitis is no different for the professional singer than for any other individual. Antibiotics, throat irritants, and gargles, along with nonaspirin-containing antipyretics are effective. The indications are the same as for tonsillectomy in the nonsinger. If a tonsillectomy is to be performed, extreme care is taken to preserve as much of the anterior and posterior tonsilar pillars as possible. Great care is taken to avoid injury to underlying musculature in the tonsilar bed.

Some adults develop chronic tonsillitis with a great deal of tonsilar cryptal debris. This may cause halitosis. For most individuals, this can be managed by irrigating the tonsils with a bulb syringe or electric-powered throat irrigator. Occasionally, a cotton-tipped applicator can be used to remove the cryptal debris. For the professional singer who is performing close to others, persistent halitosis may be disconcerting and a tonsillectomy warranted.

VOCAL CORD POLYP

Vocal cord polyps (see Appendix B, Figs. A–9, A–10, A–11) are typically unilateral and occur at the junction of the anterior and middle one-third of the vocal fold. Polyps may be broadly based or on a small pedicle. Those on a small pedicle may cause little symptoms, but occasional severe dysphonia or even aphonia can develop as the polyp gets caught between the vocal folds. While the etiology of polyps is uncertain, most can be related to a single episode or prolonged period of vocal trauma.

Smoking is a contributing factor in the etiology of vocal polyps. Smoking causes erythema, edema, and inflammation of the vocal folds. While some can easily tolerate active or passive smoking, for many professional voice users it is an irritant. The changes seen from smoking range from mild edema presenting diffusely over the vocal fold to marked polypoid change. Marijuana seems to cause an even more serious vocal reaction either because of the chemical composition or the inhalation of unfiltered smoke.[2]

Most singers with vocal polyp(s) will complain of harshness to the voice, a "double sound," or loss at the upper end of their pitch range. While some polyps will resolve with voice therapy and vocal rest, most require surgical excision. Excision should be considered relatively early after a period of conservative management, since there can be trauma to the opposite vocal fold due to contact from the polyp.

Surgical polypectomy should be done with microlaryngoscopy. While laser is a frequently chosen method for excision of laryngeal polyps, microlaryngoscopy with delicate forceps and/or scissors usually provides greater control while minimizing thermal injury to the surrounding tissue and avoiding the occasional "divot" to the vocal fold caused by the laser spot.

REINKE'S EDEMA

Reinke's edema (see Appendix B, Fig. A–8) appears as a mild redundancy of the free edge of the vocal fold within Reinke's space.[3] It is frequently associated with cigarette smoking. Other disorders to consider are vocal abuse and hypothyroidism.[4] The "myxedematous" voice of hypothyroidism is related to this disorder. Professional voice users without a great deal of formal training may develop Reinke's edema. The voice is typically harsh. Treatment should be directed toward dealing with the etiology. If this fails, surgical excision should be considered. Microlaryngoscopy may be performed on one vocal cord at a time to prevent webbing in the anterior commissure. Some laryngologists use a "laser welding" technique to seal the potential submucosal space. The laser is used at a low power density with a small spot size.

VOCAL NODULES

Vocal nodules (see Appendix B, Figs. A–5, A–6, A–7) are typically caused by overuse and abuse of the voice. This may be related to singing outside of one's capabilities, whether it be duration, range, or technical ability. More often, however, it is related to nonsinging activity such as speaking in the home, performing another job, playing a musical instrument, teaching, or conducting. While most professional singers are knowledgeable about their singing voice, many give little thought to their speaking voice, which is often the source of their problem. The conductor often tries to sing several different parts, many of which are outside the conductor's pitch range. This is frequently done at an exaggerated volume to demonstrate how the passage is to be performed. The singer who also plays a musical instrument may be doing so with poor posture and breath support, contributing to the vocal abuse. The teacher may be singing and accompanying on a piano, occasionally singing and playing the piano while standing.

Vocal abuse may occur because of the environment in which the singer must perform. Their environment may be noisy, smoky, dusty, poorly ventilated, lack proper humidity, or have poor acoustics. For some performers, especially rock singers, feedback devices should be used to monitor the volume of the accompanying music. These should be a necessity to prevent overuse of the voice by trying to overpower an overloud instrumental group. For others, appropriate amplification of voice should be available.

Vocal nodules are often asymptomatic and therefore require no treatment. Singers should be informed of their presence so that they are not alarmed if informed about them at another examination or by another laryngologist. Great care is given to the singer when discussing the presence of nodules, being certain that they know that they are neither career ending nor cancer predisposing. When symptomatic, nodules cause a harshness to the voice and loss of the upper end of the pitch range. Nodules typically appear as small bilateral swellings at the junction of the anterior one-third and middle one-third of the vocal fold. Early they may be soft and edematous looking, but become more fibrotic with time and continued abuse.

Vocal nodules are treated by speech pathologists who ideally have special expertise in the professional voice and are willing to work with the singer's vocal coach. In general, surgery is to be avoided and management is conservative. On those occasions when the nodules persist in spite of conservative vocal management for a minimum of 6 to 12 weeks, surgery is considered. If there is vocal improvement and yet the nodules persist, surgery should not be performed. Surgery should be considered for nodules that are enlarging, are irregular, or have surrounding erythroplasia, since these may be signs of a malignancy and not a benign lesion.

Surgical excision of vocal nodules is performed with microlaryngoscopy without laser. Following surgery, there is a period of absolute voice rest for 72 hours, then moderate talking in a soft voice for 1 week. The vocal folds are monitored with stroboscope to determine when the mucosal wave is returning to normal. Singing is then begun for brief periods during the day when the singer is well rested and not fatigued. Singing is confined to a narrow and comfortable pitch and volume range.

CONTACT GRANULOMATA AND VOCAL PROCESS ULCERS

Contact granulomata and vocal process ulcers typically appear at the vocal process of the arytenoid cartilage. There is frequently pain on the side of the neck in the region of the posterior aspect of the thyroid cartilage. The voice may be harsh. They are often seen in individuals who suffer from vocal abuse. Typically, these are forceful speakers who attempt to use the voice at a slightly lower pitch than is normal for them.

Another frequent cause of contact granuloma and laryngeal ulceration is laryngeal instrumentation such as intubation or bronchoscopy. When a professional singer is undergoing anesthesia with intubation, the anesthesiologist must take great care in using a properly sized endotracheal tube, avoiding trauma during intubation and avoiding "bucking" during the anesthetic. If prolonged intubation is necessary, the connecting tubes from the endotracheal tube to the respirator should be supported to prevent any pressure on the larynx from the weight of the tubes. There are those individuals who have had neither instrumentation nor use their voice inappropriately yet have contact granuloma. Other etiologies such as reflux esophagitis and pharyngitis should be sought. Reflux occurs often in professional singers who perform at night. Many do not eat before performing, but rather wait until after, eating a large meal late at night just before retiring. Many voice students keep late hours studying, working, and practicing and then have a quick dinner or snack, which contributes to reflux.

Treatment includes avoidance of the trauma or control of the reflux. If the lesion persists, microlaryngoscopy or laser excision is performed. Tissue is sent for histology and fungal and tuberculous cultures. Some physicians will attempt medical management separate from or as part of the surgical procedure. A suggested regimen includes penicillin V 250 mg four times a day for 30 days and steroids such as prednisone 10 mg four times a day for 10 to 14 days. Although not proven, this is suggested to eradicate the infection and reduce the inflammatory response producing the granulation tissue. The efficacy of zinc sulfate 220 mg three times a day continues to be anecdotal.[5] Failure of medical management may require surgical treatment. Microdissection and careful standard, or microspot, laser surgery is often effective. Recurrent granulomas may require intralesional steroid injections. Anti-reflex measures and voice therapy should follow surgery.

SUBSTANCE ABUSE

While substance abuse is a disorder that can afflict anyone, it is common in some types of singers. Hours of stress, the working environment, and the uncertainty of work are among several contributing factors. It behooves the vocal coach, speech pathologist, and laryngologist to be aware of substance abuse and willing to confront the performer. Changes in practice habits, missed rehearsals, tardy arrivals, and change in lifestyle are all warning signs.

ENDOCRINE AND REPRODUCTIVE CAUSES

While endocrine and reproductive causes of vocal disorders are discussed elsewhere in this book, there are a few aspects that pertain to the professional singer. Hypothyroidism can cause edema of the vocal fold and present with loss of the upper end of the pitch range with no other symptoms.[4] There are numerous cases reported of vocal cord hemorrhage occurring at the onset of the menstrual period, presumably due to increased capillary fragility. For these individuals, consideration must be given to voice rest just prior to the menstrual period.

Pregnancy poses special issues for the singer, with increased weight gain, fluid retention, alteration of abdominal musculature, and change in the breath support mechanism. Close vocal coaching is necessary during this time.

REFERENCES

1. Benninger MS, Finnegan EM, Kraus DH, et al: The whisper and the whistle: The role in vocal trauma. *Med Prob Perf Artists* 3:151–154, 1988.
2. Sataloff RT: *Professional Voice*. New York, Raven Press, 1991, p. 80.
3. Hirano M: Structure and vibratory pattern of the vocal folds, in Sawashima N, Cooper FS (eds): *Dynamic Aspects of Speech Production*. Tokyo, Tokyo University Press, 1977, pp 13–27.
4. Gupta OP: Nasal pharyngeal and laryngeal manifestations of hypothyroidism. *Ear Nose Throat* 56:9–21, 1977.
5. Tucker HM: *Surgery for Phonatory Disorders*. New York, Churchill Livingstone, 1981, p 40.

13

The Professional Speaking Voice

STEPHEN A. MITCHELL, MD

The professional voice user is an individual whose livelihood depends partially or wholly upon a certain voice quality. Singers and actors quickly come to mind, but we also can include clergy, attorneys, radio and television broadcasters, salespersons, teachers, auctioneers, drill instructors, and a host of others who stand to lose their professional effectiveness, their income, or their careers if a vocal disorder persists. In addition, the serious amateur is of concern. The Sunday School teacher, the community actor, and the little league coach all suffer in the quality of their life when they cannot speak normally.

Until recently, most of the voice research concerned the singing voice or the dysfunctional voice. Relatively little was known about the normal speaking voice and why some voices were normal while others were magnificent. Fortunately, this situation is being investigated, and we are learning more about format frequencies in speaking and what physical adjustments are necessary to improve them.[1]

The fundamental frequency for speaking is controlled by changing the number of times per second the vocal folds open and close. There are any number of ways to do this, as described in previous chapters. Some of these methods are healthy and some may lead to abuse of the vocal cords. The natural pitch level for speaking is in the lower part of the modal register, around 128 Hz for men and 225 Hz for women, roughly an octave apart. If the natural pitch for speaking and the habitual pitch are different, then the potential exists for vocal misuse and strain.[2]

INFLUENCING FACTORS

The speaking voice can have the same demands placed on it as the singing voice. These are described earlier in this book. Unfortunately, very few individuals study public speaking. Mimicry and the trial and error method may be the primary ways that professional speaking is learned. But, after an extended period of speaking under conditions of background noise, fatigue, illness, pollution, emotion, and demands for volume and projection, many people will become strained or hoarse. This is when they appear in the otolaryngologist's waiting rooms, hoping for an instant cure.

We learn to talk by copying the sounds and mannerisms of our parents, friends, and teachers, who usually have no training in public speaking. We grow up yelling and shouting at playmates and on the athletic field. We make school presentations with bad preparation, bad posture, and bad breath support. Now suddenly we have to teach, sell, or plead professionally, day in and day out, in sickness and in health. It is no small wonder that many people have voice problems.

A major distinction between professional speakers and singers is the lack of training in voice use obtained by many, if not most, professional speakers. Untrained vocalists are less aware of their limitations and more likely to have poor respiratory support and vocal technique and to misuse the speaking voice.[3] A second major distinction is that there is a greater tolerable margin of error in the professional speaker than is found in the professional singer. This second factor allows speakers to keep going and be professionally productive for a longer period of time than most singers with similar patterns of misuse and/or abuse. Unfortunately, this means that the time from onset of the problem until diagnosis and treatment occurs is usually longer for the speaker. An operatic baritone is likely to be forced to seek medical assistance for his vocal problems earlier than the television anchorman.

The environment is relevant in many cases. What we breathe and how loud we think we talk can adversely affect our voices. Most of us do not live and work in an antiseptic recording studio with clean, filtered, humidified air. Indeed, some of the professional recording studios I have seen are just converted houses and garages with the same dust and mold as at home. Classrooms are often old and filled with chalk dust. Courtrooms can be acoustically dead and poorly ventilated. Athletic fields are at the mercy of the weather and can have incredible background noise. Conference rooms at hotels may be permeated with smoke from the group that just left. Lecture halls can be cold, causing the speaker to shiver and take shallow breaths. Microphones are often fixed to the podium and limited in adjustment range, causing poor, ineffective posture. Slides are often projected behind the lecturer, causing him to twist and contort to one side to see the screen while leaning sideways over the podium toward the microphone. After-dinner speakers are speaking with a full stomach over the clatter of the busboys.

It is important to anticipate the environment as much as possible. Be sure the heat or air conditioning is set appropriately. Talk with the audiovisual supervisor to get the slide screen, podium, and microphone set up properly. Insist on smoke-free conference rooms in advance. Bring your own vacuum cleaner or humidifier to your classroom or work area. Nibble sparingly and skip the wine during the banquet before you speak. Never pass up the opportunity to improve the few things in your environment that you have some control over.

General health factors such as stress, smoking, drinking, and drug use are obvious detriments. Also important is quality sleep time, adequate water intake, basic nutritional needs, appropriate exercise, and taking prescribed medications. The various general influencing factors mentioned are covered in depth in other chapters of this book. We now discuss several professional fields and the problems that occur in them.

TELEVISION BROADCASTERS

One of the most visible categories of the professional voice user is the television news broadcaster. They talk to us, "face to face," often live, about something that affects our lives. Their voices and their personalities are familiar to us and even a slight illness is immediately apparent.

The work day is often extreme. If assigned to a morning show, the day may start at 3:30 AM. The evening news can keep one at the job well past midnight. Crisis situations like the Challenger Shuttle disaster or the Desert Storm War often require around the clock coverage with no chance for enough rest. Interviews take place at hours convenient to the subjects, not the reporter. Consequently, it is not uncommon to be in a perpetual state of fatigue. This will make broadcasters more susceptible to viral and bacterial upper respiratory infections. Fatigue can also cause one to become sloppy about maintaining optimal breath support, thereby increasing laryngeal strain.

The work place is often detrimental to effective vocal use. Studios may be in old, barn-like buildings that are rarely dusted and the air filters may be changed infrequently. Small shreds of paper waste from the newscopy machines permeate the air, irritating the nose and throat. The photoflood lights required for color television are several orders of magnitude more than is comfortable to the eye and may cause a photochemical injury to the retina, generalized discomfort, drying of the eye, and tearing.[4] The eye strain and pain, particularly in novices, can make it difficult to see the monitors and cause stress that affects vocal technique. People on television should wear sunglasses off camera whenever possible.

Ozone is a toxic byproduct of nitrogen oxides and organic emissions. Ozone is a serious pollutant that causes respiratory damage similar to cigarette smoking. The host of high voltage equipment required by a studio also produces ozone. If the broadcaster suffers from a preexisting bronchial asthma or hyperreactivity, occupational asthma or vocal fold inflammation could occur if they spend too much time around this equipment.[5,6]

Television announcers were shown in one study to have an increased number of chromosomal aberrations in their peripheral blood cells and an increased reproduction failure rate (females).[7] There is some suspicion that the azo dyes in the cosmetics may have a role in this, but it is unconfirmed.[7,8] Whether the reproduction failure rate in this case is associated with hormonal changes is unknown. It is of concern, though, because the hormone imbalances that occur during menstruation or estrogen therapy in females can result in tone-altering vocal cord swelling and even vocal cord hemorrhage.[9,10]

Normal subconscious habits like swallowing are restrained while on camera. Often the quantity and quality of saliva will cause tension and abnormal breathing patterns as the announcer tries to read long phrases without choking and without the viewers seeing them swallow. Most will try to drink lots of water, but not immediately before going on the air. Certain foods also must be avoided that have lots of spice, sugar, milk, or carbonation. One of our patients reports that she finds that pickles will cause her to salivate excessively. Peanuts are notorious for causing a mild chemical irritation of the tracheobronchial tree with resultant cough and hypersecretion.

Female television announcers have their own particular problems. As noted earlier, in some individuals the days during and before menses can alter voice quality and make the vocal cords more prone to small hemorrhages. The news broadcasts are regular, 5 days a week, and cannot be scheduled around menstrual flow cycles. Pregnancy causes its own hormonal effects, but also can markedly reduce vital capacity during the last trimester, especially in the sitting position. Female news broadcasters are the norm now, and many work until a week or two before delivery. The reduction in respiratory support for the voice in the final phases of pregnancy can cause significant laryngeal strain.

Interestingly, the microphones tend to pitch voices higher and thus the lower pitched voice is more marketable for this line of work. This will cause some men and women artificially to pitch their voice abnormally low, causing neck muscle tension, vocal fatigue, and vocal dysfunction.[11]

RADIO BROADCASTERS

In many ways the radio broadcasters have less to contend with than their colleagues in television. The sound booths are small and easier to clean. The background noise is minimal. They can dress comfortably and do not need to worry about make-up or intense lights. They are, however, very restricted in body and neck position, as the microphones are usually very directional and it is necessary to keep the relative position of the mouth and microphone constant.[12]

The cost per minute for air time on the radio is many orders of magnitude cheaper than for television. Consequently, it is possible to have a talk show format that can go on for 3 or 4 hours straight with only brief commercial breaks. Prolonged talking in an improper sitting position can lead to unsupported respiratory support and vocal stress. Also, loud or forceful talking for over an hour by untrained vocalists can lead to vocal abnormalities and deterioration.[13]

It is easier to smoke in the radio booth than on a television set. Because of the influence on audience acceptance, it is rare to see smoking on TV unless required by an acting role. The smoking, the posture, and the long hours of talking can all set the stage for serious vocal dysfunction and pathology.

Except for these points, the problems of radio and television broadcasters are very similar. Both types of broadcasters may get formal professional training in speech and public speaking from their colleges or from workshops sponsored by their station.

CLERGY

Ministers, priests, and rabbis usually receive training in homiletics, preparing a religious message. The training in public speaking is not always satisfactory. The tendency for young clergy to sound more authoritative often leads them to pitch their voice artificially lower and can lead to severe vocal strain.[11,12] Delivery style can vary widely as well. Some prefer the "Harry Emerson Fosdick" deep sepulchre sound, others the "Reverend Ike" excited shout method. When examining clergy in the office, it is vital to hear what they really do with their voice when they work. It may not be what one expects. The quiet, dignified scholar in your examination chair may undergo a metamorphosis in the pulpit and become a screaming "fire and brimstone" evangelist.

Clergy may not be able to rest their voices. It is common to teach a class, preach a sermon, greet and counsel between services, preach again, converse over a church lunch, meet with officers, and then make house calls and hospital calls with no break. An hour of loud talking with an untrained voice can result in measurable deterioration of vocal function.[13] In addition, the desire to sacrifice reduces the odds that they will forego helping others to take care of themselves. Clergy can be the most apologetic and least compliant patients.

The acoustics of the buildings where preaching occurs are variable, but often not good. Monitor speakers, high quality microphones, well-designed sound systems, and sound technicians are unusual. Calling the parishioners to prayer is often done with an unamplified voice, whether in a sanctuary, over a banquet table, or in a cemetery.

STAGE ACTORS

Actors are usually trained before they venture on the professional stage. Yet the training can never stop because the demands on the larynx never remain the same. Each role requires a different dialect or accent, different mannerisms, and sometimes a different voice sound. Actors may need to talk like children or like octogenarians. Certain roles may require stuttering, loud coughing, throat clearing, sobbing, or stage whispering. The technique required is not the same for a falsetto voice, or a Scottish accent, or a scream. Use of incorrect technique night after night of rehearsals and performances can result in vocal abuse and laryngeal pathology. Even comedians can benefit from time with a voice therapist to help switch from one voice style to another.[14,15]

The instinct that "the show must go on" often forces the actor to perform in spite of illness, even laryngitis, sometimes with career-shattering results. Much like the professional singer, the actor is in a field where the law of supply and demand is working against her. Actors who miss performances are viewed as "risky" and may have problems getting work.

The phrase "starving actor" is also based on reality. Except for a frightfully few stars, acting is not well-paying and usually requires a day job that may not have medical insurance benefits. Consequently, actors often treat each other and frequently share medication to save money. Physicians who treat actors should not be surprised if the prescription for an $80 third generation cephalosporin goes unfilled. An actor's dietary habits can be very irregular and reduce general resistance to infection and slow healing.

Although AIDS has gotten much notoriety as a disease that kills artistic individuals, suicide is the proportional mortality leader in the acting profession.[8] Actors tend to be emotionally "tightly strung," very labile, and often feel insecure. The roles they play may require them to dig deep into their own personalities as well as their character's. The mental strain of becoming Hamlet, Macbeth, or Willie Loman night after night might prove too much for some.

Actors will become very depressed if the most important tool of their trade, their voice, is not well. Dealing with the mental aspect is just as important as the speech therapy. Mention of the words "vocal nodules" can cause a suicidal depression physicians would not anticipate in their other patients. Caution and time should be taken when presenting diagnoses to these patients.

The tragedy of AIDS has emotionally affected many people in one way or another, and they now live in fear, fear of catching the virus from having intimate relations, taking drugs, or working around the sick or injured; fear of losing jobs and friends or of developing the disease if tested positive for the HIV antigen; fear of a horrible, painful death. The bohemian lifestyle that used to be part of the charm of the theater has proved to be potentially lethal. Fortunately, education and changes in that lifestyle are helping to decrease the spread of AIDS. Once contracted, actors on medication can still function for some time.

The theater environment is usually dusty, moldy, and either too hot or too cold. Make-up powder permeates the air, irritating eye, nose, and throat. Dust mites and mold flourish in the old ill-fitting costumes. The adhesive holding the fake beard restricts jaw motion. The drinking fountain is far from the stage, assuming it works at all. Dramatic scenes may use dry ice or vaporized oil particles to create fog and mist. The acoustics of the theater for the performances are totally different and uniformly worse than those for the rehearsals.

After the stress of the performance comes the backstage greeters followed by the late night dinner or, worse yet, the cast party. These events all conspire to wear out and injure an already stressed larynx. Talking over the background din of talkers, it is easy to push the voice into yelling without realizing it until attempting to talk the next morning.

The road show adds new problems. Like the singer on tour, the travel between jobs provides very little quality rest or sleep. The diet often consists of fast food and very little water. Any free time before the performance is often spent promoting the show to schools, reporters, or on talk shows. Conversations on the bus, boat, and plane involve the "Lombard effect" whereby the speaker inadvertently talks louder as the background noise increases. This results in excessive volume while sitting with poor posture.

If the actor does not have a voice coach, it is wise to urge him or her to retain one. If there already is a coach, the clinician should request permission to talk and work with the coach as a team member in the patient's therapy. This will go far to keep the individual's voice healthy.

TEACHERS

Teachers, like clergy, require a tone of voice of authority. They need to inspire students to follow instructions, without question. Sometimes the stress of the job can cause the voice to become strained and tense, especially if discipline is a problem. Work-related stress can be correlated with a desire to leave the profession and with drug use. In one study, two-thirds of the teachers surveyed wanted to quit, and there was a higher than the national average of lifetime alcohol, amphetamine, and tranquilizer use. This suggests significant stress, as well as secondary damage from alcohol consumption, that can adversely affect vocal function.[16] These vital parts of the medical history will usually not be volunteered and must be pursued.

In a study of teachers referred for dysphonia, 96% suffered from vocal fatigue, 86% had vocal lesions (usual nodules), and 85% had faulty vocal technique.[17] Unfortunately, most teachers receive no instruction in proper voice use or public speaking or even stress management.[12] The physician must help the teacher get the necessary instruction in these areas to effect a cure.

The classroom environment is extremely variable. Although chalk dust is the usual problem one thinks of, the chemistry teacher has chemical fumes, the biology teacher has formalin, the botany teacher has pollen, and the gym coach has the gym and the out-of-doors. Learning what kind of duties the teacher has may help to determine the etiology of the vocal problem. Teachers of mentally retarded students have an additional problem of a 2.6% per year hepatitis B virus infection rate.[18] Hepatitis is an extremely dangerous and debilitating disease that weakens the patient and sets the stage for other opportunistic infections. It could also propose a risk to the health care worker if not suspected.

A special kind of teacher is the aerobics instructor. Many aerobics instructors were former cheerleaders and thereby already prone to dysphonic episodes.[19] These teachers are shouting instructions to their students over the loud background music while dancing or contorting themselves. The 30 to 60 minute sessions are almost nonstop, and several classes may be scheduled in a row with little rest. Although the aerobics instructors are probably the most physically fit individuals to sit in the otolaryngologist's examination chair, they also have a very high rate of vocal abuse that is extremely hard to resolve. Although microphone and amplifier systems exist for aerobics, they are expensive, some feel it is difficult to exercise with them, and few instructors make the investment. Their vocal enthusiasm and hyperactivity permeate their whole lives and require extensive long-term speech therapy for any improvement.

COACHING

Coaching is a mixture of teaching, preaching, commanding, and threatening. Whether little league or NBA basketball, coaching is performed in the heat of emotion, in a stressful, noisy environment, and without regard to acoustics or posture. The coaches almost never learn public speaking skills, belting techniques, or even basic vocal hygiene. In spite of this, they are expected to lecture to civic groups, shout intelligible instructions, and move the minds and hearts of men and women.

Young coaches usually receive no voice training in school. Instead, they will often try to emulate a Marine drill instructor or a famous successful coach. Unfortunately, both of the professions they are copying have a high level of vocal abuse and laryngeal pathology.[20,21] These individuals use load, short bursts of words to carry the power and authority to their charges. They have to motivate, reward, and terrify across a basketball court or football field surrounded by hundreds or thousands of screaming fans. Rather than a megaphone, the glottal attack is the usual technique used and is the etiology of a host of chronic laryngeal pathology.[22]

Dedicated members of this profession keep long hours, eat unbalanced diets, travel extensively, and are under constant stress. Their careers are often tenuous and can be ended after a single lost game. Voice rest is impossible. Secondary school coaches are usually required to teach a classroom subject daily. University and professional level coaches participate in endless administrative and booster club meetings as well as recruiting trips, civic group lectures, radio talk shows, and paid advertisements on television and radio.

When signs of hoarseness and vocal nodules occur, they usually do not seek medical care unless pain or aphonia are present. If instructed to receive speech therapy, they usually will not make the time for follow up visits and often fail to apply what they learned. I have found that the long-term success rate in treating hyperfunctional dysphonia and the related laryngeal pathology in coaches is dismal.

OTHER CAREERS

The problems associated with salesmen are similar to those of teachers except that the rigors of travel that affect coaches are frequently present as well. Travel by car and plane is associated with dehydration of the throat and thickening of the mucus secondary to dry air and inadequate water intake. The ever-present background noise also brings the Lombard effect into play, and the travellers often talk much louder than they think.

Traders in the stock and commodity markets need to shout and scream over the frantic commotion of the trading pit. The personality traits that enable them to succeed in their job usually carry over off the job. They will talk just as loud and animated at sporting events and social gatherings.

Politicians and trial lawyers incorporate an interesting mix of problems. Much like the clergy and salesmen, they travel, preach, and sell. The frequent parties and receptions make alcohol abuse a real issue for politicians.

CONCLUSION

Professional speakers use their voices, like surgeons use their hands, to make a living. Here and there, individual otolaryngologists emerged who took time to listen and learn and share their knowledge with their colleagues. Until recently, appreciation of the significance of subtle dysphonias was not widely taught to residents. Care for the professional voice user is usually a nonsurgical, time-intensive endeavor that is ego satisfying but not exceptionally remunerative. Now through organizations such as the Voice Foundation, the Performing Arts Medicine Association, and the American Academy of Otolaryngology—Head and Neck Surgery, conferences and workshops are available to fill this void.

REFERENCES

1. Sundberg J: Vocal tract resonance, in Sataloff RT (ed): *Professional Voice: The Science and Art of Clinical Care*. New York, Raven Press, 1991, pp 49–68.
2. Boone DR: *The Voice and Voice Therapy*, Englewood Cliffs, NJ, Prentice-Hall, 1971, pp 89–101.
3. Teachey JC, Kahane JC, Beckford NS: Vocal mechanics in untrained professional singers. *J Voice* 5:51–56, 1991.
4. Hietanen MT, Hoikkala MJ: Ultraviolet radiation and blue light from photofloods in television studios and theaters. *Health Phys* 59:193–198, 1990.
5. Lee HS, Wan YT, Tan KT: Occupational asthma due to ozone. *Singapore Med J* 30:485–487, 1989.
6. Leonard RJ, Charpied GL, Faddis B: Effects of ambient inhaled ozone on vocal fold mucosa in bonnet monkeys. *J Voice* 5:304–309, 1991.
7. Kucerova M, et al: The possible mutagenic effect of the occupation of TV announcer. *Mutat Res* 192:59–63, 1987.
8. Depue RH, Kagey BT, Heid MF: A proportional mortality study of the acting profession. *Am J Ind Med* 8:57–66, 1985.
9. Lin PT, Stern JC, Gould WJ: Risk factors and management of vocal cord hemorrhages: An experience with 44 cases. *J Voice* 5:74–77, 1991.
10. Sataloff RT: Care of the professional voice, in Sataloff RT, Brandfonbrener AG, Lederman RJ (eds): *Textbook of Performing Arts Medicine*. New York, Raven Press, 1991, p 242.
11. Koufman JA, Blalock PD: Vocal fatigue and dysphonia in the professional voice user: Bogart-Bacall syndrome. *Laryngoscope* 98:493–498, 1988.
12. Brodnitz FS: *Keep Your Voice Healthy*, 2nd ed. Boston, College Hill Press, 1988, pp 45–51.
13. Gelfer MP, Andrews ML, Schmidt CP: Effects of prolonged loud reading on selected measures of vocal function in trained and untrained singers. *J Voice* 5:158–167, 1991.
14. Roch JB: The phoniatrician and the actor. *Rev Laryngol Otol Rhinol Bord* 111:379–380, 1990.
15. Raphael BN: Actors and their voices. Workshop given at the *Care of the Professional Voice Symposium*, 1991.
16. Watts WD, Short AP: Teacher drug use: a response to occupational stress. *J Drug Educ* 20:47–65, 1990.
17. Calas M et al.: Vocal pathology of teachers. *Rev Laryngol Otol Rhinol Bord* 110:397–406, 1989.
18. Remis RS, Rossignol MA, Kane MA: Hepatitis B infection in a day school for mentally retarded students: transmission from students to staff. *Am J Public Health* 77:1183–1186, 1987.
19. Greene MCL, Mathieson L: *The Voice and Its Disorders*, 5th ed. San Diego, Singular, 1989, pp 118–119.
20. Sapir S, Atias J, Shahar A: Symptoms of vocal attrition in women army instructors and new recruits: results from a survey. *Laryngoscope* 100:991–994, 1990.
21. Brodnitz FS: *Keep Your Voice Healthy*, 2nd ed. Boston, College Hill Press, 1988, p 53.
22. Prater RJ: Voice therapy, techniques and applications. *Otolaryngol Clin North Am* 24:1075–1091, 1991.

14

Medical Disorders in the Vocal Artist

MICHAEL S. BENNINGER, MD

MEDICAL PROBLEMS IN VOICE

To produce sounds in speaking or singing, four elements are involved: (1) respiration, (2) phonation, (3) articulation, and (4) resonance.[1] A disruption due to general medical conditions of any of these may result in abnormalities of speech or sound production. This chapter is devoted to the most common medical problems encountered in the voice professional. It is not meant to be inclusive but addresses most conditions.

The care of performing vocalists requires a thorough understanding of the many medical conditions that can affect the quality of the voice. Although many problems are laryngeal in origin, often vocal dysfunction may be secondary to disorders of other areas of the head and neck or other body systems. A complete history is necessary to guide the physical examination and direct further investigation, if necessary. The initial assessment by the medical voice team of otolaryngologists and speech–language pathologists may need to be followed by referrals to general medical or surgical practitioners or to therapeutic specialists.

GENERAL HEALTH

Performing or professional vocalists in many ways can be thought of as vocal athletes. The strength, endurance, and fine motor skills necessary to optimize voice production is not dissimilar to other athletic endeavors. As other athletes work to maintain a high level of general physical fitness so is it necessary for vocalists to work for similar conditioning to be "on top of their game." The mystique relating the quality of the singing voice to obese or overweight opera singers has been refuted as a better understanding of the mechanism of voice production evolves. Furthermore, with the ever-present role of the media and the visibility of most high level performers, attractive body type is more conducive to career development.

Proper diet and body weight has been an area of emphasis in most athletic arenas. Muscle glycogen is the body's chief source of energy, and this is especially true during moderate to high levels of activity for prolonged periods of time.[2] After prolonged exercise, glycogen synthesis is directly related to dietary carbohydrate intake.[2] Although in many vocal endeavors such endurance may not play a role, it can be an integral part of performance particularly for song and dance, musicals, rock and roll, or rhythm and blues singers. Furthermore, low fat, high fiber and carbohydrate diets have been found to be associated with decreased heart disease and life prolongation.[3] A higher incidence of certain cancers, diabetes, and increased cardiovascular disease has been found to be present in individuals with high fat, low carbohydrate diets.[4] General exercise conditioning will improve overall fitness, improve muscle tone and breath support, and decrease risks related to cholesterol such as heart disease or even cancer.[5,6] General conditioning appropriate for age, sex, and size or body weight results in feelings of well-being, decreased fatiguability, and increased vigor, which are crucial to optimizing performance.

Some concerns have been raised regarding rapid weight change adversely affecting performance. As with other fine motor activities requiring sensitivity and finesse, minor changes can upset the delicate balance of a highly specialized, fine-tuned instrument. Although weight loss in overweight vocalists is preferred, quick changes should be avoided. Small gradual weight reductions over long periods of time under closely monitored weight loss programs are recommended.[7]

Eating disorders may be associated with voice dysfunction. Anorexia nervosa and bulimia are occasionally present in the performing voice community, although they tend to be less common than in other artistic fields such as classical dance, where body physical appearance may have a more prominent role. Nonetheless, such disorders can have drastic effects on the voice. Anorexia often leads to fatigue and unpredictable weight changes. Bulimia, with forced vomiting behaviors, is frequently associated with chronic laryngeal and pharyngeal inflammation and edema from chronic gastric acid irritation of the susceptible mucosa. The underlying psychological and emotional problems that lead to and are consequences of these behaviors result in additional stress and anxiety that can disrupt the delicate psyche so important to a performance. Such eating disorders should be recognized and treated early with assistance from psychiatric practitioners and nutritionists.

Sleep Disorders

Regimented sleep–wake cycles may be difficult for many performing vocalists due to the rigors of touring and the timing of performances. Often the singer's agenda is full from early in the morning to late at night with rehearsals, performances, and social engagements. Many performers find it difficult to allow time for relaxation. Chronic problems with sleep deprivation may occur and can result in excessive physical and emotional strain with diminishing quality of performance.

Sleep can be thought of as an active physiologic process. It is generally described as both rapid eye movement (REM) and nonrapid eye movement sleep. The nonrapid eye movement sleep is broken into four stages, from stage 1 or light sleep to stage 4 or deep delta sleep. In normal individuals there is a cyclical alteration between REM and non-REM sleep, with REM accounting for approximately one-fourth to one-fifth of total sleep time.[8] Sleep time does not change in general as one ages but sleep can become less efficient. The time it takes to fall asleep or sleep latency will lengthen and awakenings occur more frequently. Many conditions can predispose to alterations in sleep. These include certain medications, gastroesophageal reflux, obesity, anxiety or stress-related disorders, and poorly controlled sleep–wake cycles. Obtaining a careful history regarding drug use is often a good first step. Many medications can interfere with sleep and the more common of these include decongestants, alcohol, caffeine, diuretics, theophylline, steroids, and hypnotics.[8] Exercise or eating prior to bedtime can also interfere with sleep.

More significant sources of sleep disorders can be classified as central nervous system dysfunction, obstructive dysfunction, or a combination of the two. One of the common disorders that is being more frequently diagnosed is obstructive sleep apnea syndrome (OSAS).[9–12] OSAS is characterized by intermittent cessation of breathing during sleep in which obstructive apnea occurs and airflow ceases while respiratory efforts continue.[10] Collapse of the pharyngeal tissues (Fig. 14–1) can occur, resulting in inability for adequate aeration to be achieved. Desaturation of oxygen in the bloodstream and arrhythmias may occur in more significant cases, and it has even been shown that mortality rates are increased in patients with obstructive sleep apnea.[9] OSAS can be thought of as a continuum beginning with the obstructive sounds of snoring to the more significant disorders of the full-blown obstructive apnea syndrome with associated cardiorespiratory side effects. In general, OSAS occurs in obese men in their middle decades, although increasing numbers of obstructive sleep apnea patients have been found with normal body sizes. Close observation by a spouse or loved one will often assist in the diagnosis. A sleep evaluation can then be performed to verify the diagnosis and initiate treatment.

Central disorders of sleep can be found in chronic obstructive pulmonary disease, neuromuscular disorders, or primary alveolar hypoventilation. Again a daytime and nighttime sleep evaluation may be necessary to help define the etiology so that a therapy can be instituted.

In general, the treatment of sleep-related disorders is conservative. Healthy living

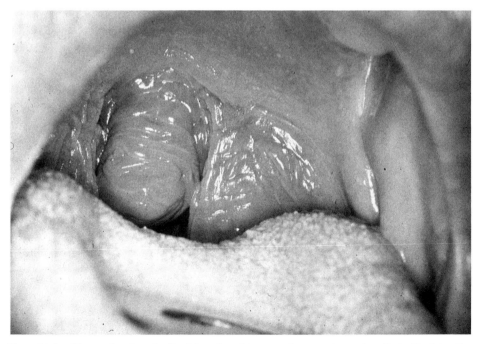

Figure 14–1.   Elongated uvula and soft palate, enlarged tongue and narrow pharynx in patient with obstructive sleep apnea syndrome (OSAS).

with weight and diet control and appropriate exercise are suggested. Regimented times to retire at bedtime and wake in the morning will help set appropriate biorhythms. Although some individuals claim that short periods of time for sleeping is all that is necessary for adequate functioning, most people still require seven to eight hours of sleep daily. Decreasing emotional stress may be difficult for the busy performer but will be helpful in reducing the amount of time needed to fall asleep and in allowing for more deep levels of sleep. Alcohol, caffeine, hypnotics, and other medications that interfere with sleep should be avoided. The bed and bedroom should be used exclusively for sleeping and not for paperwork or watching television.[8] Occasionally, a short-acting sedative such as a benzo-diazepine may be utilized, but it is preferred if these are used under close medical guidance.

In rare circumstances, functional nasal obstructive disorders such as allergic or vasomotor rhinitis or anatomic obstruction as with septal deviations may interfere with nasal breathing and result in disorders of sleep. Aggressive treatment of the nasal disorders may improve breathing. Occasionally septal or turbinate surgery may be necessary. For those with OSAS who do not respond to conservative care, nighttime utilization of continuous positive airway pressure (CPAP) or surgical care with a uvulopalatopharyngo-plasty (UPPP) have been shown to alleviate obstruction and improve sleep pattern.[13] Care must be taken in the vocalist when upper airway surgery is recommended, as it may have an effect on voice resonation (see Surgery, p. 209).

PULMONARY AND RESPIRATORY DISORDERS

As mentioned at the beginning of this chapter, respiration is necessary for normal speech and singing voice production. Controlled respiration generates a voice that is produced efficiently, providing optimal airflow for vocal fold vibration. Respiration is the process of inspiring air into the lungs and expiring it from the lungs. The respiratory system consists of essentially two parts: a gas exchange organ, or the lungs, and a pump that inflates and deflates the lungs. The pump is the chest wall, the muscles of respiration, the centers in the nervous system that control respiration, and the nerves that bring input from the nervous system to the muscles.[14] During inspiration, the diaphragm contracts downward while the intercostal muscles between the ribs contract, pulling the ribs upward and outward. The effect is to increase the chest volume in anteroposterior and lateral directions.[1] A negative pressure results, with subsequent air movement from the more positive pressure outside to more negative intrathoracic pressure.

Expiration is primarily a passive phenomenon with relaxation of the diaphragm and intercostal muscles. The elastic recoil of the ribs and muscles return the thorax and diaphragm to a resting position.[1] The intercostal muscles, which are considered muscles of inspiration, can actively contract to slow the rate of expiration.[1] The cycle of inspiration and expiration occurs from 12 to 20 times per minute at rest but can increase dramatically with the increased oxygen demands of exercise or if one wishes consciously to increase the rate.

During normal respiration at rest, inspiration lasts for 40% of the respiratory cycle while expiration accounts for 60%. During speech, inspiration occurs more deeply and for a shorter period of time to account for approximately 10% of the respiratory cycle, while expiration lasts for 90%.[1] Anything that would obstruct the airway will tend to slow inspiration, but expiration would generally remain normal.

The lungs serve to exchange gas, bringing oxygen into the bloodstream and expelling carbon dioxide. To enhance this gas exchange capability, the gradually decreasing size of the pulmonary airways ends at the alveoli, where gas exchange occurs. There are approximately 150 million alveoli to each adult lung, and if they were placed side to side the surface area of alveoli would cover a 70 m² tennis court.[15]

Disorders related to respiration can be classified according to dysfunction of the respiratory muscles, the airways themselves, the gas exchange apparatus, and the nervous control of respiration. Dysfunction of the respiratory muscles is uncommon, but prolonged, poorly trained use of the muscles of respiration (particularly on expiration) and inappropriate posture can lead to chest muscle fatigue. Training with proper chest and abdomen position will allow the muscles of respiration to function more effectively and to avoid fatigue. Obesity with significant abdominal and chest girth may prevent maximal chest excursion on inspiration through the effects on the downward movement of the diaphragm and lateral and upward movement of the chest, restricting lung volumes. Increased effort may be necessary for respiration for speaking or singing, which may result in easy fatigue.

Obstruction of airflow can occur at any level of the upper airway (Fig. 14–2). The most common sites of obstruction are in the nose, nasopharynx, and pharynx (see Disorders of Resonance, below). In particular, nasal obstruction from allergic or nonallergic rhinitis can have both direct and nondirect effects. The direct effect would be due to the inability of air to pass easily through the nose, resulting in mouth breathing. The normal humidifying, cleaning, and warming effect of nasal breathing would be lost, resulting in pharyngeal, laryngeal, and pulmonary irritation. The indirect effect is due to a nasal to pulmonary neural connection or nasopulmonary reflex whereby nasal blockage causes constriction of the small pulmonary airways and decreased oxygen absorption, with retention of carbon dioxide.[16–18]

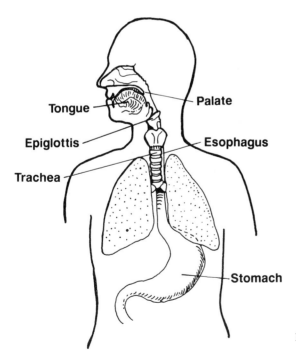

Figure 14–2. The upper aerodigestive tract.

The nasopharynx and/or pharynx are also common sites of upper airway obstruction. Hypertrophic adenoids and tonsils are common causes of upper airway obstruction in children that can affect their ability to eat and sleep. Prolonged obstruction can lead to alterations in facial development and dental abnormalities.[19–22] Surgical removal of the tonsils and adenoids may relieve the obstruction and can have far-ranging benefits for the obstructed child.[23] Although adenoid obstruction is uncommon in adults after regression of the adenoids with puberty, the tonsils may continue to be a source of obstruction in the adult. An elongated uvula with a floppy soft palate (Fig. 14–1) or enlarged tongue can also result in obstruction and is particularly common in the obese individual. Significant architectural changes can result in disorders of sleep with OSAS (see Sleep Disorders, above).

Laryngeal obstruction is usually due to disorders of the vocal folds such as edema, vocal nodules, polyps, or other vocal fold masses. These disorders are discussed in more detail in Chapter 12.

The most common obstructive disorders of the lungs are asthma and emphysema. The bronchoconstriction that occurs in the asthmatic obstructs the normal airflow and gas exchange. This can usually be reversed by the use of inhaled and/or oral bronchodilators or aerosolized steroid inhalers. Prolonged use of aerosol steroids may cause dysphonia from either a local steroid myopathy or laryngeal candidiasis.[24,25] Voice misuse can contribute to the dysphonia,[25] while reversal of the effect occurrs after cessation of aerosolized steroid use.[24]

Emphysema is a more permanent cause of obstructive pulmonary disease. Emphysema is usually the result of long and excessive cigarette smoking, but may be caused by chronic industrial or pollutant smoke exposure and inhalation. Of concern is the recent evidence that passive smoking, particularly in children, may have important effects on pulmonary function.[26] This may be of concern to the nonsmoking performer who has chronic smoke exposure from family or friends or who performs long hours in smoky environments such as nightclubs. With emphysema, the elastic structures of the lungs are destroyed so that the chronic emphysematous lung is highly distensible, highly compliant, and poorly elastic. Abnormal, reduced airflow results in abnormal ventilation–blood flow relations and secondary hypoxemia. Thickened mucus and bronchitis can develop with chronic smoking, which may further aggravate the obstruction. Some of these effects are reversible with cessation of smoking, but some may persist if the person had a long history of smoking abuse.

The most common cause of reversible obstructive pulmonary disease is the acute upper respiratory tract infection, which is usually a self-limited viral infection. Rest and adequate hydration is usually sufficient for treating viral upper respiratory tract infections. Acute bronchitis or pneumonia may occur and should be treated more aggressively with antibiotics with or without expectorants. Antihistamines may increase the viscosity of the mucus and should be used with caution.

If a pulmonary ventilatory disorder is present, historical data will usually give insight into the etiology. A thorough head and neck with pharyngeal and pulmonary examinations are needed. A pulmonary specialist may be required, although a general internist will usually be able to manage the problem. A chest x-ray may be helpful in diagnosis and in assessing the responsiveness of treatment. Pulmonary function tests with spirometry are helpful in assessing pulmonary ventilatory dysfunction, and some voice laboratories routinely perform these studies. Bronchoscopy may be needed in more refractory or complicated cases.

DISORDERS OF RESONANCE

Resonation is an important aspect of voice production. Particularly in the singer, the resonating effect of the supraglottic vocal tract is critical to voice placement and modulation. The use of nasal placement and head register are commonly utilized tools for singing voice training. Disorders of the upper respiratory vocal tract above the level of the glottis can affect the quality of voice resonation and, to a lesser degree, can actually modify pitch (see Chapter 3). Problems with resonation generally result from anatomic or functional defects of the nasal cavity or palate with inefficient control of the velopharyngeal mechanism, and from the oral cavity or oropharynx.

Nasal obstruction from chronic rhinitis due to allergic or nonallergic disorders, from anatomic deviations such as a septal deviation or turbinate hypertrophy, or from nasal mass lesions such as polyps will obstruct normal nasal airflow. In a similar fashion, adenoid tissue hypertrophy will prevent adequate airflow from the nasal passages into the pharynx. These disorders will generally result in abnormalities in the production of the nasal sounds /m/, /n/, or /ŋ/ (ng). These are the nasal consonants, and a voice that lacks proper production of nasal consonants due to obstruction is termed *hyponasal*. An absence of both nasal emissions and nasal resonance occurs in this case. This would result in production of consonant sounds that are voiced appropriately and placed appropriately for nasal sounds but are produced with oral resonance. The resulting sound substitutions would be /b/ for /m/, /d/ for /n/, and /g/ for /ŋ/.[1]

Abnormalities of the palate would result in changes in the dynamics of velopharyngeal closure. These are generally due to problems with palatal movement or structure such as in cleft palate, submucous cleft palate, palatal paresis or paralysis, foreshortened palate, and a scarred palate secondary to previous surgery, most commonly from adenoid or tonsil removal. Increased flow of air into the nasal cavities would result with increased nasal resonance and "hypernasality." All vowels and voiced oral consonants may become nasal.[1] The nasal consonants in general would be unaffected.

Disorders of resonance of the oral cavity and oropharynx is primarily due to enlarged tonsils or mucosal irritation with swelling. On a rare occasion, a large tongue or an elongated uvula may affect resonation. Even without anatomic or neurologic abnormalities, problems of resonance can occur with improper technique, training, or other functional disorders.

Although the subglottic vocal tract and lungs are generally not thought to be involved significantly in resonation, they do play some role. Therefore abnormalities of the subglottic vocal tract as well as the areas just above the false vocal folds, including the epiglottis, can affect resonation. Epiglottic inflammation or edema, secondary to chronic inflammation or acute infection, will interfere with the supraglottic airflow and change the tone generated by the vocal folds. With oral cavity or oropharyngeal changes in resonation, due to hypertrophic tonsils or inflammation, an abnormal posterior tongue positioning can occur, resulting in muffling of vowels and consonants.[1] When this is severe, a muffled, "hot potato" voice occurs, and this is usually due to significant infectious processes such as peritonsillar or uvular abscesses or Ludwig's angina.

Evaluation of changes in resonation primarily includes a thorough physical examination of the nose, oral cavity, oropharynx, nasopharynx, hypopharynx, and larynx. In most cases obvious sources of the difficulty in resonation will be present, with hypertrophic turbinates, tonsils, adenoids, or a deviated septum being the most common diagnoses. The dynamics of palatal and velopharyngeal closure cannot be adequately assessed by a straightforward examination, and measures of velopalatal movement such as cinevideo-fluorography, electromyography,[28] or nasometry are used. A flexible nasopharyngo-laryngoscope should be utilized to evaluate palatal movement from above[29] and to assess the less poorly visualized areas of the posterior nasal cavity, nasopharynx, and occasionally, the hypopharynx. Direct nasal endoscopy with rigid telescopes has recently been found to be effective in assessing various nasal disorders.[30,31]

Once the etiology has been identified, appropriate management can be directed. For most nasal conditions medical management is sufficient; however, for hypertrophic ade-noids or tonsils, septal deviation, and medically recalcitrant nasal disorders, surgery may be indicated. A close working relationship with a speech–language pathologist and a singing teacher will help the singer to maintain good nasal and pharyngeal resonation.

ALLERGIC DISORDERS

Allergic disease is very common among individuals in all developed countries. Forty-six percent of American men and 49% of American women claim to be allergic while a survey of 1,259 allergists revealed that 23% of American men and 34% of American women do have allergies.[32] The incidence of allergic nasal disease (allergic rhinitis) in America and Europe ranges from 5% to 20% of the population, accounting for over one-third of all patients with chronic rhinitis.[33] As many as one-half of all patients seen in general otolaryngology practices present with allergic complaints.[34] In 1981, 31 million people in the United States suffered from sinusitis,[35] and a strong relationship between allergic rhinitis and sinusitis has been documented.[33–37] The incidence of allergy-related disease also seems to be increasing in Japan.

Given the relative frequency of allergic disorders, it is not surprising that many professional and performing vocalists will have difficulties with allergy-related diseases. *Allergy* is defined as a hypersensitive or pathologic reaction to environmental factors present in amounts that should not affect most people. Allergy involves the release of mediators from mast cells and basophils that may be triggered by a variety of agents. Allergies are generally subdivided into atopic, which involve IgE antibody mediation, and nonatopic, which does not involve IgE.[38]

Of those Americans with allergic disease an estimated 8.9 million suffer from asthma with or without hay fever, 14.7 million have hay fever alone, and 11.8 million have other allergic manifestations such as eczema, urticaria, angioedema, or food, drug, or insect hypersensitivity.[39]

In many ways treating allergic disease in the performing vocalist may be difficult. Both the symptom complex related to the allergic disorder as well as the treatment of the allergies may have negative effects on the voice. A study of detailed vocal quality, articulation errors, and hearing disorders in 80 children and young adults with diagnosed allergies revealed that almost 50% had abnormalities in vocal quality and/or articulation and 13% had reduced auditory acuity.[40]

Allergic individuals may have many factors that may affect the voice. These include chronic cough, throat clearing, edema of the mucous membranes of the nose, pharynx, and vocal folds, large adenoids, otitis media, and an increased incidence of lesions of the vocal folds.[40–42] A previous report has suggested that 69 of 245 patients with acute or chronic laryngitis had allergy as a potential underlying cause.[43]

The major problem with allergies in the performing vocalist generally has to do with inhalant allergies and particularly allergic rhinitis. Inhalant allergies are usually secondary to organic sources such as pollens, molds, dusts, and animals. Seasonal allergic rhinitis usually involves tree pollens in the spring, grass pollens in the late spring to midsummer, and weeds, particularly ragweed, in the late summer and early fall. Ragweed has been shown to be worse in the eastern and middlewestern portions of the United States. Flower pollens for the most part are large particles and rarely cause allergy.[39]

Nonseasonal (perennial) allergic rhinitis is usually due to dust, animal danders, and molds. Dust contains lint, mites, danders, insect parts, fibers, and other particulate matter all of which may be a potential source of allergic inflammation. Singers and actors who are repeatedly exposed to set constructions and dusty theaters particularly may be affected should they have dust allergies.

When these airborne particles are present in a susceptible host and there is repeated exposures, IgE antibody production is stimulated. On repeat exposure of the sensitized respiratory mucous membranes to the specific allergens, allergen reactions with the antibody result. Subsequent release of histamine and other mediators of inflammation from mast cells and basophils occurs. These mediators produce swelling, tissue edema with fluid accumulation, and irritation. The effects of these are the typical symptoms of hay fever with itchy eyes, sneezing, nasal congestion, runny nose, and, in vocalists, a change in voice.

The mechanism of allergic laryngitis is primarily associated with edema formation that involves portions of the larynx. In more severe episodes, the entire larynx including the epiglottis, arytenoids, and vocal folds may be involved.[44] In some cases, laryngeal swelling and edema may be the only symptom of hypersensitivity to salicylic acid (aspirin) and other substances.[45] With less severe allergic reactions the swelling and edema accumulation occurs in the more susceptible areas of the true vocal folds with Reinke's space edema. Some feel that allergic manifestations in the larynx occur more often than has been generally noted in the literature.[44]

Asthma can also be an allergy-mediated disorder. The incidence of asthma in patients with allergies appears to be greater than in the general population.[46] This is particularly true in the context of aspirin hypersensitivity, sinusitis, nasal polyps, and asthma, which can be present in some individuals as an associated complex. Asthma can alter the production of airflow necessary for proper phonation or singing. Bronchial constriction with wheezing can prevent adequate pulmonary support of the voice. On rare occasions, vocal cord dysfunction may be confused with wheezing and exercise-induced asthma.[47]

The effect of allergies on the nasal mucosa results in the typical symptoms of allergic rhinitis with nasal congestion and runny nose (rhinitis). Persistent nasal congestion can affect the resonating qualities of the voice. The rhinitis itself, without the direct effect of the allergens on the larynx, is unlikely to result in much laryngeal dysfunction unless purulent sinusitis is simultaneously present.

In some individuals who do not have any evidence of allergic disease, ongoing nasal problems can occur and is referred to as *perennial nonallergic rhinitis* or *vasomotor rhinitis*. In these circumstances nasal congestion and drainage can occur and are secondary to nonspecific inflammation rather than true allergies. These reactions are often associated with irritation from pollution, changes in barometric pressure, temperature, or humidity, smoke or other various external irritants. Vasomotor rhinitis can cause problems similar to those that would be expected with allergic disease. Although these irritants generally affect the nasal mucous membranes where they are filtered, on occasion external irritants and pollution in the air can result in laryngeal dysfunction.[48]

Infectious sinusitis has been found to be more common in patients with allergic disorders. The generalized symptoms of allergic or vasomotor rhinitis are compounded by a purulent posterior nasal drainage, midfacial pressure, and, occasionally, fever. Purulent nasal drainage may affect laryngeal function directly from resultant laryngeal irritation, and the systemic effects due to the infectious process with fatigue and fever will have an adverse effect on the vocalist's ability to perform. The management of sinusitis should be more aggressive than with allergic or vasomotor rhinitis and should include antibiotic therapy. It is uncommon for vasomotor rhinitis alone, without allergic disease, to affect the voice directly. If a chronic laryngeal irritation is present in the absence of allergic disease or purulent sinusitis, then it is unlikely that the nasal drainage is the etiology. This has been suggested as far back as 1887 in a symposium presented by the American Laryngological Association concerning the treatment of laryngitis in professionals.[49] If such symptoms are present in the absence of allergies, even if there is an associated vasomotor rhinitis, then other sources of laryngitis should be fully investigated before being ascribed to perennial nonallergic rhinitis.

The assessment of a patient with an allergic disorder of the upper airways relies on an appropriate history to determine if there is antecedent exposure to potential allergens. Once a thorough history has been obtained, obvious sources of allergies may be determined. In some cases patients are allergic to more than one allergen, or the substance that is causing the problem cannot be easily elucidated by history.

Based on the historical information, an appropriate physical examination should be performed with examination of the ears, the nose, the upper airway, larynx, and lungs. Laboratory studies can then be initiated to evaluate possible allergens. The standard of allergic testing is careful skin testing.[39] Blood tests with in vitro analysis (such as the RAST test) have been found to be beneficial in many circumstances. Many allergists use a combination of skin testing and RAST or other in vitro tests. Other blood tests, such as blood IgE counts, and nasal smears may also be helpful.

Once a diagnosis of allergic rhinitis or laryngitis is made, treatment is initiated. The hallmark of treatment of allergic disorders is removal, if possible, of the allergic precipitant. In some instances, particularly in the situation of animal dander allergies, removal of the animal from the home is sufficient to alleviate symptoms. In those patients with seasonal allergies, appropriate treatment may be initiated only at the time of or just prior to their allergy season. In patients with perennial disease, treatment may be more difficult, particularly if they are allergic to substances that are somewhat ubiquitous such as dust and molds.

One of the concerns in treatment of allergic disorders in the professional vocalist is that many of the medications that are utilized to treat allergies can have an adverse effect on the voice. Standard allergic management with antihistamines and decongestants can result in drying of the mucous membranes and thickening of the mucus, which is not preferred in a vocalist. Most common antihistamines are noted to have a significant drying effect. With the development of newer nonsedating antihistamines such as Seldane and Hismanal, less drying effects have been noted, although some feel that these antihistamine effects are less potent. Decongestants tend to have less drying effect. Entex is a medication that the author prescribes for many of these professionals. Iodinated glycerol (Organidin) has been shown to help relieve the mucous-related symptoms of chronic pulmonary disease and has been used safely for treatment of chronic upper airway problems.[50] Oral expectorants, terpinhydrate, and inorganic iodides have all been successful in treating abnormal or thick mucus.[51] In addition, Guaifenesin has been utilized for the treatment of thick mucus or dryness in acute or chronic sinusitis, asthma, bronchitis, laryngitis, and cough.

Balanced physiologic saline or salt water nasal sprays alone have proved to be effective in controlling symptoms of nasal blockage and nasal drainage in patients with chronic rhinitis of various etiologies, including allergic rhinitis.[52] Over-the-counter preparations of saline are available and can be purchased in most pharmacies or can be mixed at home with a combination of one quart of clean or boiled tap water per tablespoon of salt. The utilization of nasal decongestant sprays may occasionally be necessary, but should be used with caution since prolonged use of such sprays results in rebound nasal congestion or rhinitis medicamentosa. In some instances, steroid nasal sprays such as Beconase, Vancenase, and Nasalide can stabilize the nasal mucous membranes, resulting in decreased swelling, diminished drainage, and alleviation of symptoms.[53,54] There is no evidence of long-term negative effects of these medications nor do they have any significant systemic effects. This is of particular interest to the vocalist for whom androgen steroids are contraindicated. Corticosteroids of this type do not have any effect directly on the voice. However, steroid nasal sprays, particularly the older nonaqueous preparations, can have a drying effect in the nose that can diminish the humidifying effect of nasal airflow. Therefore, as with all medications, steroid nasal sprays should be used with caution by a singer.

In individuals who are resistant to allergic treatment with elimination of the allergens and medications, allergy immunotherapy or allergy shots may be initiated. Particularly in those with severe allergies, this will often provide significant relief. From the perspective of the voice and upper airway, no negative effects are expected with this treatment regimen. Prolonged therapy is often necessary, and singers must be cautioned that immunotherapy may take some time before it becomes effective.

The treatment of nasal allergic problems in the singer or speaker emphasizes the need for close cooperation between patients and the medical professionals involved with their treatment. This may include an otolaryngologist, allergist, or pulmonary medicine specialist. Tempering the side effects of the medication with alleviation of symptoms may be difficult, and experimentation may be necessary to fine tune the treatment so that the allergies are under good control without adverse effects on the voice. With the introduction or change in dosing of any medication, it is important to be cautious and to balance the benefits of the treatment with the side effects with respect to the effects on performance. With an appropriate history, evaluation, and treatment regimen, allergic disorders in the performing vocalist may be well controlled to allow for continuous, generally uninterrupted, activity.

XEROSTOMIA

Xerostomia refers to a dry mouth. Since adequate moisture is necessary to the voice both to maintain normal vocal fold vibration and to prevent irritation, xerostomia has major implications for the performing vocalist. Although temporary dry mouth may occur in many performers in association with pre-performance anxiety and "flight or fight" nervous system responses to performance, it tends to be self-limited and responds well to hydration and relaxation. More severe and persistent problems with xerostomia can occur and should be investigated.

Causes of xerostomia can be broken into two major groups: local and systemic. Local disorders are uncommon in the vocalist and is most often attributed to oral, salivary gland, or ear (where the chorda tympani nerve may be injured) surgery or irradiation of the area for tumors.

Systemic causes of xerostomia are much more common in this group and are listed in Table 14–1.[55] Certain medications are particularly important causes of xerostomia and are discussed in more detail in Chapter 15. Anemia should be ruled out, particularly in the female vocalist in reproductive age groups.

Of interest, despite its irritative effect, smoking generally results in increased saliva production, but decreased mucociliary transport will occur. It is not until smoking is prolonged and heavy that a dry, atrophic mouth occurs.

Sjögren syndrome is a disease characterized by xerostomia, dryness of the eyes (xerophthalmia), and rheumatoid arthritis or one of the other connective tissue diseases such as systemic lupus erythematosus or scleroderma.[56] The degree of xerostomia can be severe with resultant dental caries, salivary duct blockage, and retrograde salivary gland infections or mucous membrane ulcerations. This disease is treated with both systemic steroid treatment and local care.

Once the etiology of xerostomia is detected and treatment of the direct cause has been initiated, further care is directed toward increasing the moisture in the mouth. Saliva substitutes, sugar-free acid or glycerin drops or lemon juice, hydration, appropriate dental care, and elimination of drying drugs such as antidepressants and antihistamines may all improve oral moisture and hydration.[57]

DENTAL–PERIODONTAL DISEASE AND TEMPORAL MANDIBULAR JOINT DYSFUNCTION

Dental hygiene is necessary to prevent mouth irritation, infection, and to promote normal saliva flow. Dental caries is a localized, progressive destruction of the tooth initiated by acid dissolution of the outer tooth surface.[58] Caries can result in mucosal irritation and discomfort. The tooth discoloration that occurs may be detrimental to the physical image important for the performing vocalist. Prevention is the key to caries treatment. Oral and tooth hygiene with brushing and flossing and fluoride have all been shown to decrease

Table 14–1   Systemic Causes of Xerostomia

Dehydration
Anemia
Drugs (antihistamines, antidepressants, nicotine, atropine)
Sjögren syndrome
Chronic mental stress or anxiety
Debilitation
Infection
Advanced age
Chronic mouth breathing

dental caries. Careful and routine dental examination and cleaning will control present caries and decrease the risk of further caries.

Periodontal disease may impact the performer more than dental caries. Periodontal disease is a collection of several diseases of the hard and soft tissue surrounding the teeth. The most common are irritation of the gums (gingivitis) and inflammation and destructive changes of the bone and soft tissues that support the teeth (periodontitis).[59] Chronic periodontitis can result in tartar formation and make it harder to keep the area clean.[59] Periodontal disease can lead to discomfort, mucous membrane irritation, and tooth loss. Frequent cleaning of dental plaque by combined personal and professional care are the keystones of the care and prevention of periodontal disease.

Since articulation is one of the key areas necessary for proper voice production both in singing and speaking, any abnormalities of teeth alignment that can interfere with proper articulation would be expected to have an adverse effect for the singer. Fortunately, severe abnormalities must be present to have a significant effect on speech articulatory function. The physical appearance of the teeth if misaligned, however, may be of more importance to the performing vocalist because of facial and body image.

The temporomandibular joint is a joint space where the mandible (jaw) comes to lie just in front of the external ear canal in the glenoid fossa. Most temporomandibular joint disorders are secondary to trauma or to the excessive stresses being placed on the joint by the strong muscles that attach to the jaw for creating forces for chewing (muscles of mastication). Chronic microtraumas secondary to stress-induced functional oral habits such as bruxism or teeth grinding and emotional stress or tension with secondary muscle contractions can result in chronic irritation and discomfort in the joint space. These are enhanced by predisposing occlusal neuromuscular or psychogenic factors.[60]

Definitional symptoms of temporomandibular joint dysfunction include one or more of the following: (1) pain and tenderness in the joint or the muscles of mastication, (2) grating sound or crepitance with temporomandibular joint movement, and (3) limitations in movement of the jaw.[61] The pain can radiate to other areas of the head, neck, shoulders, or arms and may be associated with trigger points. Headaches usually in the temples or frontal or occipital areas can occur. Ear pain with tinnitus and vertigo have also been reported to be related to temporomandibular joint dysfunction.[61]

Temporomandibular joint dysfunction is a common disorder, although among performing musicians it may be more common in brass and woodwind instrumentalists.[62] The incidence in vocalists has not been established. Nonetheless, given the relative frequency in the general population, it would be expected to affect a large number of vocalists. The discomfort and associated head, neck, and shoulder musculotension can cause excessive stresses and early fatigue to the muscles of the larynx and jaw. Limitations in jaw movement will alter resonance, and a chronic effect can alter the psychological nuances of performance.

The diagnosis of temporomandibular joint dysfunction is established by a strong history supporting the disorder substantiated by a confirmatory physical examination. A dental consultation should be considered if simple methods of treatment are not successful. Limitations in movement of the jaw and crepitance or tenderness on palpation of the joint during jaw movement may be found. Plain x-rays and video arthrography are used for corroboration. CT scan or MRI may hold promise in the diagnosis of temporomandibular joint disease.

The treatment of temporomandibular joint dysfunction can be broken into initial, provisional, and definitive. In most cases, until the cause of the dysfunction is identified, initial conservative treatment may be both therapeutic and diagnostic.[61] Soft diet, warm compresses, and nonsteroidal antiinflammatory agents will provide relief for most individuals so that no further intervention is needed. Provisional treatment by the reestablishment of the normal maxillomandibular relationship, and altering joint loading with orthotic appliances or bite plates is usually effective in those with more significant problems. These often can be used at night and removed during the day. In rare circumstances with significant joint derangements, definitive surgical treatment can be performed.

MUSCULOSKELETAL DISORDERS

The musculoskeletal system provides support for respiration and phonation. Although neck, jaw, and shoulder tension are most prominently recognized as affecting the voice, the entire musculoskeletal system must be considered should a voice disorder occur. Since appropriate posture is necessary for efficient and controlled voice production, acute or chronic leg or back disorders can inhibit the ability to support the voice adequately. In particular, common problems of low back pain and dysfunction that increase in frequency with age may be a problem for the aging singer. Those vocal performers who are also dancers are prone to the stress-related injuries to the joints of the spine, ankles, and knees. Appropriate conservative care with stretching, rest, ice, and antiinflammatory agents are indicated. An orthopaedic, sports medicine, or dance medicine referral for assessment and treatment may be necessary. Vocalists should be aware of the problems that can occur due to such disorders and adjust to optimize their vocal use.

Laryngeal tension-fatigue syndrome[63] and *muscle tension dysphonia*[64,65] are terms used to describe dysphonia secondary to muscle tension disorders. The laryngeal, perilaryngeal, suprahyoid, neck, and jaw muscles may be involved. Increased muscular tension in the neck and larynx has been found to be associated with palpable increased muscle tension in the suprahyoid and perilaryngeal muscles during phonation, elevation of the larynx with increased pitch, an open posterior glottic chink on phonation, and associated vocal fold abnormalities such as nodules or chronic laryngitis.[64] The nodules may be more fleshy than those seen with other disorders.

Under mild conditions, alterations in pitch and easy fatigue may be present and chronic intermittent dysphonia may occur.[63] With more significant musculotension dysfunction, the voice may become breathy and harsh to variable degrees.[65] Such muscular tension-related disorders are often noted in professional speakers. Some feel that the perceived desirable low-pitched voice used by some men and women, coined by Koufman and Blalock[63] as the Bogart-Bacall syndrome, may be secondary to low pitching of the voice. These problems are functional in nature and usually respond to appropriate speaking and singing therapy. A scalloped tongue, where the teeth leave indentations on the tongue from constant tongue thrusting, may be noted on physical examination (Fig. 14–3). Relaxation techniques, appropriate neck and shoulder positioning, and instruction for efficient voice use is recommended and is discussed in more detail in Chapter 20. Nonsteroidal antiinflammatory agents, physical therapy, warm compresses, and massage of both the neck and larynx may help chronic neck, jaw, and perilaryngeal muscular tension dysfunction.

Forced whispering can result in musculotension-type dysfunction. Sound production during loud whispering results in turbulence of rapid airflow unlike the regular pulsations of

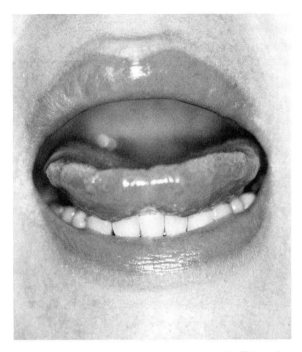

Figure 14–3. Scalloped tongue secondary to tongue thrusting against teeth. This can be seen in musculotension dysphonia.

airflow that occur in voicing of sound.[66] A frictional sound may be produced as outgoing air passes through the glottis, particularly through a posterior glottic chink.[67] It has been suggested that whispering produces excessive strain or hyperfunctioning of the laryngeal mechanism.[68] Benninger et al[69] have shown variable degrees of vocal fold adduction while whispering. In the majority of subjects evaluated there was a potential for a harmful effect to the vocal mechanism by whispering, particularly in the previously traumatized larynx.[69] A quiet whisper, however, may not result in any potential injury to the vocal folds.[70,71] It is therefore generally recommended that loud or forced whispering be avoided, particularly in the previously injured or traumatized larynx.

HEARING LOSS

Phonation involves the sequential function of three neurologic control systems: prephonatory tuning, acoustic monitoring, and reflex modulation.[72] The importance of acoustic voice monitoring can be seen in the flat, unmodulated voices of those with long-standing and profound neurosensory deafness. Delayed acoustic feedback has been shown to affect vocal performance in normal speakers and singers.[72]

Vocalists depend on their hearing for development of their musical abilities, ongoing music education, and performance. Auditory feedback is critical to allow the individual to monitor his/her sound production, refine pitch and volume production, and blend with surrounding accompaniment or voices. Hearing loss in the vocalist can affect both musical ability development if occurring in early ages or may prevent appropriate feedback for performance optimization in older age groups.

To understand the dynamics of hearing, a foundation in anatomic and physiologic principles are important. The ear can be thought of as having three separate parts with a fourth if one includes the auditory nerve pathways in the brain (Fig. 14–4). There is an outer ear, which includes the visible ear or auricle, and the ear canal (external auditory canal). The outer ear is separated from the middle ear by the eardrum (tympanic membrane). The external ear acts as a cone to bring sound into the ear canal so that it can reach the eardrum. It also allows protection for the delicate structures of the middle and inner ears.

The middle ear is a space that contains the three bones of hearing or ossicular chain and the eustachian tube that connects to the nasopharynx to allow equalization of pressure on both sides of the tympanic membrane. The ossicles are the malleus (hammer), incus (anvil), and stapes (stirrup), the latter of which comes in contact with the oval window into the inner ear. These structures along with the size difference between the tympanic membrane and oval window, increase sound volume reaching the inner ear by 22 times.[73] Any process that will decrease movement of the ossicular chain or fill the middle ear will diminish the sound reaching the inner ear.

The inner ear has two separate portions (Fig. 14–4): the cochlea, or organ of hearing, and the semicircular canals, utricle, and saccule, which are organs of balance. The inner ear structures are fluid-filled cavities with sensitive neurostructures to detect movement of the fluid. The cochlea converts the acoustic transducer energy of the middle ear to electrical impulses which then travel via the acoustic nerve (eighth cranial nerve) to the brain. Similar movement of fluid causes the vestibular or balance portion of the ear to respond to acceleration, deceleration, rotation, or gravity.

Sound is defined by both intensity and frequency. Intensity or loudness is the power or

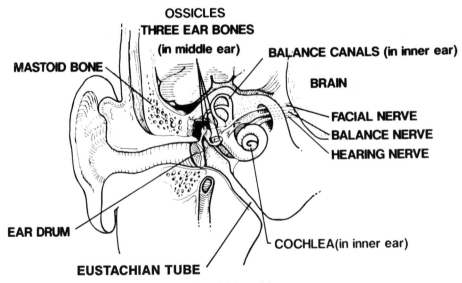

Figure 14–4.   Outer, middle, and inner ear with eighth cranial nerve.

Table 14–2   Sound Pressure Levels of Common Sounds

SOUND	dB
Rocket launching pad	180
Jet plane	140
Automobile horn	120
Punch press	100
Subway	90
Busy traffic	75
Conversational speech	66
Soft whisper	30

pressure of the sound and is measured in decibels (dB). Decibels are logarithmic so that a tone that is 10 dB more intense is perceived as twice as loud. Common sound pressure levels of various sounds are listed in Table 14–2,[74] while those of various musical instruments are shown in Table 14–3.[75] The loudest sound a normal human ear can tolerate is 10 million times the softest it can hear.[74] This wide variation allows the ability to detect, discriminate, and identify the myriad of inputs we hear.

Hearing is necessary for the development of language and speech. Deaf children can develop language, but speech rarely is normal. In a similar fashion musical abilities and voice would also be expected to be decreased in hearing impaired children. An investigation by Klajman et al[76] of musical abilities in hearing impaired and normal-hearing children revealed (1) 50% of hearing impaired children and 80% of normal-hearing children had a good ear for music; (2) there were only small differences in the musical abilities in children in both groups who had a good ear for music; (3) developing musical abilities in hearing-impaired children through musical exercises is possible; (4) improvement of musical abilities of hearing-impaired children by musical exercises may affect a positive influence on rehabilitation.[76] The degree of hearing loss would be expected to play a role in a child's musical abilities and voice, but musical and voice development should be encouraged as part of the hearing impaired child's growth.

Any process that would affect hearing can result in problems for the singer or speaker. These disorders could be broken up into those of the external, middle, or inner ears. The

Table 14–3   Sound Pressure Levels of Different Musical Instruments

INSTRUMENT	dB
Trombone	85–114
Piccolo	95–112
Flute	85–111
French horn	90–106
Clarinet	92–103
Violin	84–103
Oboe	80–94
Xylophone	90–92
Cello	84–92
Bass	75–83

most common cause of decreased hearing in the external ear is ear wax (cerumen) impaction. In general, large amounts of cerumen need to be present, and complete occlusion of the ear canal is usually necessary for any change in hearing to be detectable. Should this occur, it is important that attempts at self-removal be avoided, as this can worsen the impaction or cause inflammation of the ear canal. Rather, cerumen removal by a medical professional is preferred. The role of wax softeners such as Cerumenex are debated but in some cases may be used. A more attractive approach in those individuals with recurrent cerumen problems is prevention of impaction by the installation of a small amount of hydrogen peroxide intermittently in the ears.

External ear infections or "swimmer's ear" may occur. This is usually found in warm or humid environments and associated with frequent water exposures such as with swimming. Tenderness of the ear with decreased hearing are hallmarks of this disorder, and it is treated with antibiotics with or without steroid ear drops. Prevention, again, is preferred for those who have recurrent problems, with dry ear precautions or ear plugs and the placement of a few drops of a mild acetic acid solution or vinegar.[77]

Middle ear disorders are less common in adults than in children, who are predisposed to recurrent ear infections or middle ear fluid. Most middle ear problems are associated with eustachian tube dysfunction in which the middle ear is unable to be aerated. The eustachian tube normally remains closed but opens every time one chews, yawns, or swallows. If it remains closed, then a negative pressure is created and fluid may accumulate, preventing adequate sound conduction through the middle ear. Often this can be treated by inflation of the ears by pinching the nose, closing the mouth, and blowing to overcome the eustachian tube resistance, as is frequently done by scuba divers. Pressure-equalizing tubes can be placed if blockage persists. Disorders of the ossicular chain can also occur but are uncommon.

Disorders of the inner ear most commonly affect the hearing of the performing vocalist. Age-related changes in hearing or presbycusis and noise-induced hearing loss are predominant. Loss of hearing with age frequently occurs, but the degree of loss is variable. The characteristic of presbycusis is a very gradual sloping high frequency hearing loss (Fig. 14–5). With the gradual mild loss that can occur in the years of peak performance, the hearing loss may not adversely affect voice or music production. If more significant changes occur, there can be a substantial effect.

The more significant hearing disorder that might result in hearing loss in the performing vocalist is "noise-induced" hearing loss. Chronic exposure to loud noises can result in temporary hearing loss or temporary threshold shift (TTS) with recovery some time after exposure or in permanent hearing loss or permanent threshold shift (PTS) without recovery in hearing (Fig. 14–6). OSHA has established guidelines for exposure to noise for the work place. While 8 hours of 90 dB noise has been found permissible, only 2 hours of 100 dB and 15 minutes of 115 dB noise is permissible in the work place without hearing protection. These guidelines have been developed for constant noise levels, while the pulsatile noise normally present with music does not directly correlate with the OSHA guidelines. Karlsson et al[78] have suggested "that the sound exposure criteria for industrial noise are not valid when discussing such sounds as are produced by acoustic instruments in a symphonic environment." Nonetheless, prolonged exposure to musical instrument noise levels could potentially result in a hearing loss.

Many studies have been reported assessing the role of prolonged musical instrument exposure to hearing loss.[75,78–81] Studies have shown that noise-induced hearing loss can

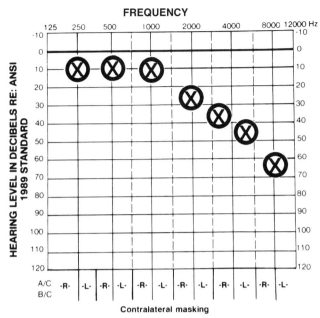

FREQUENCY

Figure 14–5. Age-related high frequency hearing loss. Normal hearing is considered to be between −10 to 20 dB.

occur in orchestral musicians,[78,79,82] with up to 43% of musicians showing worse hearing than would be expected for their age.[75] Evidence of noise-induced hearing loss has been found in 15.5%[80] to 33.8%[79] of classical orchestral musicians. The type of music hall, instrument type, duration of exposure, previous musical background, and position on the stage have all been raised as possible sources of hearing loss.[75,79,82]

The amount of instrument sound exposure has been found to vary widely by experience, age, and instrument type.[82] Although older musicians tend to practice fewer hours per week, the average practice/performance time of orchestral musicians is about 33 hours per week with a range of 12 to 56 hours.[82] Longer exposure times might be expected to have a greater effect on hearing. Individuals with a previous background of participation in military bands and exposure to gun fire are particularly prone to decreased hearing.[75] Orchestral pit musicians may have a more pronounced hearing loss than stage musicians.[75]

The role of instrumental music as an etiology for hearing loss is controversial, as some investigators have not detected any difference in hearing among orchestral musicians than would be expected in the general population.[78,82] A similar controversy has been raised with regard to hearing loss and different instrument types. Brass wind instruments have been implicated for greater hearing losses, and violinists have been reported to have worse hearing on the left than the right.[75] Others, however, have not found any difference in hearing among different instrument types or stage positions.[82]

Regardless of the controversy, it would seem to be prudent for musicians to be aware of the potential risks to their hearing by prolonged exposure to high intensity noise from

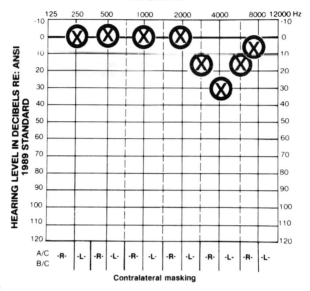

A

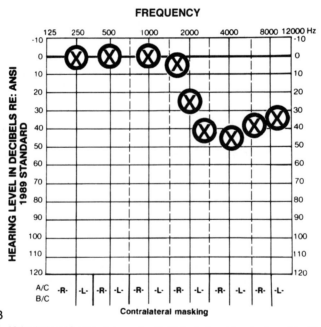

B

Figure 14–6. **A,** Noise-induced hearing loss, early; **B,** Noise-induced hearing loss, late. Typical hearing dip greatest at 4,000 Hz.

their music or any other source. In response to these issues, many musicians and some orchestras have instituted measures for hearing protection at least during practice conditions. Larger spaces for practice rather than the more confined settings and head shields to divert sound from behind the musicians will decrease sound exposure. Sound can be attenuated or reduced by 3 to 14 dB with cotton, 11 to 30 dB with ear plugs, and 28 to 47 dB with fluid-sealed muffs, depending on the frequency of sound.[74]

Rock and roll musicians, or those who are exposed to significant sound amplification, are particularly prone to noise-induced hearing loss.[83–85] With amplification, sound intensity levels can be far in excess of those to which musicians are normally exposed. Temporary changes in hearing (TTS) are common while permanent loss of hearing (PTS) can occur. One-half of rock musicians studied were found to have TTS, and almost one-fourth had a PTS.[84] The amount of hearing loss in this group, however, is lower than expected given the sound intensity level and length of exposure.[85] This may be due to two factors: (1) the dominant frequencies of pop music are low, with 250 to 500 Hz being maximally amplified, which may be less damaging to the ear; and (2) the presentation of music with frequent pauses or interruptions might allow short periods of rest and recovery.[85] Nonetheless, the magnitude of the exposure has resulted in some prominent pop and rock vocalists developing significant noise-induced hearing loss.

Another area for concern is for studio musicians or those who spend significant amounts of time utilizing headphones. Although interest in this area has only recently been generated by the popularity of individual stereo radios, stereo headphones have had a longer duration of utilization since becoming popular in the 1960s. A recent study of intensity levels of 14 consumer available headphone brands revealed maximum outputs in the range of 102 to 128 dB,[86] which are above levels that can result in noise-induced hearing loss. In a similar fashion, home amplifiers can deliver 700 W into each of two channels,[86] and a recent national newspaper article discussed a man who has a car stereo with sound outputs in excess of 150 dB, which is beyond the threshold for pain.[87]

Other, more unusual, sources of hearing loss that can occur is beyond the scope of this chapter. Many infections (syphilis, mumps, measles), autoimmune and metabolic (hypothyroidism, diabetes, renal failure, and multiple sclerosis) disorders, as well as certain ototoxic medications can result in either temporary or permanent hearing loss.

The best treatment for hearing loss in the vocalist is dependent on the underlying cause. Aggressive treatment of medical disorders and avoidance of ototoxic drugs, if possible, should be achieved. Noise-induced hearing loss is best treated by avoidance of noise, proper hearing protection, and a controlled environment.

If a hearing loss should occur, the amount of intervention necessary will depend on the severity of the hearing loss and on the hearing demands of the individual. Hearing aids can be used to assist the hearing-impaired musician. One of the problems with hearing aids for the musician is that hearing aids have been designed primarily to improve speech intelligibility and since speech sounds may be in a lower frequency range than music, aids that augment speech may not provide the best sound quality for music.[88] New hearing aids with wider and more selective frequency augmentation will likely improve the sensitivity of hearing for the performing artist.

Even before hearing aids were available, some individuals have been able to overcome severe hearing disabilities to remain prominent members of the music community. Most notable of these is Ludwig von Beethoven, who had a severe progressive hearing loss but even when nearly deaf was able to compose his 7th, 8th, and 9th symphonies. Some feel that his best works were created at the end of his career.[89]

GASTROINTESTINAL DISORDERS

Abdominal musculature plays a critical role in the support of the voice. Any medical problem that affects abdominal control can adversely affect the voice. In general, abdominal dysfunction is usually temporary and is the result of an acute infectious gastrointestinal condition. Viral enteritis with diarrhea or vomiting is a self-limited disorder, best treated with conservative therapy, adequate hydration, and rest. In many cases, such episodes may preclude performance often due to the associated systemic symptoms of fever and malaise that accompany the intestinal symptoms. Fortunately, such episodes tend to be of short duration, and resumption of normal activity occurs quickly. If the episode is mild and the vocalist wishes to proceed with performing, hydration is very important as mild dehydration often occurs with gastrointestinal dysfunction.

Constipation can be a more chronic problem for many singers and speakers. Active lifestyles, touring, and socialization can lead to irregular meals that are often of high fat, low carbohydrate composition. Such dietary habits can lead to decreased intestinal transit times, harder and more-formed stools, and constipation. Sensations of bloating, pressure, or cramping can occur. In general, dietary control with regimented timing of meals, increased carbohydrates (particularly complex carbohydrates), and decreased fats can relieve the constipation. Occasionally utilization of a bulk laxative may be needed. Prolonged use of laxatives, particularly nonbulk ones, should be used with close physician monitoring, as electrolyte and fluid abnormalities may occur.

Probably the most common and most underdiagnosed gastrointestinal problem affecting vocalists is gastroesophageal (GE) reflux. This may be a substantial cause of voice dysfunction. Up to 7% of the adult population experiences symptoms of GE reflux at least once daily.[90] As mentioned previously, performing vocalists are prone to dietary difficulties that can stimulate stomach acid production. Many singers prefer to eat little prior to a performance and, if they perform in the evening or at night, eat after the performance within a short period before bedtime. Such behaviors lead to increased acidic production for digestion, and the gravitational forces that help to prevent reflux are lost when the individual assumes a recumbent position to sleep. Alcohol, which may be used prior to retiring, directly inhibits resting lower esophageal sphincter tone with resultant increased reflux. High fat diets[91] and smoking[92] also have been shown to decrease lower esophageal sphincter pressure.

A thorough history of eating habits and laryngeal symptoms will usually allow the practitioner to suspect GE reflux. Vocalists only occasionally relay symptoms referable to reflux without questioning. Although symptoms of heartburn or acid reflux into the pharynx may be present, the absence of such symptoms does not exclude GE reflux. More commonly, vocalists complain of a scratchy or "foreign body" sensation in the laryngeal area, a bitter taste in the mouth particularly in the morning, a worse voice in the morning that improves as the day progresses, or gradual lengthening of the time of vocal warm-up. Frequent throat clearing despite minimal mucus production is common. Many individuals feel that this is a chronic sinus-related problem, but in the absence of any other nasal or sinus symptomatology and with a normal sinus work-up this would suggest that the problem is laryngeal in origin and not due to chronic nasal sinus drainage. The author has found that one-fourth of patients referred for nasal–sinus problems were found to have laryngeal etiologies for their chronic nasal sinus symptoms. Half of these patients were found by further investigation to have GE reflux and/or a hiatal hernia. Atypical chest pain, particularly after meals, or nocturnal cough may be present with GE reflux.[93] Dysphagia or a chronic cough may also be present.[94] Symptoms may be more prominent after large meals or when bending, lifting, or straining. An associated hiatal hernia may be present, and, although some reports suggest no direct association between hiatal hernia and GE reflux,[93] most feel that a hiatal hernia may predispose to reflux symptoms.

Physical examination of patients with reflux laryngitis will reveal edematous or erythematous, sometimes "cherry red" arytenoids,[95] although such findings may be subtle. Small, early contact ulcers on the vocal processes of the arytenoids may be present if chronic throat clearing or aggressive vocalization accompanies the laryngeal irritation caused by reflux. In addition, marked thickening of the posterior commissure with a more grayish color to the mucosa is often seen. Rarely does the edema or erythema extend into the anterior two-thirds of the vocal folds, but a small amount of Reinke's space edema may be present.

The diagnosis of reflux laryngitis is most commonly made by a thorough history and physical examination. A successful trial of conservative therapy is confirmatory. General measures for the treatment of GE reflux are listed in Table 14–4. Such a list may be given to patients at the time of an office visit. With night performances, having larger meals at breakfast or lunch with a small meal of rapidly absorbing complex carbohydrates a couple of hours before a performance may be well tolerated. Aerobic athletes frequently eat complex or simple carbohydrates a short time before or during activity without adverse side effects and with improved performance.[96] Antacids taken between meals or before bedtime may diminish symptoms.

If response to conservative treatment is not effective, diagnostic studies are indicated. A barium esophogram with fluoroscopy, esophageal pH monitoring, the acid infusion test (Bernstein test),[97] a standard acid reflux test,[98] or endoscopy may be performed. Combined hypopharyngeal and esophageal pH monitoring is useful in the diagnosis of reflux-induced hoarseness.[94,98] Other, more significant, functional or anatomic conditions can therefore be ruled out, while better direction for therapy can be determined.

Symptoms refractory to general reflux measures and antacids may be treated with H_2-receptor antagonist antihistamines. Ranitidine has been shown to decrease heartburn symptoms markedly and significantly improve the endoscopic appearance of the esophageal mucosa in patients with GE reflux.[99] Cimetidine has also been used for the treatment of GE reflux.[100] The hydrogen-potassium-ATPase inhibitor omeprazole has been used for esophagitis, and metoclopramide may increase gastric emptying and increase lower esophageal sphincter pressure.[101]

Table 14–4   Treatment of Gastroesophageal Reflux

Reduce, if overweight
Eat smaller, if necessary, more frequent meals
Do not eat within 3 hours of bedtime
Elevate the head of bed at night 6–12 inches by placing supports under the mattress
Do not lie down after eating
Do not smoke
Eat lower fat, higher carbohydrate/protein meals
Avoid foods that regularly cause heartburn (alcohol, chocolate, coffee, citric juices)
Decrease stress
Wear loose clothing
Minimize heavy lifting and bending

It is critical to emphasize to the vocalist that adequate hydration, proper diet, and avoidance of throat clearing is necessary if ongoing gastroesophageal reflux occurs. In addition, having water available to drink rather than clearing the throat may be necessary. If the above measures are unsuccessful and assessment does reveal evidence of persistent GE reflux, then a consultation with a gastroenterologist for further intervention would be recommended. It is important to suspect GE reflux in any individual who has persistent posterior glottic erythema or edema and chronic throat clearing without evidence of other laryngeal pathologies.

NEUROLOGIC DISORDERS

The nervous system forms the groundwork for normal voice production both through coordinated muscular activity of the chest, lungs, larynx, and upper supraglottic resonating cavities and through the proprioceptive sensation that is integral to fine tuning the voice. The vocalist requires coordinated fine movements, strength, speed, and endurance which are moderated by the central and peripheral nervous systems. The kinesthetic or proprioceptive feedback mechanism is important to control the phonatory process both from an automatic reflex and conscious active action. It becomes apparent therefore, considering the critical role of the nervous system in coordinating phonatory activity, why disorders of the nervous system can have significant impact on the vocalist. An indepth discussion of the myriad of neurologic disorders that can occur in the vocalist is beyond the scope of this chapter, and therefore isolating a few of the more common disorders is attempted. Dysfunction of the nervous system is easily divided into broad categories of those dealing with sensation, those involved with neuromuscular control, and a combination of these two.

Histologic examination of the larynx has revealed receptor end-organs in the mucous membranes.[102] In addition, muscle spindles and spiral nerve endings have been identified in the larynges of animals and humans, and afferent nerve discharges have been recorded in the recurrent laryngeal and superior laryngeal nerves by the stimulation that occurs during phonation.[103] Such nerve fibers and afferent input are thought to be necessary for appropriate proprioception, which allows normal laryngeal function to occur. There is strong support for the concept that kinesthetic control is closely related to the quality of vocal function.[103] Any disruption in the normal afferent nerve impulses and sensation to the larynx may interfere with normal phonatory control.

As was discussed in Chapters 2 and 3, the primary sensory nerve input supply to the larynx is from the internal branch of the superior laryngeal nerve, which innervates the upper portion of the glottis, and into the supraglottic region and from the recurrent laryngeal nerve in the lower glottis and subglottic region. In addition, the ninth and tenth cranial nerves help to innervate the more superior and posterior aspects of the pharynx. Selective injury to the motor and sensory nerves usually occurs secondary to trauma such as penetrating neck injuries or following surgery. However, idiopathic injury can occur, and this is particularly prominent with superior laryngeal nerve paralyses.[104,105] Involvement of the superior laryngeal nerve diminishes sensation to the upper portion of the larynx and can result in mild aspiration and is usually associated with a simultaneous injury to the motor branch of the superior laryngeal nerve to the cricothyroid muscle. This can cause a shift of the posterior glottis to the side of injury and an asymmetric level of the vocal folds with an associated dysphonia.[105]

With more significant effects on sensation caused by injury to other cranial nerves, both phonation and swallowing can be affected. Such significant loss of proprioception would only be expected under circumstances of severe neurologic impairment as in a stroke or a progressive degenerative disease. Minor changes in proprioception can occur in areas of inflammation or edema.

Neuromuscular disorders are uncommon problems in the general population and in performers. As in proprioceptive disorders, trauma or postsurgical injury to the nerves of phonation or articulation can result in difficulties with normal speech or song production. Injury to the recurrent laryngeal nerve would result in paralysis of a unilateral vocal fold, which can leave the voice somewhat breathy with loss of a normal mucosal wave on that side. Some accommodation generally occurs, but it would not be expected that completely normal sound production would return. The most common sources of recurrent laryngeal paralyses are previous surgery (particularly thyroid surgery), idiopathic paralysis that is generally felt to be due to a viral neuropathy, trauma, and certain tumors.[106] A large number of acute onset viral or idiopathic vocal fold paralyses would be expected to resolve spontaneously, and it is generally thought that a waiting period of 6 to 12 months is preferred prior to any permanent intervention. During that time period, vocal fold adjustments can be made by injecting temporary agents such as Gelfoam; however, with permanent paralyses laryngeal framework surgery with silastic implantation,[107,108] nerve implantation,[109,110] collagen injection,[111] or Teflon injections may be utilized to medialize the vocal fold. A speech–language pathologist is very valuable in working with patients to improve their voices when a vocal fold paralysis has occurred.

Injury to other cranial nerves, including the ninth and twelfth cranial nerves, will likely affect the resonating and articulatory function necessary for normal voice and speech production. These can be affected by motor neuropathies, including amyotrophic lateral sclerosis, meningeal processes, or idiopathic neuropathies. Certain muscular dystrophies (such as oculopharyngeal) seem preferentially to affect muscles of phonation.

Tremor can be a significant problem for some vocalists. This may be due to essential tremor or to a tremor of another etiology such as Parkinson disease. On rare occasions, the tremor can be primarily associated only with phonation and is referred to as a *vocal tremor*. A careful physical examination will reveal the tremor component, and it is important not to confuse a vocal tremor with other voice disturbance such as spasmodic dysphonia, particularly since some patients with spasmodic dysphonia also have an associated vocal tremor. In general, mild tremors that are associated with vocalization and with no evidence of a more significant systemic tremor disorder can be treated with beta-adrenergic blockers with good results.[112]

Myasthenia gravis is a disease characterized by easy fatiguability of muscles, weakness, and gradual return of muscle strength. It can affect any striated muscle but especially those innervated by cranial nerves, most frequently from the oculomotor, facial, and vagus nerves.[113] This disorder occurs in approximately 10 per 100,000 of the population with a 2:1 male predominance. Interestingly, the peak incidence of onset for females is in the third decade, while for men it is in the sixth or seventh decades of life.[113] Although the most common initial symptom of myasthenia gravis is ptosis, dysphonia or dysarthria can occur in 6% to 25% of individuals, while generalized fatigue can occur in 6%.[114]

The hallmark of voice change with myasthenia gravis is vocal fatigue. Upon prolonged voice utilization, the voice will become weak and breathy. Physical examination during that time may show sluggish movements of both vocal folds. With adequate rest, normal vocal fold mobility and normal voice production may return. Weakness of the muscles of the lips, tongue, and jaw may result in problems with articulation, and palatal fatigue can result in velopharyngeal dysfunction and hypernasality. Laryngeal function has been found to be abnormal in 60% of patients with myasthenia gravis.

Diagnosis is dependent on an appropriate history of muscle fatiguability and can be corroborated by the tensilon test in which intravenous edrophonium chloride restores muscle strength or intramuscular injections of neostigmine will relieve the weakness. Electromyography demonstrates fatigue on repetitive electrical stimulation or increased jitter on single fiber examination.[113] The treatment of myasthenia gravis includes use of acetyl cholinesterase inhibitors, thymectomy, and steroids. Plasmapheresis is utilized in rare occasions, and curare-like drugs should be avoided.

Multiple sclerosis is a disease of undetermined etiology that is characterized by demyelination of the white matter of the periventricular region, brainstem, cerebellum, and spinal cord and may present with intention tremor, dysarthric speech, and nystagmus known historically as the *Charcot triad*. Multiple sclerosis can affect many functions of the head and neck, as it causes both sensory and motor disturbances. Alterations in smell, loss or disturbances of vision, decreased sensation particularly in distribution of the trigeminal nerve, facial weakness, changes in hearing and balance function, and dysarthric-type speech are all well documented.[116] Unlike most progressive neurologic disorders, multiple sclerosis generally involves a younger age group and therefore may have greater impact on the performing voice community. The prevalence of multiple sclerosis appears to be greater in the higher latitudes of both the northern and southern hemispheres and can be as high as 80 per 100,000 in some regions of the United States.[116] Seventy percent of cases develop between the ages of 20 and 40 years, with men being affected more commonly than women.[117]

The hallmark of multiple sclerosis is recurring episodes of focal disorders of the central nervous system. These remit and recur and often may have long latency periods.[113] The diagnosis of multiple sclerosis is made through history of associated intermittent symptoms and is corroborated by evidence of demyelination on MRI scanning and characteristic spinal fluid abnormalities. The treatment of multiple sclerosis is largely symptomatic. Speech and physical therapy, audiologic amplification, prosthetics, parenteral nutrition, and psychiatric support all play a role in treating the multiple sclerosis patient.[113] The use of adrenocorticotropic hormone and adrenocorticosteroids is controversial but appears to be effective during the active phases of disease and can lead to remission. Tremor medications such as beta-blockers may also be utilized. In general, the clinical course is associated with resolution and remission of symptoms, although after each exacerbation progression may occur to the point that fixed neurologic deficits may be present.[116]

A discussion of dysarthria is beyond the scope of this chapter. Nonetheless, it is important to mention *dysarthria* as a term to describe a group of speech disorders resulting from disturbances in muscular control of speech due to damage of the central or peripheral nervous system. A number of neurologic disorders can result in dysarthria, and appropriate neurologic consultation is necessary for evaluation and treatment.

Neurologic and general medical assessment is paramount in the evaluation of any individual with a potentially neurologically mediated voice disorder. The exception is the individual cranial nerve paralysis such as recurrent laryngeal nerve paralysis. In many cases, the dysfunction will be self-limited, and no aggressive neurologic intervention may be necessary. However, a progressive neurologic disorder should be ruled out. In those who have no other symptoms that might suggest a systemic neurologic disease, investigation of the larynx with videostroboscopy and laryngeal electromyography may be critical for diagnosis and subsequent care. In some cases of myasthenia gravis, multiple sclerosis, and amyotrophic lateral sclerosis, a voice-related complaint may be the primary or only complaint at the time of presentation.

ENDOCRINE DISORDERS

The mass of the vocal folds is affected by the amount of fluid content extracellularly. An increase in fluid accumulation primarily within the loose connective tissue of the lamina propria deep to the mucosa of the vocal folds results in increased mass and alterations in pitch. This may be minimal with limited fluid shifts, but can result in substantial decreases in pitch and loss of the normal mucosal wave of the free edge of the vocal fold when fluid changes are more significant. Many endocrine-related effects on the vocal folds are related to alterations in fluid concentration.

Thyroid Disorders

The thyroid gland has a primary role in the production of thyroid hormone, which is instrumental in helping to control a number of metabolic and physiologic processes. Its principal role is to regulate tissue metabolism and protein synthesis and is required for normal growth and bone maturation.[117]

Thyroid disease is very common. Approximately 4% of adults in the United States have thyroid nodules, 1.4% of women are hypothyroid with greater percentages found in elderly women, and almost 2% of women will develop Graves disease.[118] Hypothyroidism can present with weakness, dry skin, lethargy, cold intolerance, menorrhagia, constipation, paresthesia, or muscle cramps, while hyperthyroidism results in nervousness, heat intolerance, fatigue, palpitations, weight loss, weakness, and hyperdefecation.[118] Muscle weakness can occur in both hypothyroidism and hyperthyroidism, and thus either can affect the voice.

Disorders of thyroid function can alter the voice, and although the mechanism is not clearly understood it does appear to be mostly related to alterations in the fluid dynamics of the vocal folds. Although hyperthyroidism can be a cause of vocal dysfunction, it tends to have minimal effects until significant increases in thyroid hormone levels and thyrotoxicosis occur. In patients with thyrotoxicosis, the quality of the voice is affected due to alteration of tone, and frequently the volume of voice is diminished. In severe cases there can be changes that may result from mild bulbar muscle dysfunction.[119] Preoperative assessment of patients with nontoxic goiter or medically pretreated toxic goiter have been shown to have impaired voice function based on stroboscopy, electroglottography, phono-oscillometry, and determinations of voice range, phonation time, pitch, and peak flow. These voice dysfunctions improve following surgical correction of the thyroid disorder.[120]

In contrast to hyperthyroidism, relatively minor decreases in circulating thyroid hormone with hypothyroidism is not only more common but result in earlier and more noticeable voice changes. Although in severe hypothyroidism with myxedema alteration in vocal function can occur due to the effect on muscular strength or even vocal fold paralysis, hypothyroidism primarily causes hoarseness from a purely vocal fold effect.[121] Both human and animal studies have revealed accumulation of acid mucopolysaccharides in the submucosa of the true and false vocal folds with hypothyroidism. This is most marked in patients with myxedema.[121] In association with the acid mucopolysaccharide accumulation, increased fluid content will occur. The secondary increased mass of the vocal folds will affect vocal vibration and diminish vocal pitch.

Slight to significant changes in fluid concentration within the vocal fold with Reinke's edema may become apparent with hypothyroidism. In performers without other obvious causes of Reinke's space edema, a thyroid evaluation may be warranted. An assessment of thyroid function can be easily achieved by a standard assessment of circulating thyroid hormone, thyrotropin-releasing hormone, and thyroid-stimulating hormone. Hyper- and hypothyroidism can therefore be diagnosed.

The treatment of hypothyroidism is directed at finding the underlying etiology and subsequent thyroid replacement, with levothyroxine most commonly being used. In most cases, thyroid supplementation alone is all that is necessary to maintain good vocal physiology in the patient with hypothyroidism. Close monitoring should be maintained while patients are being treated, and an endocrinologist may be needed in the difficult to treat hypothyroid patient.

The treatment of hyperthyroidism can be more complex and multiple treatment modalities may be considered, including thyroid suppression with the use of antithyroid drugs, thyroid ablation, or surgical removal of the thyroid. An otolaryngologist or another thyroid surgeon and endocrinologist are often necessary for adequate evaluation and treatment of hyperthyroidism.

Diabetes

Diabetes mellitus is a disorder of carbohydrate metabolism that generally involves absolute or relative insulin deficiency, insulin resistance, or both. Multiple etiologic factors may be involved, but all lead to hyperglycemia (high levels of glucose in the blood), which is the hallmark of the disease.[122] Chronic microvascular disease can occur with secondary polyneuropathy, retinopathy, and neuropathy. Patients have also been found to have accelerated atherogenesis and cardiovascular disease.

While most endocrine abnormalities result in vocal dysfunction primarily through alterations in vocal fold fluid accumulation, diabetes mellitus appears to have a different mechanism. Diabetes results in microvascular disease with gradual vascular occlusion. With prolonged affect, muscle wasting may occur. In addition, xerostomia and zerophonia[123] can occur with diabetes likely due to decreased mucus production secondary to changes in glandular innervation.

The major effect of diabetes on the voice may be due to gradually progressive diabetic neuropathy. While early in the disease there may not be detectable voice changes, gradual loss of fine neuromuscular coordination may occur. In an organ such as the larynx in which fine neuromotor manipulations need to occur, minor changes in neuromuscular control can have perceptible alterations in voice, particularly in performing voices. With more advanced disease, progressive diabetic neuropathy can result in vocal fold paralysis with subsequent weak, breathy voice.[124] The rates of vocal changes that occur usually parallel the progression of the disease systemically.

In chronic diabetes, diminished sensation can occur that can affect the proprioception necessary for refined phonation. Weight loss and fatigue are common in diabetics, and such systemic and general health problems may also affect phonation. These patients are also at increased risk of infections that can result in inflammation, tissue edema, swelling, and irritation.

In many, particularly in those with adult onset diabetes, noticeable alterations in voice may never occur. Unfortunately, aggressive treatment in those with progressive disease may not significantly alter the rate of insidious progression. Voice modification and instruction with voice teachers and speech–language pathologists will help with maintenance of good vocal performance, especially with early changes. Hydration, humidification, salivary substitutes, and salivary stimulants will decrease the effects of diabetic-induced xerostomia. Aggressive treatment of pharyngeal or pulmonary infections should be undertaken. General measures to decrease weight loss and fatigue are also valuable.

In general, diabetics should be closely monitored and treated as needed by either an internist or an endocrinologist. With newer oral antihypoglycemic agents, satisfactory treatment may be accomplished without the need for insulin therapy; however, insulin is utilized in those with more refractory disease.

Sex Hormones

Voice alterations with changes in sex hormone levels can be significant. The most obvious changes in voice occur at puberty, particularly in males and to a less extent with aging. Although sex hormone-associated voice changes can occur with both sexes, problems associated with the sexual hormones are more common in the female vocalist.[123]

Sex Hormone Dysfunction

There are two phases to the cyclical ovarian cycle. The first is the follicular stage, which lasts for the first 14 days of the cycle, begins with the menstrual period, and ends just prior to ovulation. During this phase there are minimal levels of progesterone throughout with gradually increasing estrogen levels. At ovulation, peak estrogen levels are reached but progesterone remains at a relatively low level. In the luteal phase, after ovulation, gradually increasing progesterone levels occur, peaking in the midluteal phase, and there is a secondary minor estrogen peak premenstrually. It is during the secondary estrogen peak during the luteal phase that the premenstrual syndrome occurs.[125]

Estrogens in synergistic action with progesterone act as potent smooth muscle relaxants that result in vasodilation, increased blood volume, and decreased gastric motility. In addition, these in combination with aldosterone can result in increased salt and water retention.[126] It is suggested that the vasodilation and water retention effects of estrogen and progesterone are what results in the increased vocal fold swelling that occurs during the times of ovulation and premenstrually. In addition, the vasodilation that occurs with increases in these steroids results in nasal congestion and can change upper airways resonance.

The effect of the menstrual cycle on the voice has been an area of much debate and investigation. Epithelial characteristics may vary depending on whether estrogen or progesterone is predominant, with estrogen stimulation resulting in a thickened superficial epithelium of the vocal folds while progesterone has been found to be associated with development of the intermediate layer of the vocal folds. The voice changes that occur are usually due to water retention, edema, and dilation of mucosal veins.[127]

Some traditional, classical music and opera groups have allowed singers to be excused from performance during the premenstrual and early menstrual cycle. The term *laryngopathia menstrualis* is commonly used to describe the adverse effects on voice that occur in the immediate premenstrual period.[123] Even if hormonally related changes in voice occur, controversy exists as to whether more dysfunction occurs at ovulation or premenstrually.[128–133] Most studies have suggested that voice changes occur in the premenstrual portion of the menstrual cycle due to edema with subsequent increase in mass of the vocal folds.[128,130,131] An evaluation of voices of 38 women showed that the 22 with premenstrual vocal syndromes had evidence of luteal insufficiency by laryngeal smears while only two of sixteen had abnormal smears with no menstrual voice changes.[127]

In young women with no voice training, premenstrual hoarseness is uncommon.[128] Data are lacking to extrapolate such findings to the trained vocalist and therefore should not be generalized to the professional vocalist.[129,132] One recent study showed more significant changes in voice occurring at ovulation rather than premenstrually.[133]

Such conflicting reports make recommendations with regard to performances at various times during the menstrual cycle difficult. If a dysfunctional voice should occur, it will most likely be in the premenstrual period. Whether a noticeable change in voice will occur that would alter performance will have to be predicted individually. If concerns are raised, then objective voice assessments (see Chapters 8 and 10) can be made at varied times through the menstrual cycle. Such an evaluation will give information to the female vocalist as to whether performance schedules should be adjusted to suit the voice demands. If extreme voice changes are present that correlate with regular times during the menstrual cycle, then an endocrinologic assessment may better define if these are hormonally mediated. Hormonal therapy may be beneficial in some individuals.

In a similar context, exogenous hormones may be a cause for concern. Androgen hormones in female vocalists are regarded as contraindicated[123] unless medically indicated. Deepening in voice with lowering of the fundamental frequency with changes in timbre can occur.[134–136] Female body builders who use androgen steroids to increase muscle mass have been found to develop deepening voice, increased facial hair, increased aggressiveness, clitoral enlargement, and menstrual irregularities.[135]

The role of birth control pills and their effects on voice is somewhat less well established. Although evidence is present suggesting changes in voice due to birth control pill use,[123] many performers use birth control pills without noting adverse effects to their performances. As with any medication utilized by a performer, they must be used with caution and must be individualized to the situation. Birth control pills have differing androgen effects depending on the type of progesterone used. If a woman wishes to use these to prevent an unwanted pregnancy or to treat a sexual hormone endocrine dysfunction, it is prudent to assess the effects these may have at a time distant from an important performance. As with any new medication, all factors that are important to performance should be considered (see Chapter 5). Once birth control pills are taken regularly, quick changes in dosing or intermittent missed doses should be avoided. Again, the role of the objective voice laboratory to quantitate voice effects from birth control pills may gain valuable insight as to whether they should be used.

Irrespective of direct changes in voice that may occur, other problems may be associated with the menstrual cycle that can affect performance. Two significant problems are known to occur: dysmenorrhea and premenstrual syndrome (PMS). Dysmenorrhea, or painful menstruation, occurs to some degree in one-half of postmenarcheal women, and 10% of women may be incapacitated for 1 to 3 days each month.[137] In some populations, dysmenorrhea has been reported in as many as 72% of women.[138] It has been estimated to be the greatest cause of time lost from work and school.[139] The symptoms of dysmenorrhea include tiredness, nausea and vomiting, low back pain, nervousness, abdominal cramping, dizziness, diarrhea, and headaches. Estrogen stimulates uterine contraction, which results in abdominal cramping. Since progesterone inhibits uterine contraction it has been postulated that dysmenorrhea may be secondary to abnormalities in the estrogen/progesterone ratio during the luteal phase before menstruation, but no absolute data have been found to support this. Cramping can result in loss of abdominal support, which can affect the strength and control of the voice.

The treatment of dysmenorrhea includes symptomatic treatment with heat, exercise, reassurance, and, on rare instances, psychotherapy. Since there appears to be a significant prostaglandin effect, prostaglandin inhibition with aspirin or nonsteroidal antiinflammatory agents may diminish symptoms, although these should be used cautiously in vocal performers. Narcotics can be given if there is severe pain. Combined oral contraceptives have been utilized.

The other significant problem associated with the menstrual cycle is PMS, which is defined as a menstrual-related mood disorder that includes cyclical symptoms with relationship to menses that interfere with some aspects of life.[140] Many potential causes of PMS have been suggested, with most having to do with the physiologic effects of the changes in estrogen and progesterone concentrations. At present, evidence that supports a psychologic basis for menstrual-related mood disorders is lacking.[141]

Symptoms of PMS are those of an altered emotional state with anxiety, irritability, emotional liability, depression, some behavioral changes, decreased concentration, somatic complaints including headache, backache, and muscle pain, fatigue and lethargy, change in appetite, abdominal bloating and edema, change in coordination and dizziness, and autonomic nervous system disorders with nausea, diarrhea, and palpitations. In addition, the increased estrogen response results in increased retention of water and sodium.

As with dysmenorrhea, therapy for PMS has been directed toward symptomatic and pharmacologic treatments. With both dysmenorrhea and PMS, such effects on general well being can affect the quality of performance. Water retention may have a direct effect on the vocal fold vibration. Nausea, vomiting, and somatic complaints such as a backache and muscle pain can affect abdominal and skeletal support of the voice. The altered emotional states, behavioral changes, and decreased concentration along with the change in appetite and difficulty sleeping can affect the focus and fine motor tuning necessary for optimal voice production.

Menopause

Menopause is a hypoestrogenic state with signs and symptoms of hormonal insufficiency noted in tissues containing estrogen receptors. Hot flushes occur in 80% of all women.[142] These can alter REM sleep with sleep deprivation during periods of hot flushes.[143] Genital atrophy, cardiovascular disease, osteoporosis, and psychological symptoms also occur. The postmenopausal ovary secretes androgens but virtually no estrogen,[144] and masculinization of the voice can occur. Other symptoms in association with menopause, such as fatigue, nervousness, headaches, insomnia, dizziness, and decreased concentration, possibly may affect the performance. Many of these changes are transient but, if permanent, estrogen supplementation may result in alleviation of symptoms.

Pregnancy

Pregnancy may be a major concern to the performing female vocalist. Increased estrogen and progesterone secretions occur throughout pregnancy. Since estrogens in synergistic action with progesterone are potent smooth muscle relaxants, marked vasodilation with decreased peripheral vascular resistance and increased blood volume can occur.[126] Blood volume may increase as much as 40% to 55%.[125] Estrogen and progesterone along with aldosterone can result in increased salt and water retention. These factors can result in increased fluid retention, peripheral edema, or Reinke's space edema. The direct voice changes that occur with pregnancy are known as *laryngeopathia gravidarum*.[123] The increased vascularity may make the larynx more susceptible to traumatic injury from vocal overuse and misuse.

Decreased gastrointestinal motility can occur with a gradual increase in gastric emptying times and subsequent constipation. This, along with the gradually enlarging size of the uterus with subsequent compression of the thorax, can result in loss of some abdominal–pulmonary support of the voice via decreased lung capacity. GE reflux can result in reflux-related laryngitis. The extra weight can also have an effect on support, as it alters the mechanics of musculoskeletal stability.

Pregnancy represents a 725 mg iron drain to the mother and occasionally can result in anemia if not well supplemented.[126] These changes, along with the gradual increasing fatigue that occurs, can all affect the mother's ability to perform.

Pregnancy in itself is not a contraindication to performance; however, it is important for the performer to realize there may be changes that are not preventable. During these times conservative care of the voice seems paramount with appropriate behavioral changes to avoid voice injury.

Sex Hormones and the Male Voice

Hormonal changes in the male voice are restricted largely to periods of voice maturation. The cultivation of the postpubertal male soprano via castration has only historical context at this time. The adult male soprano endured from the 16th century until 1903, when Pope Pius X formally banned the practice of castrati.[145,146] Although sex hormonal dysfunction is less common and probably plays a lesser role in the male vocalist, except in unusual syndromal disorders, the thoughtful approach to a dysfunctional male voice should consider such problems in the differential diagnosis.

Sex Hormone Summary

The treatment of sex hormone dysfunction will require the assistance of medical specialists with expertise in this area. Although a primary care physician may be able to manage straightforward problems, more than likely a reproductive endocrinologist will be needed. By evaluating hormonal levels and comparing them to normal values, disturbances may be detected and hormonal treatment initiated.

SURGERY

The surgical approach to disorders of the larynx are discussed in some detail in Chapter 21. Surgery may be considered for a multitude of problems in the performing vocalist, and care must be taken to understand the implications of the surgical treatment upon performance and potentially on the vocalist's career. This care must be taken both by the performer and the treating surgeon to understand the indications for surgery and to establish the potential urgency of the operation. If there is a medical urgency in performing the operation, particularly if there is potential life- or limb-threatening adverse effects should it not be performed immediately, then accommodation may need to be made following surgery to reestablish the best environment for vocalization. However, in most cases operations are not performed on an urgent basis, and the timing of the operation can be selected according to the performer's schedule. In nonlife-threatening and, particularly, in purely elective surgical procedures the potential risks to the voice must be weighed and addressed prior to proceeding.

Surgery in the pharynx, oral cavity, nasopharynx and nose can affect subsequent resonation. The most common problems that might require surgical intervention include recurrent infectious processes such as chronic or recurrent sinusitis or tonsillitis. Functional or obstructive problems such as adenoid, tonsil, or turbinate hypertrophy, recurrent turbinate swelling, or a nasal–septal deviation might be present without any significant documented evidence of problems with resonation. In the author's practice, tonsillectomy has been performed for recurrent or acute tonsillitis in a number of vocalists without any perceivable long-term effect on their voices. With surgery of the upper airways, however, care must be taken to protect the function of the vocal tract.[147] Careful surgical dissection should be directed toward avascular and appropriate planes in as atraumatic a manner as possible. Avoidance of excessive scarring and maintenance of the normal anatomic–physiologic relationship is critical. Surgery in the oral cavity, teeth, or temporomandibular joint area may affect articulation, and therefore caution must be taken in these areas.

Surgery to structures in the neck may affect the voice by postsurgical scarring, which can occur in the soft tissues of the neck or perilaryngeal muscles. The vertical motion of the larynx may subsequently be inhibited. Neck surgery in and around the nerve supply to the larynx, particularly the close relationship of the thyroid gland and the recurrent laryngeal nerves, may predispose to injury to those structures. The surgeon and vocalist must be well aware of the potential risks, and these must be weighed in lieu of the underlying surgical–medical disorder and the career of the individual.

Since the lungs and chest are necessary for adequate respiration for vocal function, surgery to the chest or lungs can be a significant hazard to the performing vocalist. Resection of portions of the lung or partial lobectomies are sometimes medically indicated, and therefore the main concern is appropriate rehabilitation to increase lung volume and respiratory support. Surgery to the ribcage or chest wall may also interfere with respiration.

Surgery involving the musculoskeletal system, particularly the neck, back, and legs, will affect the support of the voice. The singer must be aware of the potential risks with potential increased fatiguability from inadequate support and improper posturing following such surgery. Physical therapy and thorough voice instruction will minimize the side effects.

The abdomen plays a prominent role in respiratory support. Surgery in the abdomen will involve incisions through the abdominal musculature and can result in significant postoperative pain. It has been recommended that the surgeon be cautioned to minimize damage to the muscular structures.[148] Postabdominal surgery rehabilitation is critical for the establishment of appropriate vocal support. It has been recommended that the abdominal musculature should be restrengthened prior to reassuming aggressive vocal activity. Sataloff recommends that singers be able to perform 10 sit-ups before resuming singing following abdominal or thoracic surgery.[149]

Performing voice users are often in a position of high visibility where not only their voices but their general physical appearance is critical for career development. In some cases this might cause the singer to evaluate his or her appearance to determine if surgical alteration in appearance or cosmetic surgery might be beneficial. In the aging singer or speaker, who is also often very aware of the role of personal appearance, plastic or cosmetic surgery is often considered.

As with all surgical procedures, the vocalist must be aware that there are potential risks associated with these procedures. In elective surgery, such as cosmetic surgery, the risk to benefit ratio must be weighed carefully to determine if the potential benefits from the cosmetic appearance change is worth the potential risks. In all cases, the history of performance scheduling should be taken into consideration to make sure that any acute effects following surgery have had time to resolve and the individual has had adequate ability to compensate for them. Such concerns are addressed in detail in the chapter on the vocal history (Chapter 5). Most facial cosmetic operations should not result in long restrictions in voice use and would not be expected to alter vocalization significantly.

Facelift surgery, or rhytidectomy, can affect the ability to relax the upper neck and facial muscles. If done properly and in an appropriate surgical plane, this should resolve in a short period of time. Nasal or rhinoplastic surgery is often performed in conjunction with a septoplasty. In most regards, this would be expected to improve the nasal breathing; however, changes in resonation for a short period of time might be expected. It is generally felt that facial cosmetic surgery is not contraindicated in the vocalist and should not have any long-term effects. Spiegel et al[150] have recommended from 0 to 6 weeks of voice restriction following various cosmetic surgical procedures.

With most surgical procedures, some anesthesia must be utilized. This can vary between a small amount of local anesthetic, a combination of local anesthesia and intravenous sedation, or general anesthetic depending on the type and character of the operation. Anesthesia itself has its own risks. In elective surgical procedures, anesthetic risks must be taken into account. With many surgical procedures that require endotracheal intubation, potential injury to the larynx can occur. It is prudent for the surgeon and the vocalist to inform the anesthesiologist of the importance of nontraumatic intubation and if possible the utilization of smaller endotracheal tubes. In some situations, a small amount of systemic corticosteroids may be utilized during or at the completion of the operation to minimize potential vocal fold swelling. Postanesthesia nausea and vomiting can occur that also irritates the delicate mucosa of the larynx. With more prolonged intubation there is a possibility of small ulcerations or granulomas on the vocal processes of the arytenoids.

Appropriate caution by both the surgeon and anesthesiologist will minimize such risks. In instances in which either a local or general anesthetic may be administered it might be preferred to elect the local anesthetic to diminish the potential risks associated with intubation. Fortunately, in most instances minimal laryngeal trauma occurs with general anesthesia and laryngotracheal intubation.

The keys to surgery in the performing vocalist rely on appropriate assessment of the risk-benefit relationship of the potential surgical procedure, appropriate selection of a surgeon and anesthesiologist who are aware of the unique risks associated with surgery to the performing vocalist, and proper preoperative and postoperative care. If voice activity needs to be minimized for some period of time around the time of the surgical procedure, the vocalist should be aware that muscular changes can occur within 2 to 3 weeks of minimal voice utilization. Therefore a gradual progressive strengthening program should be initiated at the resumption of singing or speaking activities. The help of a speech–language pathologist or voice teacher may be critical in working with the individual during the time of postsurgical voice resumption.

SUMMARY OF MEDICAL PROBLEMS

As can be seen, multiple medical problems can have an effect on vocalization. In the performer whose voice does not improve despite general intensive measures with vocal hygiene, hydration, and adequate speech and singing instruction, other medical disorders should be investigated. On occasion obvious laryngeal abnormalities such as vocal nodules, polyps, Reinke's space edema, and contact ulcers may not be due to the type or amount of vocal activity but rather to a systemic cause. Appropriate awareness of these potential etiologies, adequate assessment, and referrals to medical and surgical specialists may allow for a quick diagnosis and institution of treatment. It is fortunate that most of the medical problems that can affect the voice are readily diagnosable and treatable if they are considered as sources of dysfunction and diagnosed in a timely fashion.

REFERENCES

1. Hasbrouk JM, Kenevan R: *Speech Physiology for the Head and Neck Surgeon.* Alexandria, VA, American Academy of Otolaryngology Head and Neck Surgery, 1991, pp 1–108.
2. Sherman WM: Carbohydrate, muscle glycogen, and improved performance. *Phys Sports Med* 15:157–164, 1987.
3. Council on Scientific Affairs, American Medical Association: Dietary fiber and health. *JAMA* 262:542–546, 1989.
4. Consensus Conference, National Institutes of Health: Lowering blood cholesterol to prevent heart disease. *JAMA* 253:2080–2086, 1985.
5. Tran ZV, Weltman A: Differential effects of exercise on serum lipid and lipoprotein levels seen with changes in body weight: A meta-analysis. *JAMA* 254:919–924, 1985.
6. Blair SN, Kohl HW, Paffenbarger RS, et al: Physical fitness and all-cause mortality: A prospective study of healthy men and women. *JAMA* 262:2395–2401, 1989.
7. Sataloff RT: Professional singers: The science and art of clinical care. *Am J Otolaryngol* 2:251–266, 1981.
8. Weinstein CE: Managing sleep disorders in the elderly patient. *Cleve Clin J Med* 56:666–667, 1989.
9. Jiang H, et al: Mortality and apnea index in obstructive sleep apnea: Experience in 385 male patients. *Chest* 94:9–14, 1988.
10. Thawley SE: Obstructive sleep apnea. *Insights Otolaryngol* 1:1–8, 1986.
11. Millman RP: Sleep apnea and nasal patency. *Am J Rhinol* 2:177–182, 1988.

12. Hall JB: The cardiopulmonary failure of sleep-disordered breathing. *JAMA* 255:930–933, 1986.
13. Katsantonis GP, Miyanzaki S, Walsh JK: Effects of uvulopalatopharyngoplasty on sleep architecture and patterns of obstructed breathing. *Laryngoscope* 100:1068–1072, 1990.
14. Roussen C, Macklem PT: The respiratory muscles. *N Engl J Med* 307:786–800, 1982.
15. Greenberg SD: The lungs and their response to disease. *Res Staff Phys* 29:28–35, 1983.
16. Patow CA, Kaliner M: Nasal and cardiopulmonary reflexes. *Ear Nose Throat* 63:22–28, 1984.
17. McFadden ER. Nasal-sinus-pulmonary reflexes and bronchial asthma. *J Allergy Clin Immunol* 78:1–3, 1986.
18. Drettner B: Pathophysiological relationships between upper and lower airways. *Ann Otol Rhinol Laryngol* 79:499–503, 1970.
19. Rubin RM: Effects of nasal airway obstruction on facial growth. *Ear Nose Throat* 66:44–53, 1987.
20. Meredith GM: The airway and dentofacial development. *Ear Nose Throat* 66:7–16, 1987.
21. Kline JC: Nasal respiratory function and craniofacial growth. *Arch Otolaryngol Head Neck Surg* 112:843–849, 1986.
22. Principato JJ: Upper airway obstruction and craniofacial morphology. *Otolaryngol Head Neck Surg* 104:881–890, 1991.
23. Polsic WP, Pasquasiello PS, Baranak CC, et al: Relief of upper airway obstruction by adenotonsillectomy. *Otolaryngol Head Neck Surg* 9:476–480, 1986.
24. Williams AJ, Baghat MS, Stableforth DE, et al: Dysphonia caused by inhaled steroids: recognition of a characteristic laryngeal abnormality. *Thorax* 38:813–821, 1983.
25. Toogwood JH, Jennings B, Greenuay RW, Chuang L: Candidiasis and dysphonia complicating beclemethasone treatment of asthma. *J Allergy Clin Immunol* 65:145–153, 1980.
26. Tager IB, Weiss ST, Munoy A, et al: Longitudinal study of the effects of maternal smoking on pulmonary function in children. *N Engl J Med* 309:699–703, 1983.
27. Sachs F, Lee KJ: The chest, in Lee KJ (ed): *Essential Otolaryngology.* New York, Medical Examination Publishing, 1987, pp 775–797.
28. Niimi S, Bell-Berti F, Harris KS: Dynamic aspects of velopharyngeal closure. *Folia Phoniatr* 34:246–257, 1982.
29. Benninger MS, Carwell MA, Finnegan EM, et al: Flexible direct nasopharyngolaryngoscopy in association with vocal pedagogy. *Med Prob Perf Art* 4:163–167, 1989.
30. Levine HL: The office diagnosis of nasal and sinus disorders using rigid nasal endoscopy. *Otolaryngol Head Neck Surg* 102:370–373, 1990.
31. Benninger MS, Mickelson SA, Yaremchuk K: Functional endoscopic sinus surgery: Morbidity and early results. *Henry Ford Hosp Med J* 38:5–8, 1990.
32. America's allergists underestimate their allergic patient potential, in *Frontline.* Abbott Laboratories, 1991.
33. Zeiger RS: Allergic and nonallergic rhinitis: Classification and pathogenesis. Part I. Allergic rhinitis. *Am J Rhinol* 3:21–47, 1989.
34. King WP: Allergic disorders in the otolaryngolic practice. *Otolaryngol Clin North Am* 18:677–690, 1985.
35. Slaven RG: Sinusitis in adults and its relation to allergic rhinitis, asthma, and nasal polyps. *J Allergy Clin Immunol* 82:950–955, 1988.
36. Norman PS: Allergic rhinitis. *J Allergy Clin Immunol* 75:531–545, 1985.
37. Druce HM, Koliner MA: Allergic rhinitis. *JAMA* 259:260–263, 1988.
38. Rosenberg P: Allergy and immunology, in Lee KJ (ed): *Essential Otolaryngology Head and Neck Surgery.* New York, Medical Examinations Publishing, 1987, pp 759–773.
39. Matthews KP: Respiratory atopic disease. *JAMA* 248:2587–2610, 1982.
40. Baker BM, Baker CD, Le HT: Vocal quality, articulation and audiological characteristics of children and young adults with diagnosed allergies. *Ann Otol Rhinol Laryngol* 91:277–280, 1982.
41. Clemis JD, Derlacki EL: Allergy of the upper respiratory tract. *Otolaryngol Clin North Am* 3:265–276, 1970.
42. Pang LQ: Allergy of the larynx, trachea, and bronchial tree. *Otolaryngol Clin North Am* 7:719–734, 1974.
43. Brodnitz FS: Allergy of the larynx. *Otolaryngol Clin North Am* 4:579–582, 1971.
44. Williams RJ: Allergic laryngitis. *Ann Otol* 81:558–565, 1972.
45. Hillerdol GG, Lindholm H: Laryngeal edema as the only symptoms of hypersensitivity of salicylic acid and other substances. *J Laryngol Otol* 98:547–548, 1984.
46. Settipane GA, Chaffee FH: Nasal polyps in asthma and rhinitis. A review of 6,037 patients. *J Allergy Clin Immunol* 59:17–21, 1977.
47. Kivity S, Bibitt, Schwartz Y, et al: Variable vocal cord dysfunction presenting as wheezing and exercise-induced asthma. *J Asthma* 23:241–244, 1986.
48. Haapanen ML: Provoked laryngeal dysfunction. *Folia Phoniatr* 42:157–169, 1990.
49. Solis-Cohen J: The treatment of laryngitis in professionals unable to rest, in *Transactions of the Ninth Annual Meeting of the American Laryngological Society.* New York, D. Appleton and Company, 1888, pp 155–160.

50. Petty TL: The national mucolytic study. Results of a randomized, double-blind, placebo-controlled study of iodinated glycerol in chronic obstructive bronchitis. *Chest* 97:75–83, 1990.

51. Ziment I: Help for an overtaxed mucociliary system: Managing abnormal mucus. *J Respir Dis* 12:21–33, 1991.

52. Nuutenen J, Halopainen E, Haahtela T, et al: Balanced physiological saline in the treatment of chronic rhinitis. *Rhinology* 24:265–269, 1986.

53. Delafuente JC, Davis TA, Davis JA: Pharmacotherapy of allergic rhinitis. *Clin Pharmacol* 8:474–485, 1989.

54. Siegel SC: Topical intranasal corticosteroid therapy in rhinitis. *J Allergy Clin Immunol* 81:984–991, 1988.

55. Shemen LJ: Salivary glands: Benign and malignant disease, in Lee KJ (ed): *Essential Otolaryngology Head and Neck Surgery*. New York, Medical Examinations Publishing, 1987, pp 449–473.

56. Snaith ML: Sjögren's syndrome, in Scott JT (ed): *Copeman's Textbook of Rheumatic Diseases*. Edinburgh, Churchill Livingstone, 1986, pp 1386–1403.

57. Klestow AC, Webb J, Latt D, et al: Treatment of xerostomia: A double-blind trial in 108 patients with Sjögren's syndrome. *Oral Med Oral Surg* 51:594–599, 1981.

58. Green JC, Louie R, Wycoff SJ: Preventive dentistry I. Dental caries. *JAMA* 262:3459–3463, 1989.

59. Green JC, Louie R, Wycoff, SJ: Preventive dentistry II. Periodontal diseases, malocclusion, trauma, and oral cancer. *JAMA* 263:421–425, 1990.

60. Rugh JD, Solberg WK: Psychological implications in temporomandibular pain and dysfunction. *Oral Sci Rev* 7:3–30, 1976.

61. Bronstein SL: Update on temporomandibular joint problems: Diagnosis and treatment. *Res Staff Phys* 34: 71–87, 1988.

62. Howard JA: Temporomandibular joint disorders, facial pain and dental problems in performing artists, in Sataloff RT, Brandforandbrener AG, Ledermen RJ (eds): *Textbook of Performing Arts Medicine*. New York, Raven Press, 1991, pp 111–169.

63. Koufman J, Blalock PD: Vocal fatigue and dysphonia in the professional voice user: Bogart-Bacall syndrome. *Laryngoscope* 98:493–498, 1988.

64. Belisle GM, Morrison MD: Anatomic correlation for muscle tension dysphonia. *J Otolaryngol* 12:319–321, 1983.

65. Morrison MD, Rammage LA, Belisle GM, et al: Muscular tension dysphonia. *J Otolaryngol* 12:302–306, 1983.

66. Minifie FD, Hixon TJ, Williams F (eds): *Normal Aspects of Speech Hearing and Language*. Englewood Cliffs, NJ: Prentice Hall, 1973, pp 143–144.

67. Boone DR: *The Voice and Voice Therapy*, 2nd ed. Englewood Cliffs, NJ, Prentice Hall, 1973, pp 23–31.

68. Brodnitz F: Vocal rehabilitation in benign lesions of the vocal cords. *J Speech Hear Disorders* 23:112–117, 1958.

69. Benninger MS, Finnegan EM, Kraus DH, et al: The whisper and whistle: The role in vocal trauma. *Med Prob Perf Art* 3:151–154, 1988.

70. Hufnagle J, Hufnagle K: Is quiet whisper harmful to the vocal mechanism? A research note. *Percept Motor Skills* 57:735–737, 1983.

71. Pressman JJ, Keleman G: Physiology of the larynx. *Physiol Rev* 35:506–554, 1955.

72. Kirchner Penn JP: Voice and speech patterns of the hard of hearing. *Acta Otol Laryngolog* [Suppl] 124:1–69, 1955.

73. Hughes GB, Nordar RH: Physiology of hearing, in Hughes GB: *Textbook of Clinical Otology*. New York, Thieme-Stratton, 1985, pp 71–77.

74. Albright M, Lee KJ: Audiology, in Lee KJ (ed): *Essential Otolaryngology Head and Neck Surgery*. New York, Medical Examination Publishing, 1987, pp 27–72.

75. Axellsson A, Lindgren F: Hearing in classical musicians. *Acta Otolaryngol [Suppl]* 371:1–74, 1981.

76. Klajman S, Koldej E, Kowalska A: Investigation of musical abilities in hearing-impaired and normal-hearing children. *Folia Phoniatr* 34:229–233, 1982.

77. Benninger MS: Treating swimmer's ear. *Triathlon Today* July:37, 1990.

78. Karlsson K, Lundquist PG, Olaussen T: The hearing of symphony orchestra musicians. *Scand Audiol* 12: 257–264, 1983.

79. Westmore GA, Eversden ID: Noise-induced hearing loss and orchestral musicians. *Arch Otolaryngol* 107: 761–764, 1981.

80. Flach M: The musician's hearing seen by the otologist. *Msch Ohrhk* 106:424–432, 1972.

81. Grycznska D, Czyzewski I: Damaging effect of music on the hearing organ in musicians. *Otolaryngol Polska* 31:527–532, 1977.

82. Johnson DW, Sherman RE, Aldridge J, Lorraine A: Effects of instrument type and orchestral position on hearing sensitivity for 0.25 to 20 kHz in the orchestral musician. *Scand Audiol* 14:215–221, 1985.

83. Nodar RH: The effects of aging and loud music on hearing. *Cleve Clin Q* 53:49–52, 1986.

84. Speaks C, Nelson D, Ward WD: Hearing loss in rock and roll musicians. *J Occup Med* 12:216–219, 1970.

85. Axellson A, Lindgren F: Hearing in pop musicians. *Arch Otolaryngol* 85:225–231, 1978.
86. Goodman RS: Output intensity of home stereo headphones. *Ear Nose Throat J* 59:330–333, 1980.
87. *USA Today*, 1988.
88. Franks JR: Judgments of hearing aid processed music. *Ear Hearing* 3:18–23, 1982.
89. Chalot NI: Some psychologic aspects of deafness: Beethoven, Goya, and Oscar Wilde. *Am J Otolaryngol* 1: 240–246, 1980.
90. Nebel OT, Forbes MF, Castell DO: Symptomatic gastroesophageal reflux: Incidence and precipitating factors. *Am J Dig Dis* 21:953–956, 1976.
91. Nebel OT, Castell DO: Lower esophageal sphincter pressure changes after food ingestion. *Gastroenterology* 63:778–783, 1972.
92. Dennish GW, Castell DO: Inhibitory effect of smoking on the lower esophageal sphincter. *N Engl J Med* 284:1136–1137, 1971.
93. Meyer GW, Castell DO: Evaluation and management of diseases of the esophagus. *Am J Otolaryngol* 2: 336–343, 1981.
94. Koufman JA: The otolaryngologic manifestations of gastroesophageal reflux (GERD): A clinical investigation of 225 patients using ambulatory pH monitoring and an experimental investigation of the role of acid and pepsin in the development of laryngeal injury. *Laryngoscope [Suppl]* 53:1–78, 1991.
95. Sataloff RT: Common diagnoses and treatments in professional singers. *Ear Nose Throat* 66:28–46, 1987.
96. Cantwell JD: Carbohydrate loading. *JAMA* 256:3024, 1986.
97. Bernstein LM, Baker LA: A clinical test of esophagitis. *Gastroenterology* 34:760–781, 1958.
98. Katz PO: Ambulatory esophageal and hypopharyngeal pH monitoring in patients with hoarseness. *Am J Gastroenterol* 85:38–40, 1990.
99. Sontag S, Robinson M, McCallum RW, et al: Ranitidine therapy for gastroesophageal reflux disease. *Arch Intern Med* 147:1485–1491, 1987.
100. *Drug Facts and Comparison*. St. Louis, MO, Facts and Comparisons, Inc, 1991, pp 291–326.
101. Behar JN, Ramsley G: Gastric emptying and antral motility in reflux esophagitis. *Gastroenterology* 74: 253–256, 1978.
102. Konig WF, vonLeden H: The peripheral nervous system of the human larynx I. The mucus membrane. *Arch Otolaryngol* 73:1–14, 1961.
103. Kirchner JA: Laryngeal afferent systems in phonatory control. *ASHA Rep* 11:31–35, 1981.
104. Ward PH: Superior laryngeal paralysis: An often overlooked entity. *Laryngoscope* 84:78–89, 1977.
105. Abelson T, Tucker HM: Laryngeal findings in superior laryngeal nerve paralysis: A controversy. *Otolaryngol Head Neck Surg* 89:463–470, 1981.
106. Tucker HM: Vocal cord paralysis—1979: Etiology and management. *Laryngoscope* 90:585–590, 1989.
107. Isshiki N, Okamura H, Ishikawa T: Thyroplasty type I (lateral compression) for dysphonia due to vocal cord paralysis or atrophy. *Arch Otolaryngol* 80:465–473, 1975.
108. Koufman JA: Laryngoplasty for vocal cord medialization: An alternative to Teflon. *Laryngoscope* 96:726–731, 1986.
109. Crumley RL: Update: Ansa cervicalis to recurrent laryngeal nerve anastomosis for unilateral laryngeal paralysis. *Laryngoscope* 101:384–388, 1991.
110. Tucker HM: Reinnervation of the unilaterally paralyzed larynx. *Ann Otol Rhinol Laryngol* 86:789–794, 1977.
111. Ford CN, Bless DM: Clinical experience with injectable collagen for vocal fold augmentation. *Laryngoscope* 96:863–869, 1986.
112. Hallett M: Classification and treatment of tremor. *JAMA* 266:1115–1117, 1991.
113. Garfinkle TJ, Kimmelman CP: Neurologic disorders: Amyotophic lateral sclerosis, myasthenia gravis, multiple sclerosis, and poliomyelitis. *Am J Otolaryngol* 3:204–212, 1982.
114. Grob D: Myasthenia gravis. *Arch Intern Med* 108:615–638, 1961.
115. Rontel M, Rontel E, Leuchter W, Rolnick M: Voice spectrography in the evaluation of myasthenia gravis of the larynx. *Ann Otol Rhinol Laryngol* 87:722–728, 1978.
116. Boucher RM, Hendrix RA: The otolaryngic manifestations of multiple sclerosis. *Ear Nose Throat* 70:224–233, 1991.
117. Scheinberg L, Smith CB: Rehabilitation of patients with multiple sclerosis. *Neurol Clin* 5:585–598, 1987.
118. Larson PR: The thyroid in Wyngaarden JB, Smith LH (eds): *Cecil's Textbook of Medicine*, 18th ed, vol 2. Philadelphia, W.B. Saunders, 1988, pp. 1315–1344.
119. Malinsky M, Chevrie-Muller, Cerceau N: Clinical and electrophysiological study of voice changes in thyrotoxicosis. *Ann Endocrinol (Paris)* 38:171–172, 1977.
120. Watt-Boolsen S, Blichert-Toft M, Boberg A: Influence of thyroid surgery on voice function and laryngeal symptoms. *Br J Surg* 66:535–536, 1979.
121. Ritter FN: The effect of hypothyroidism on the larynx of the rat: An explanation for hoarseness associated with hypothyroidism in the human. *Ann Otol Rhinol Laryngol* 73:404–416, 1964.
122. Olefsky JM: Diabetes mellitus, in Wyngaarden JB, Smith LK (eds): *Cecil's Textbook of Medicine*, 18th ed, vol 2. Philadelphia, W.B. Saunders, 1988, pp 1360–1381.

123. Sataloff RT: Endocrine dysfunction, in Sataloff RT (ed): *Professional Voice. The Science and Art of Clinical Care*. New York, Raven Press, 1991, pp 201–205.

124. Vaughan CW: Diagnosis and treatment of organic voice disorders. *N Engl J Med* 307:863–866, 1982.

125. Hume RF, Killan AP: Maternal physiology, in Scott JR, Disaia PJ, Hammond CB, Spellacy WN (eds): *Danforth's Obstetrics and Gynecology*, 6th ed. Philadelphia, J.B. Lippincott, 1990, pp 93–100.

126. Rovisky JJ: Maternal physiology in pregnancy, in Sciarro JJ (ed): *Gynecology and Obstetrics*, vol II. Philadelphia, J.B. Lippincott, 1990, pp 1–19.

127. Abitbol J, deBrux J, Millot G, et al: Does a hormonal vocal cord cycle exist in women? Study of vocal premenstrual syndrome in voice performers by videostroboscopy glottography and cytology on 38 women. *J Voice* 3:157–162, 1989.

128. Silverman E, Zimmer CH: Effect of menstrual cycle on voice quality. *Arch Otolaryngol* 104:7–10, 1978.

129. Brodnitz FS: Menstrual cycle and voice quality. *Arch Otolaryngol* 105:300, 1979.

130. Smith FM: Hoarseness, a symptom of premenstrual tension. *Arch Otolaryngol* 75:66–68, 1962.

131. Brodnitz F: Hormones and the human voice. *Bull NY Acad Med* 47:183–191, 1971.

132. Silverman EM: Letter in reply. *Arch Otolaryngol* 105:300, 1979.

133. Higgin MB, Sarman JH: Variations in vocal frequency perturbation across the menstrual cycle. *J Voice* 3:233–243, 1989.

134. Damste PH: Virilization of the voice due to anabolic steroids. *Folia Phoniatr* 16:10–18, 1964.

135. Strauss RH, Liggett MT, Lanese RR: Anabolic steroid use and perceived effects in ten weight-trained women athletes. *JAMA* 253:2871–2873, 1985.

136. Damste PH: Voice changes in adult women caused by virilization agents. *J Speech Hear Disord* 32:126–132, 1967.

137. Wentz AC: Dysmenorrhea, premenstrual syndrome and related disorders, in Jones HW, Wentz AC, Burnett LS (eds): *Novak's Textbook of Gynecology*. Baltimore, Williams & Wilkins, 1988, pp 240–262.

138. Andersch B, Milson I: An epidemiologic study of young women with dysmenorrhea. *Am J Obstet Gynecol* 144:655–660, 1982.

139. Bergso P: Socioeconomic implications of dysmenorrhea. *Acta Obstet Gynecol Scand (Suppl)* 87:67–68, 1979.

140. Rubinov DR, Roy-Byrne P: Premenstrual syndromes: Overview from a methodologic perspective. *Am J Psychiatry* 141:163–172, 1984.

141. Gannon L: Evidence for a psychological etiology of menstrual disorders: A critical review. *Psychol Rep* 48:287–294, 1971.

142. Anderson E, Hamburger S, Liu JH, Rebar RW: Characteristics of menopausal women seeking assistance. *Am J Obstet Gynecol* 156:428–433, 1987.

143. Mezrow G, Rebar RW: The menopause, in Sciarra JJ (ed): *Gynecology and Obstetrics*, vol II. Philadelphia, J.B. Lippincott, 1990, pp 1–22.

144. Judd HL, Judd GE, Lucas WE, et al: Endocrine function of the postmenopausal ovary concentrations of androgens and estrogens in ovarian and peripheral vein blood. *J Clin Endocrinol Metab* 39:1020–1024, 1974.

145. Smith AM: Eunuchs and castrations: JAMA faces the music. *JAMA* 266:655–656, 1991.

146. Walker T: Castrato, in *The New Grove Dictionary of Music and Musicians*. London, Macmillan, 1980, pp 875–876.

147. Gould WJ: Surgery in professional singers. *Ear Nose Throat* 66:35–42, 1987.

148. Gould WJ: Some specific medical problems of professional operatic singers. *Cleve Clin Q* 53:45–47, 1986.

149. Sataloff RT: Care of the professional voice, in Sataloff RT, Brandfonbrener A, Lederman R (eds): *Textbook of Performing Arts Medicine*. New York, Raven Press, 1991, pp 229–286.

150. Spiegel JR, Sataloff RT, Haukshaw WM: Facial plastic surgery in professional voice users, in Sataloff RT: *Professional Voice. The Science and Art of Clinical Care*. New York, Raven Press, 1991, pp 301–308.

15

Medications and Their Effects on the Voice

ROBERT THAYER SATALOFF, MD, DMA
VAN L. LAWRENCE, MD
MARY J. HAWKSHAW, RN, BSN
DEBORAH C. ROSEN, RN, MS

Nearly every medication has some laryngeal effect, although in most cases the effects are so minor as to be clinically insignificant. However, many common medications have significant impact on the voice and larynx, and all physicians caring for professional voice users should be familiar with drug-induced phenomena that can alter vocal function.

In discussing medications, one must remember that substantial biologic variability exists in response to a given "recommended dose." In addition to individual response tendencies, medication effects and side effects may be influenced by age, metabolic status, sex, body composition, concurrent use of other medications, and other factors. A "recommended dose" is the amount of drug usually necessary to produce the desired pharmacologic effect in most patients, while minimizing the occurrence of serious side effects. Recommended doses are only guidelines. Optimizing the relationship between desired effects and undesirable side effects requires individualization in all patients, and especially in professional voice users for whom many "minor" side effects may be disabling.

In this chapter, we discuss medications used to treat many problems commonly encountered in professional voice users, as well as voice complications from medications used for ailments outside the head and neck.[1]

ANTIBIOTICS

In professional voice users, when antibiotics are used, high doses are recommended to achieve therapeutic blood levels rapidly, especially if important performances are imminent. When patients have no pressing engagements, antibiotic use should be based on culture results whenever appropriate (e.g., throat infections), as with patients who are not voice professionals. However, in the common situation in which a performance must proceed and when there is clinical evidence of bacterial infection, antibiotics should be instituted after cultures are taken without waiting for the results. The potential damage of delayed treatment in an active performer is greater than the potential harm of antibiotic use for an unproven organism.

ANTIVIRAL AGENTS

A few antiviral agents are now available. Acyclovir is used specifically for herpes and may be appropriate in patients with herpetic recurrent superior laryngeal nerve paralysis. Amantadine appears useful against influenza A.[2–5] It may also have some beneficial effects against other viruses. If a performer must work in an area in which there is a flu epidemic, it may be reasonable to use this drug. However, agitation, tachycardia, and extreme xerostomia and xerophonia may occur. When these side effects are present, they are generally severe enough to require cancellation of a performance.

ANTIHISTAMINES

Normal phonation requires uninhibited movement of the vibratory margin of the vocal folds, and normal mucosal secretions are exceedingly important. If vocal tract lubrication is impaired, aberrations in phonation occur. When singers or public speakers develop thick, viscous vocal fold secretions during performance, the effects can be catastrophic. Excessive drying of the upper respiratory tract is the vocal complication associated with the largest number of medications, and it is especially prominent following antihistamine ingestion.

Antihistamines may be used to treat allergies. However, virtually all antihistamines can exert a drying effect on upper respiratory tract secretions, although severity varies widely from drug to drug and from person to person. In addition, antihistamines are often combined with sympathomimetic or parasympatholytic agents that further reduce and thicken mucosal secretion and may reduce lubrication to the point of producing a dry cough. This may be more harmful to phonation than the allergic condition itself. Often the laryngologist will find that a patient has self-medicated with an over-the-counter (OTC) antihistamine preparation. The majority of antihistamine agents are acetylcholine antagonists, and this parasympatholytic activity probably accounts for the increased viscosity of secretions. Interestingly, antihistamines used to treat allergies do not act to block the stimulant effects of histamine upon gastric acid secretions, but do affect salivary glands and mucous-secreting membranes of the respiratory tract. They may also have sedative effects that impair sensorium and disturb performance. They are different from the effects achieved by antihistamines used to treat other conditions such as gastroesophageal reflux (cimetidine, ranitidine, and other H_2-blockers). Mild, newer antihistamines such as Seldane (Merrill Dow) produce less drowsiness and often less dryness; but in many people they are also less effective than drugs with more disturbing side effects. Mild antihistamines in small doses, or pediatric doses for adults, may be helpful for performers with intermittent allergic symptoms, but the medications should be tried between, not immediately prior to performances. When medication is needed for an acute allergic response shortly before performance, oral or injected corticosteroids usually accomplish the desired result without causing significant side effects.

Clinically, the most commonly encountered antihistamines are those belonging to the alkylamine or chlorpheniramine family. Because they have been recently deregulated by the FDA, these agents are being used with increasing frequency. Diphenhydramine is also present in some OTC sleep aids. Some of these aids also include scopolamine (which has a significant drying effect), presumably for its sedative effect. Promethazine is contained in several antitussive mixtures and can dry glottic secretions. Meclizine, an OTC antihistamine used for dizziness and motion sickness, is also commonly used. All anti-histamines provide some degree of relief from motion sickness, and to a greater or lesser degree all cause drying.

MUCOLYTIC AND WETTING AGENTS

Viscosity of the patient's upper respiratory tract secretions is affected significantly by environmental dryness. Feder[6] has described the drying effects of airplane flight and the resultant irritation of respiratory tract mucosa. Similar problems occur when mountain climbing or traveling to cities located at high altitudes. The coaching staffs of athletic teams have long been aware of the deleterious effects of dehydration upon general body function. These well-known factors may impinge on the vocal professional as a result of recreational practices, such as jogging, especially if done in hot or dry environments, or as a consequence of strenuous rehearsal and performance.

Viscosity of upper respiratory secretions is directly related to the availability of body water, assuming that no metabolic or pharmacologic agents have been interposed. The ideal wetting agent for respiratory tract secretions is water in the form of increased fluid intake and an elevated environmental humidity. Other wetting agents often used for dry respiratory tract secretions are expectorants or mucolytics. Although these agents are less effective than water and subject to individual variation, dry mucous membranes will usually respond favorably. Iodinated glycerol (Organidin, [Wallace]) is an older mucolytic expectorant that helps to liquify viscous mucus and increase the output of thin respiratory tract secretions. Entex (Baylor) is a useful expectorant and vasoconstrictor that increases and thins mucosal secretions. Guaifenesin also thins and increases secretions. Humibid (Adams) is currently among the most convenient preparations available.

These drugs are relatively harmless and may be very helpful to singers who complain of thick secretions, frequent throat clearing, or "postnasal drip." Postnasal drip is often caused by secretions that are too thick rather than too plentiful.

DIURETICS AND OTHER NONSTEROID MEDICATIONS FOR EDEMA

Transudation of body water from the vascular system producing edema and subsequent swelling of soft tissues of the respiratory tract is a commonly encountered phenomenon. Physical trauma to the mucous membranes, as with inappropriate voice use or abuse, is frequently etiologic in vocal fold edema. All laryngologists recognize glottal edema and distortion secondary to overenthusiastic cheering at an athletic event. Highly trained voice users rarely have vocal fold edema as a result of their occupations (i.e., the operatic singer), but even these persons sometimes experience edema as a result of direct trauma to the laryngeal mucosa from inappropriately loud singing or yelling. Such problems are encountered much more commonly in performers without extensive voice training, including many pop and rock singers and young students whose training may not be sufficient for the tasks assigned to school musical productions. Specific agents that provoke edema of the vocal folds include all of the respiratory allergens and some endocrine hormones, primarily the estrogens.

In response to a variety of stimuli, water leaves the circulatory system and enters the submucosal spaces of the vocal tract, including areas in the vocal folds and in the air passages themselves. Under most circumstances, edema of the vocal folds will be caused by protein-bound water.[7] As such it will not be ameliorated by diuretic agents commonly prescribed for tissue edema. Diuretic use for premenstrual voice changes is common but inappropriate because they do not alleviate protein-bound edema in Reinke's space, but may produce undesirable dehydration. Professional voice users taking diuretics for any disease condition must be monitored closely for adverse effects of diuretics caused by drying. Corticosteroid medications may affect protein-bound water directly. They are discussed later in this chapter.

Another group of pharmacologic agents used for soft tissue edema in the respiratory tract are the topical or systemic decongestants. Their primary action involves reduction in the diameter and volume of vascular structures in the submucosal area. These decongestants include norepinephrine used as an inhalant and pseudoephedrine. Topical decongestants may produce "rebound" phenomena with increased congestion after use. Effects of sprays are discussed below.

CORTICOSTEROIDS

Corticosteroids are extremely effective antiinflammatory agents and may be helpful in managing acute inflammatory laryngitis. Occasionally, they may also be appropriate for use in infectious laryngitis when extraordinary performance obligations supervene. Appropriate steroid dosing is controversial. Additional study is necessary to establish valid recommendations. Care must be taken not to prescribe steroids indiscriminately. They should be used only if there is a pressing, professional commitment that is being hampered by vocal fold inflammation. If an infectious origin is suspected, antibiotic coverage is recommended.

Corticosteroids may have adverse effects. Although they are not generally seen following the short-term steroid use appropriate for acute voice problem, they may occur in any patient. The more common corticosteroid side effects include gastric irritation with possible ulceration and hemorrhage, insomnia, mild mucosal drying, mood change (euphoria, occasionally psychosis), and irritability. Long-term effects such as muscle wasting and fat redistribution are generally not encountered following appropriate short-term use of steroids in professional vocalists. Another potential problem peculiar to professional voice users is steroid abuse. Because side effects are uncommon and steroids work extremely well, there is a tendency (especially among singers) to overuse or abuse them. This practice must be avoided.

SPRAYS, MISTS, AND INHALANTS

Diphenhydramine hydrochloride (Benadryl [Parke-Davis]), 0.5% in distilled water, delivered to the larynx as a mist may be helpful for its vasoconstrictive properties, but it is also dangerous because of its analgesic effect and is not recommended by the present authors. However, Punt[8] advocated this mixture and several modifications of it. Other topical vasoconstrictors that do not contain analgesics may be beneficial in selected cases. Oxymetazoline hydrochloride (Afrin [Schering]) applied by large-particle mist to the larynx is particularly helpful in treating severe edema immediately prior to performance, but it should be used only under emergent, extreme circumstances. Five percent propylene glycol in a physiologically balanced salt solution may be delivered by large-particle mist and can provide helpful lubrication, particularly in cases of laryngitis sicca following air travel or associated with dry climates. Such treatment is harmless and may also provide a beneficial placebo effect. Water, saline, or other balanced fluid delivered via a vaporizer or steam generator is frequently effective and sufficient. This therapy should be augmented by oral hydration, which is the mainstay of treatment for dehydration. A singer can monitor his/her state of hydration by observing urine color. He/she should be instructed to "pee pale."

Most inhalers are not recommended for use in professional voice users. Many people develop contact inflammation from sensitivity to the propellants used in inhalers; and propellants may also cause mucosal drying. Steroid inhalers used for prolonged periods may result in candida laryngitis. In addition, dysphonia occurs in up to 50% of patients using steroid inhalers, related to the aerosolized steroid itself rather than to the Freon propellent.[9] Prolonged steroid use such as is common in asthmatics also may cause wasting of the vocalis muscle.

ANTITUSSIVE MEDICATIONS

Cough suppressant mixtures often include agents that have a secondary drying effect on vocal tract secretions,[10] especially those preparations containing codeine.[11] Antihistamines are also common ingredients in antitussives. Dextromethorphan has pharmacologic effects similar to those of codeine and is encountered in a variety of OTC preparations. Generally, preparations that contain dextromethorphan and a wetting agent such as guaifenesin work well for voice professionals.

ANTIHYPERTENSIVE AGENTS

Almost all of the current antihypertensive agents have some degree of parasympatho-mimetic effect and thus dry mucous membranes of the upper respiratory tract. They commonly are used in combination with diuretic agents that also promote dehydration. In some circumstances, the laryngologist may find this drying effect substantial enough to merit recommending that the patient's internist prescribe another antihypertensive agent. The authors have frequently noted dryness with reserpines and agents of the methyldopa group.[12]

GASTROENTEROLOGIC MEDICATIONS

Antispasmodic agents are well known for their ability to reduce pain and motility arising from smooth muscles, especially those of the gastrointestinal tract. H_2-blockers have revolutionized the treatment of gastric ulcers and have proved very useful in laryngology for the treatment of gastric acid reflux laryngitis. Although drying of the laryngeal mucosa is not a major side effect of the H_2-blockers, it does occur and must be considered. Other gastric medications include phenobarbital, prochlorperazine, isopropamide, and propantheline bromide. Members of the belladonna alkaloid group including scopolamine and atropine are widely used and prescribed for their antispasmodic effects. All of these agents have significant drying effects on secretions in the vocal tract.

VITAMIN C

Not infrequently, the laryngologist may encounter a patient who consumes large amounts of vitamin C (ascorbic acid) in an effort to maintain health or to prevent the occurrence of a common cold. In some patients, a drying effect similar to that of a mild antihistamine occurs when vitamin C is taken in large doses.[13] Additionally, a patient with less than optimal renal function may produce an acidic urine and possibly form calculi.

SLEEPING PILLS

In general, sleeping pills should not be necessary for healthy people. Occasionally the stresses of a tour and the aggravations of travel, along with frequent changes in time zone, can disturb sleeping patterns. Sleeping pills should be used with great caution. However, especially when going on tour for the first few times, a small supply of mild sleeping medication such as Halcion [Upjohn] is appropriate. Performers should avoid using Benadryl [Parke-Davis], an antihistamine frequently also used as a sleeping medication. It is a safe drug and works well, but it produces excessive drying, which may impair singing.

ANALGESICS

Aspirin and other analgesics frequently have been prescribed for relief of minor throat and laryngeal irritations. The platelet dysfunction caused by aspirin predisposes to hemorrhage, especially in vocal folds traumatized by excessive voice use in the face of vocal dysfunction. Mucosal hemorrhage can be devastating to a professional voice, and aspirin products should be avoided altogether in singers. Acetaminophen is the best substitute, as even the most common nonsteroidal antiinflammatory drugs such as Ibuprofen may interfere with the clotting mechanism. Caruso used a spray of ether and iodoform on his vocal folds when he had to sing with laryngitis.

Nevertheless, the use of analgesics is dangerous and should be avoided. Pain is an important protective physiologic function. Masking it risks incurring significant vocal damage that may be unrecognized until after the analgesic or anesthetic effect wears off. If a singer requires analgesics or topical anesthetics to alleviate laryngeal discomfort, the laryngitis is severe enough to warrant canceling a performance. If a strong analgesic is for headache or some other discomfort not intimately associated with voice production, symptomatic treatment should be limited as much as possible until singing commitments have been completed.

HORMONES

Hormone medications may cause substantial changes in voice quality due to alterations in fluid content or to structural changes. Structural alterations in laryngeal architecture seldom occur as the result of pharmacologic influences, but androgens are an exception. They may produce permanent lowering of the fundamental frequencies, especially in females, and coarsening of the voice.[14–19] Androgenic agents are frequently used in the treatment of endometriosis and as part of chemotherapy regimens for breast cancer. Professional voice users should be informed of potential voice changes before these medications are employed, and their use should be avoided whenever possible.

Birth control pills with relatively high progesterone content are most likely to produce androgen-like changes in the voice. Most oral contraceptives marketed in the last several years have had appropriate estrogen-progesterone balance, and voice changes are seen in only about 5% of women who use birth control pills (Christine Carroll, MD, Arizona State University at Tempe, personal communication with Dr. Hans von Leden).[20–27] These changes generally are temporary, abating when oral contraceptive use is discontinued. Estrogen replacement is helpful in forestalling the typical voice changes that follow menopause. Sequential hormone replacement is mostly physiologic. Unless medical contraindications are present, professional voice users should be offered hormone replacement under appropriate medical supervision at the time of menopause.

Other endocrine medications may also affect the voice, often beneficially. Thyroid replacement may restore vocal efficiency and "ring" lost with even a mild degree of hypothyroidism. Agents used to treat maladies in any part of the diencephalic pituitary axis should be presumed to have laryngeal effects and warrant close monitoring of voice function.

BRONCHOACTIVE MEDICATIONS

Vocal function depends on the availability of a powerfully supported airstream passing between the vocal folds. Impairment of pulmonary function can cause severe problems for professional voice users. Pulmonary function is affected deleteriously by bronchoconstricting agents. Bronchodilators are often helpful, especially for patients with reactive airway disease, although inhaled bronchodilators may produce laryngitis, as discussed above in the section on other inhalers. Clinically, inhaled cromolyn sodium appears to cause fewer problems than most of the other agents commonly used in the treatment of asthma. The most commonly used bronchodilator is epinephrine and its related compounds including xanthines (aminophylline, for example). They can be used to counter the bronchoconstrictive effects of such environmental factors as house dust, pollen, other allergenic agents, and common air pollutants produced by our increasingly industrialized society. Active bronchoconstriction or asthma may occur with allergic reactions. These conditions may seriously hamper or prevent vocal performance unless recognized and treated properly.

BETA-BLOCKERS

Within the last few years, propranolol and other beta-blockers have been designated in the literature as useful for stage fright. Although British investigators[28] found that instrumental musicians given this potent beta-blocker did in fact exhibit less anxiety during performance, a unanimous response in voice professionals was not seen.

A subsequent study appears to indicate that propranolol, given for pre-performance anxiety, lessened anxiety and also produced an increase in salivation.[29] This investigation was conducted by measuring the weight increase in saliva-saturated dental rolls of cotton placed in the mouth during performance. This indicated that the problem of upper respiratory tract secretion dryness had been avoided and that some of the parasympathomimetic effects of performance anxiety had been negated. Even with such information, the laryngologic community generally agrees that these drugs should not be used for singers. They are potentially dangerous, affecting heart rate, blood pressure, and provoking asthma attacks in susceptible patients. In addition, when given in doses sufficient to ameliorate stage fright, they produce a lackluster performance.[12] Moreover, any professional voice user who requires an ingested substance to perform the daily activities for his or her chosen profession is revealing a significant problem. Physicians should refer such a patient for appropriate counseling and treatment of the *cause* of the problem, not merely medicate the symptom. (See Chapter 18.)

CENTRAL NERVOUS SYSTEM STIMULANTS

Central nervous system stimulants, such as cocaine, amphetamines, "diet pills," and other vasoconstrictor agents are to be regarded skeptically. An idiosyncratic response to a vasoconstrictor such as a pseudoephedrine, or an overdose of such an OTC medication, may manifest itself as acute central nervous system stimulation. Added to the "adrenalin high" of performance in the actor or musical performer, the combination of effects may very well be deleterious.

CENTRAL NERVOUS SYSTEM DEPRESSANTS

Use of central nervous system depressants is also questionable in people who use their voices in a competitive way. In this category are alcohol, barbiturates, sedative–hypnotics, and marijuana. Alteration of sensory input either by a stimulant or a depressant is potentially hazardous in a voice professional. The patient who is unaware of these effects should be apprised of them promptly by the laryngologist.

OTHER PSYCHOACTIVE MEDICATIONS

As the clinical syndromes associated with depression become better recognized, treatment of depression becomes more frequent. Biologic variation between persons is prominent, but some of the antidepressants (such as imipramine, amitriptyline, and amoxapine) now in clinical use can have undesirable laryngeal drying effects. The laryngologist may wish to suggest to the prescribing physician that an alternate compound be employed.

Rarely, we encounter a professional voice user for whom antipsychotic agents or the "major" tranquilizers are prescribed. The majority of these patients are either institutionalized or at least under fairly close supervision by their primary physician or psychiatrist. The authors have encountered well-known voice professionals who are touring successfully and performing while taking antipsychotic medications or tranquilizers. Certainly their use does not preclude professional voice use. Some of the "major" tranquilizers or antipsychotic medications can produce a parkinsonlike syndrome, with resultant voice tremor. Indeed the extrapyramidal effects of thorazine are well documented. Some of the more common major tranquilizers are chlorpromazine thioridazine, and haloperidol. These medications produce drying effects on the laryngeal mucous membranes. When this is perceived by the laryngologist or patient as constituting a problem, it is appropriate to consult with the prescribing physician directly to advocate use of antipsychotic agents less likely to cause drying effects. Some of these agents may also cause tremor, which is problematic if audible during singing.

CONCLUSION

Only a small number of the pharmacologic agents that may have laryngeal side effects were reviewed in this chapter. Virtually all pharmaceutical and chemical agents may have adverse effects on the voice. It is essential for laryngologists to be familiar with the vocal effects of any substance ingested by a professional voice patient and to educate voice professionals about the potential vocal problems associated with even prescribed medication use.

Acknowledgments—The authors express their appreciation to Raven Press for permission to reprint material from Sataloff RT: *Professional Voice: The Science and Art of Clinical Care,* New York, New York, 1991; and to the International Publishing Group for permission to republish material from Van Lawrence L: Common medications with laryngeal effects. *ENT J.* August, 66: 318–322, 1987.

REFERENCES

1. Sataloff RT: *Professional Voice: Science and Art of Clinical Care.* Raven Press, New York, 1991.
2. Davies WL, Gunert RR, Hoff RF, et al: Antiviral activity of 1-amantanamine (Amantadine). *Science* 144:862–863, 1964.
3. McGahen JW, Hoffmann CE: Influenza infections of mice. 1. Curative activity of amantadine HCl. *Proc Soc Exp Biol Med* 129:678–681, 1968.
4. Wingfield WL, Pollock D, Gunert RR: Therapeutic efficacy of amantadine-HCl and rumantidine-HCl in naturally occurring influence A_2 respiratory illness in man. *N Engl J Med* 281:579–584, 1969.
5. Council on Drugs: The amantadine controversy. *JAMA* 201:372–373, 1967.
6. Feder RL: The professional voice and airline flight. *Otolaryngol Head Neck Surg* 92:251–254, 1984.
7. Sataloff RT: Professional singers: The science and art of clinical care. *Am J Otolaryngol* 2:251–266, 1981.
8. Punt NA: Applied laryngology—Singers and actors. *Proc R Soc Med* 61:1152–1156, 1968.
9. Toogood JH, Jennings B, Greenway RW, Chuang L: Candidiasis and dysphonia complicating beclomethasone treatment of asthma. *J Allergy Clin Immunol* 65:145–153, 1980.
10. Martin FG: Drugs and vocal function. *J Voice* 2:338–344, 1988.
11. *Nursing '89 Drug Handbook.* Springhouse, PA, Springhouse Corporation, 1989, p 236.
12. Gates GA, Saegert J, Wilson N, et al: Effects of beta-blockade on singing performance. *Ann Otol Rhinol Laryngol* 94:570–574, 1985.
13. Lawrence VL: Medical care for professional voice, in Lawrence VL ed: *Transcripts From the Annual Symposium: Care of the Professional Voice,* vol 3. New York, The Voice Foundation, 1978, pp 17–18.
14. Damste PH: Virilization of the voice due to anabolic steroids. *Folia Phoniatr* 16:10–18, 1964.
15. Damste PH: Voice changes in adult women caused by virilizing agents. *J Speech Hearing Disorders* 32:126–132, 1967.
16. Saez S, Francoise S: Recepteurs d'androgenes: mise en evidence dans la fraction cytosolique de muqueuse normale et d'epitheliomas pharyngolarynges humains. *CR Acad Sci* 280:935–938, 1975.
17. Vuorenkoski V, et al: Fundamental voice frequency during normal and abnormal growth, and after androgen treatment. *Arch Dis Child* 53:201–209, 1978.

18. Arndt HJ: Stimmstorungen nach Behandlung mit androgenen und anabolen Hormonen. *Munch Med Wochenschr* 116:1715–1720, 1974.

19. Bourdial J: Les troubles de la voix provoques par la therapeutique hormonale androgene. *Ann Otolaryngol* 87:725–734, 1970.

20. Dordain M: Etude Statistique de l'influence des contraceptifs hormonaux sur la voix. *Folia Phoniatr* 24: 86–96, 1972.

21. Pahn V, Goretzlehner G: Stimmstorungen durch hormonale Kontrazeptiva. *Zentralb Gynakol* 100:341–346, 1978.

22. Schiff M: "The pill" in otolaryngology. *Trans Am Acad Ophthalmol Otolaryngol* 72:76–84, 1968.

23. Brodnitz F: Medical care preventive therapy, in Lawrence V (ed): *Transcripts of the Seventh Annual Symposium, Care of the Professional Voice*, vol 3. New York, The Voice Foundation, 1978, p 86.

24. Bausch J: Effects and side effects of hormonal contraceptives in the region of the nose, throat and ear. *Wirkung Nebenwirkung Horm Antikonzeptiva Bereich Nase* 31:409–414, 1983.

25. Kunnen contraceptiva met progestatieve werking stemveranderingen veroorzaken? [Could contraceptives with progestation effect cause voice changes?] *Ned Tijdschr Geneeskd* 119:1726–1727, 1975.

26. Krahulec I, Urbanova O, Simko S: Prispevok kstudiu zmien hlasu pri hormonalnej antikoncepcii. [Voice changes during hormonal contraception.] *Cesk Otolaryngol* 26:234–237, 1977.

27. Wendler J: Zyklusabhangige Leistungsschwankungen der Stimme und ihre Beeinflussung durch Ovulations-hemmer. [Cyclicly dependent variations in efficiency of the voice and its influencing by ovulation inhibitors.] *Folia Phoniatr* 24:259–277, 1972.

28. James IM: The effects of oxprenolol on stage fright in musicians. *Lancet* 2:952–954, 1977.

29. Brantigan CD: The effect of beta blockage and beta stimulation on stage fright. *Am J Med* 72:88–94, 1982.

16

Voice Education and Health Care for Young Voices

LEON THURMAN, EdD
CAROL A. KLITZKE, MS

A nine-year-old youngster is seen for a "hoarse voice." The next day, a 14-year-old male in the peak of voice change appears with the same vocal symptom. They are both singers-actors in a professional children's theatre company. Are you as confidently prepared to help these young people as you are to help adults? Is your approach to them as "routine" and up-to-date as it is for adults?

"Professional voice users" sometimes are thought of exclusively as performers in the speaking and singing arts. A broader definition of "professional voice user" would include all people who use their voices extensively and/or vigorously as an integral part of earning their livelihood. Wilson[1] includes "singers, actors, ministers, teachers and lecturers, salespersons, attorneys, telephone operators, . . . radio and television personalities, school class leaders and public officials." A complete list would include many more career categories.

Nearly all of the people who are employed in those livelihood-earning careers are adults. Children and adolescents comprise a small percentage of people in those careers. The likelihood is high, however, that most youngsters will *become* "professional voice users" in the broader sense.

During childhood and adolescence, many young people use their voices extensively and vigorously, and the health of many young voices will be at risk. They may talk loudly and hyperfunctionally in a loud-talking home environment; have a high-stress "family" and social life; yell frequently on the school playground; be a cheerleader; play sports; cheer at sports events; sing in school, church, and community choirs; act and sing in school and community theatre productions; sing daily with recorded popular music for 1 to 2 hours; sing in a "garage band"; have a high-profile, high emotional stress, talkative school social life; and ingest "recreational" drugs like tobacco and alcohol.

Several studies[2-6] have described the incidence of vocal dysphonia in various populations of school age children. The percentage of children who showed a dysphonic voice ranged from 6% to 17.4%. In 1985, von Leden[7] estimated that 3.5 million of the 60 million kindergarten through grade 12 students in the United States may display dysphonic voice.

Instead of limiting one's expertise to the very few youngsters who are professional voice users, can clinicians approach *all* children and adolescents with the same heightened concentration and state-of-the-art care given to adult performing arts professionals? Children's career choices are in their future. Preserving the health and expressive skill of their voices will enable them to perform the vocal communication requirements of their eventual career choices. This chapter is oriented to the children and adolescents from the families, schools, religions and performing groups in all communities who use their voices extensively and vigorously, whether or not they are paid to do so.

YOUNG-VOICE TREATMENT AND EDUCATION TEAMS

Multidisciplinary "teams" can provide the most comprehensive, "whole person" voice care and education to patients and clients. Current custom is to ally laryngologists, private practice or hospital speech–language pathologists, and teachers of solo singing skills to help professional singing and speaking artists. Presently, teams tend to focus on treating adults who already have out-of-health voices.

How can clinicians best provide the most beneficial care and effective prevention of voice disorders in young people? Identifying the chronologic age range of "young," and examining who may be candidates for effective team members may be a way to begin.

We propose that the age range that identifies "the young" begins when prenatal auditory processing begins, and ends when laryngeal and vocal tract anatomy have assumed adult dimensions—about age 20 to 21 years. To have a unified reference point, "young" may be categorized into the following developmental groups:

1. Prenatal: onset of auditory processing to birth
2. Infancy: birth to 2 years
3. Early childhood: 2 to 5 years
4. Middle childhood: 5 to 9 years
5. Late childhood: 9 years to onset of puberty
6. Early adolescence: puberty, usually 12 to 15 years
7. Middle adolescence: 15 to 18 years
8. Late adolescence: 18 to 21 years

Voice teams are made up of members who primarily contribute treatment for disorders and members who primarily contribute voice education. The goal of treatment is to return voice-producing tissues and function to a condition in which *optimum* voice function is *possible*. Optimum voice function may vary according to the vocal demands of each patient's circumstances. The goal of voice education is to provide to the patient

1. Voice disorder prevention methods
2. Increased physical and acoustic efficiency in expressive voice skills, while preserving the vocal "output" that is necessary for continued professional potential.

Core members of a voice treatment and education team may be those with specific training in treating disordered young voices or educating young voices. In addition to a laryngologist and a school, hospital, or private practice speech pathologist, a young-voice team needs someone who is trained in the teaching of age-appropriate, self-expressive voice skills in the speaking and singing arts to children and adolescents. In most cases, singing teachers who are trained in traditional vocal pedagogy are not qualified to fill this core team role. There is great need for a category of voice professional who might be labeled a "voice educator." This team member would be trained in voice anatomy and function, effects of voice use and disease states on voice, trained and experienced in methods of teaching physically and acoustically efficient speaking and singing skills and the prevention of voice problems, and age-appropriate forms of communication.

Auxiliary members of a voice treatment team can be anyone who has a special-interest relationship with a particular youngster and is willing to provide vocal help. Candidates for these roles may be parents, peers, school teachers, singing teachers, music educators, and choral conductors.

Treating children and adolescents and providing preventive education requires adaptation of our adult and professional communication patterns to the less evolved patterns of young clients. It requires the use of repertoires of treatment techniques that generally have not been part of a voice team's training and experience. In addition to traditional training within each voice team member's field, all members need

1. Deep, current knowledge about vocal macro- and microanatomy and morphology; the function and acoustics of vocal sound making, speaking, and singing coordinations in young voices from birth to age 21 years; the nature, etiology, and restoration of out-of-health voices
2. Direct experience with the extent of vocal capabilities in young people (skill potential or talent in speaking and singing) through personal observation; the relationship between vocal capabilities and their realization into vocal abilities
3. Personal voice skills in speaking and singing that enable modeling of basic efficient and inefficient vocal characteristics
4. Knowledge of and experience with current psychosocial contexts in which young people grow up and the effects of same on voice function
5. The use of the preceding background in establishing a communicative relationship of mutual trust with young people
6. Knowledge and experience with teaching and learning processes that are consistent with conscious and other-than-conscious learning capabilities of children and adolescents.

A challenge for ongoing members of a young-voice team is to update continually the voice education of all the members within their own fields. Another challenge is to be very conversant with what all other team members can do and how they go about it and to exchange approaches and vocabulary. A third challenge is to ask for, respect, and use suggestions from all other team members in the performance of professional functions.

Helping young people change habitual or debilitating vocal behaviors to more beneficial ones is always challenging. Their vocal coordinations were learned and are "operated" outside their conscious awareness. To them, their vocal coordinations are part of their evolving self-identity and are necessary for their personal, everyday self-expression.

This chapter is an overview of young-voice care. It is organized into four sections: (1) anatomic morphology and voice-related function; (2) vocal capabilities and abilities in infancy, childhood, and adolescence; (3) psychosocial context for young-voice treatment and education teams; and (4) voice treatment and education processes for young vocal performers with dysfunctioning voices.

HIGHLIGHTS OF ANATOMIC MORPHOLOGY AND VOICE-RELATED FUNCTION IN THE AUDITORY SYSTEM, THE RESPIRATORY SYSTEM, THE LARYNX, AND THE VOCAL TRACT FROM PRENATAL GESTATION TO AGE 21 YEARS

All of the anatomic components that produce voice are formed during prenatal gestation, and most begin functioning in some way before birth. The macroarchitecture of voice-related anatomy is significantly smaller at birth than the adult dimension, proportional relationships are significantly different, and anatomic microarchitecture is in very early stages of maturation. Middle and inner ear structures, however, are by 5 months gestation comparable to those in adults.

The end-age parameter of the "young" voice is established by the finding of Hirano et al[8] that nearly all of the macro- and microarchitecture characteristics of adult laryngeal anatomy have been completed by about age 20 to 21 years. One important evolution of microarchitecture is not substantial until ages 28 to 32 years, that is, calcification and ossification of hyaline laryngeal cartilage. This change usually proceeds earlier in males than females.[9,10]

The Auditory System

Preparation for the neuromuscular acts of speaking and singing begins with an accumulated history of multisensory input that is predominantly auditory. By the 20th week of womb life, the cochlear system is structurally comparable to that of an adult, and the auditory nerve completes its development by the 6th month.[11] The fetal brain has been developed sufficiently to support consciousness and self-awareness sometime between the 28th and 32nd weeks of gestation.[12] In utero discrimination learning in response to sound has been experimentally demonstrated.[13–15] Maternal speech has been recorded from within the womb.[16,17] Newborn recall of mother's voice has been demonstrated in several experiments organized by DeCasper and Fifer[18] and DeCasper and Spence.[19]

The Respiratory System

Respiratory function begins prenatally as early as 21 weeks of gestation, with both "breathing" and swallowing of amniotic fluid.[20] At birth, the trachea is about one-third of adult size, the bronchi are about one-half adult size, and bronchioles about one-fourth adult size.[21] By age 8 years, the adult number of bronchioles and alveoli have developed, and subsequent tracheobronchial development is due to increases in size.[22] Through the second year of life, the ribs form largely horizontal circles and are mostly cartilaginous. As walking upright and more extensive respiratory needs develop, rib and spinal contours evolve. The thoracic cage reaches adult contour by age seven.[21]

With somatic growth, lung size and vital capacity increase. Increased aerobic activity results in increased lung size and vital capacity in children. Less aerobic activity results in comparatively less developed lung size and vital capacity.[23] The pubertal growth spurt increases lung size and vital capacity toward adult levels. Due to variability in growth rates of lung tissue and the chest wall, establishment of adult dimensions, vital capacity, and total lung volume can only be estimated to occur between the ages of 18 years to the early 20s.[22]

Until 6 to 8 months after birth, maintenance breathing almost exclusively involves diaphragmatic movement. After that time, mixtures of diaphragmatic and thoracic movement facilitate breathing. After age 7 years, thoracic movement predominates. These functional changes reflect use of larger lung size, air volumes, and amount of oxygen required for metabolic need.[21,22,24,25] Neonate breathing rate is about 87 breaths per minute compared with about 47 at age 1 year. Adults average about 16 to 20 breaths per minute for maintenance breathing. Neonate breathing is involuntary and initiated by neuronal activity in the reticular formation of the brainstem.[26] Between months 2 and 7 after birth, integration of involuntary and voluntary control of respiration takes place as cortical initiation of the neuromuscular coordinations required for speech emerge. Speech requires larger air volumes than tidal breathing and significantly longer expirations than inspirations.[27–32] Presumably, these neuromuscular coordinations evolve as infants continue to perceive adult speech and begin to learn how to produce it themselves.[33,34] Respiratory coordinations for speech become increasingly refined during childhood as speech is mastered.

To date, there has been no scientific study of the integration of respiratory function with the evolution of singing coordinations in infants and children. Hixon[35] studied respiratory functions during speaking and singing in six vocally untrained adult male subjects, three male and one female adult classical Shakespearean actors, and six male adult singers of "classical" opera. While standing upright, vocally untrained adult speakers used a typical vital capacity range of 35% to 60% in quiet conversational speech samples and softer singing. During loud speech, they typically initiated samples at 70% to 80% of vital capacity. The classical Shakespearean actors showed no significant difference in use of vital capacity from the untrained subjects. Hixon[35] speculated that the actors used vocal tract adjustments to produce a favorable acoustic advantage over the untrained speakers. The trained opera singers produced the widest variation in vital capacity use in the study's various singing tasks. When singing aria passages that involved high pitches and loud volumes and when singing passages that involved longer phrase durations in slow tempo, vital capacity use typically ranged from nearly 15% to 100%. Passages that did not involve such vocal athleticism typically used a range of 30% to 65% of vital capacity.

The Larynx

The basic elements of the larynx are formed by the 11th week of womb life but is not used in vocal function until birth. Compared with adults, infant laryngeal cartilages are (1) much smaller, (2) more rounded than angulated, (3) softer and more pliable, and (4) more compact in their connection to each other.

The cartilages assume a greater proportion of laryngeal dimensions than does the soft tissue, and the anterior areas of the thyroid cartilage and hyoid bone are almost approximate.[10,36] The vocal processes of the arytenoid cartilages assume approximately one-half the length of each vocal fold compared with the two-fifths proportion in the adult.[10,37] Infant laryngeal connective tissue is loose and highly vascular.[38] The mucosal tissues of infant vocal folds are not well defined, a vocal ligament is not developed, and laryngeal muscles are at the beginning of their maturational journey.[39,40] Morphological characteristics of infant laryngeal innervation have not been described, but von Leden's data[41] suggest that laryngeal innervation is not fully mature until age 3 years.

Laryngeal dimensions increase slowly and steadily during childhood and are correlated with overall body height, but no significant differences occur between the males and females.[42] Laryngeal cartilages increase in size and firmness, and Klock[42] observed a pattern of growth in which the greatest increase is in the anterior dimension, followed by the lateral and posterior dimensions, respectively. The glottal area also increases in length and width. Based on the sparse data available, the vocal folds increase their total length by about 6.5 mm between prepubertal ages of 1 to 12 years.[10] By age 4 years only a rudimentary vocal ligament has developed, and the mucosal tissues (lamina propria) are yet immature. Throughout childhood the fibrous connective tissues of the mucosa increase in density and structural complexity. By age 10 years, the vocal ligament and mucosal tissues are clearly developed, but become fully mature only after puberty.[8,10,39]

Puberty is the beginning of adolescence and generally is defined as the time when procreational capacity is attained. Puberty begins with the gradual appearance of secondary sex characteristics. Adolescence customarily ends with the cessation of somatic growth and generally ranges from ages 10 to 18 in females and 12 to 20 in males. The most dramatic adolescent "growth spurt" tends to occur between ages 11 to 15 years and may occur within a span of 12 to 24 months. Menarche is the clear physiologic landmark of puberty in females, with voice change and appearance of facial hair being the clearest landmarks in males.[43–45]

Prepubertal childhood laryngeal cartilages show no significant distinction between males and females. During the pubertal growth spurt, however, laryngeal cartilages become significantly larger and heavier, remarkably so in males (Fig. 16–1). Kahane[46,47] reported a study of laryngeal growth from preadolescence to adolescence to adulthood. The study was based on measurements of 20 excised human larynges ranging in age from 9 to 19 years at time of death and on measurements from a similarly designed study of adult larynges by Maue.[48] Kahane found that, during prepuberty to adulthood, the most significant proportional change of cartilage dimension was in the anteroposterior (front to back) dimension of the male thyroid cartilage. That dimension in the male thyroid cartilage underwent three times more growth than the same dimension in females (15.04 mm compared with 4.47 mm). From prepuberty to adulthood, combined weight of the male thyroid, cricoid, and arytenoid cartilages increased 10.60 g and in females that increase was 3.93 g. Approximately 50% of the increase from prepubertal weight occurred during the pubertal growth spurt and the other 50% more gradually after puberty and into adulthood. Kahane attributed the pubertal weight increase to "appositional and interstitial growth processes." He cited a study by Hately et al[9] to support his attribution of adult weight increases to "constituent changes in the cartilages, such as calcification or ossification." These processes may begin as early as age 20 years and result in a gradual stiffening of the cartilages during adulthood.

Kahane[10] also found that male vocal fold length increased by an average of 63% from prepuberty to adulthood. Female vocal fold length increased by 34% (see Table 16–1). Pubertal maturation of the laryngeal anatomy includes growth of all its muscles, particularly the adductory muscles and the cricothyroid muscles. The cricothyroid joint capsule and motor and sensory innervation also become more refined. In Japanese children between age 4 years and the onset of puberty, Hirano et al[8,39] found gradually increased definition of the connective tissue that is located between the epithelium and the vocalis portion of the thyroarytenoid muscle. During the pubertal growth spurt, however, layer definition accelerated to clearly identify the superficial and intermediate layers, with the deep layer forming a

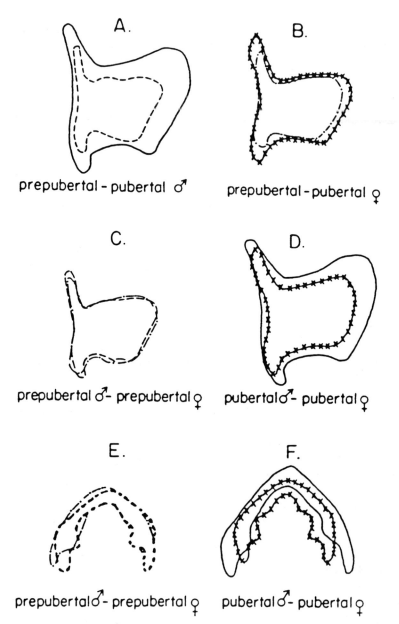

Figure 16–1.   Prepubertal and pubertal larynx. A,B, Representative lateral views of the thyroid cartilages (actual size) illustrating developmental differences within each sex. C,D, Representative lateral views of the thyroid cartilages (actual size) illustrating sex differences at each developmental stage. E,F, Representative superior views of the thyroid cartilages (actual size) illustrating sex differences at each developmental stage. Dashed lines, prepubertal male; dashed, dotted lines, prepubertal female; solid lines, pubertal male; x lines, pubertal female. (From Kahane.[46] Used by permission of the author and The Wistar Institute, Philadelphia, Pennsylvania.)

**Table 16–1   Mean Male and Female Total Vocal Fold Length (mm)
From Prepuberty Through Puberty***

	PREPUBERTY	PUBERTY	GROWTH	PERCENT INCREASE
Male	17.35	28.21	11.57	63
Female	17.31	23.15	4.16	34

*Data from Kahane.[47]

mature vocal ligament. Essential adult characteristics of the lamina propria were formed by about age 16 years.

Although the vocal folds essentially have reached adult length following the pubertal growth spurt, the connective tissues of the vocal folds may continue to increase in size and quantity into adulthood, though no study has explicitly verified such a conclusion. Data collected regarding laryngeal growth is consistent with endocrinologic data related to voice change and general body growth[49] and with data regarding general pubertal growth under hormonal influences. If thyroarytenoid muscle fibers respond similarly to bodywide muscular changes, they also may continue to increase in thickness.[50] Thyroarytenoid muscle bulk may increase with laryngeal muscle conditioning as a result of extensive and vigorous use in voicing.

The Vocal Tract

The vocal tract extends from the superior surface of the true vocal folds to the exterior surface of the lips. The infant "vocal tract" is very short, slightly curved, and so compact that the epiglottis can couple with the soft palate to enable simultaneous breathing and nursing.[10] Until age 18 to 24 months, the tongue lies entirely in the oral cavity, and then its base begins a gradual inferior progression into the pharynx. By age 4 years, the posterior one-third of the tongue is located in the pharynx, the coupling of soft palate and epiglottis is no longer possible, and the vocal tract is longer, more curved, and introduces much more variety in speech resonation.

By age 5 years the basic adult configuration, but not size, of the vocal tract is present. By age 9 years the curved contour of the vocal tract is comparable with that of an adult, but it still remains shorter and smaller.[27,51] The average dimensions of both male and female vocal tracts increase at about the same rate throughout childhood. During and following puberty, the average lengths of both male and female vocal tracts increase, but the male vocal tract becomes significantly longer and develops greater "circumference." Full adult sizes are completed at least by age 20 to 21 years. These dimensional differences are reflected in averages of the three lowest formant frequencies of all vowels. Adult females average 12%, 17%, and 18% higher than adult males, and prepubescent children (ages unspecified) average 20% higher than adult females.[52]

One indicator of vocal tract length is the location of its lower end—the larynx— relative to the cervical vertebrae of the spinal column. In infants, the inferior border of the cricoid cartilage lies adjacent to the lower border of the third cervical vertebra (C3). Under normal growth processes, the lower border of the cricoid cartilage is adjacent to the middle of C5 by age 5 years, upper to middle C6 by 10 years, the lower border of C6 following puberty, and the upper area of C7 by about age 20 years. Further downward "settling" then occurs, but the larynx remains within the C7 region throughout life.[10,53]

HIGHLIGHTS OF VOCAL CAPABILITIES AND VOCAL ABILITIES IN INFANCY, CHILDHOOD, AND ADOLESCENCE

There are some genetic predispositions and prenatal–infant–childhood experiences that provide musical and voice skill advantages to people. Only about 4% of people appear to have the neural dysfunction called *dysmelodia*.[54] The evidence to date therefore indicates that about 96% of all people who have mastered the ear–brain–voice coordinations that are necessary for speaking also can master the ear–brain–voice coordinations that are necessary for skilled, expressive singing. In short, people who have learned to speak can learn to sing, and with a high degree of skill.

Welch[55–58] integrated research findings in neuromuscular physiology and singing ability development and has proposed a theoretical "continuum of development" for the process of realizing vocal capability into vocal ability (skills). His continuum applies equally to developing voice skills in speaking and singing. Figure 16–2 is a graphic depiction of his continuum theory.

Speaking Skills

Speech acquisition begins with prenatal auditory input. "Practice" begins when visual, auditory, and kinesthetic observation of speaking by others is possible and when vocal output begins at birth.[59–61] Language acquisition and facility is enhanced when children grow up in families in which conversational talking and reading aloud is frequent. Language acquisition proceeds through cooing, babble, and then one-word, one-to-three word, and sentence stages.

Other-than-conscious vocal exploration by infants is part of the "practice" that results in language acquisition. Ries[62] sampled 146 infants and children and observed that their overall pitch range can vary from 2.3 octaves above F3 at 7 months to 2.9 octaves above F3 at 19 months. When all vocal sounds are included, Keating and Buhr[63] found a

Capability Continuum

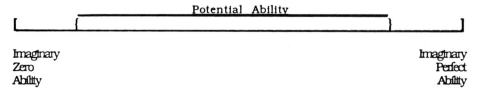

Figure 16–2. A realization of Welch's developmental continuum of vocal ability. (From Thurman.[133] Used by permission of the author and The VoiceCare Network.)

frequency range in the first 3 years from a low of 30 Hz to a high of 2,500 Hz. As language is acquired and customary social behavior is learned, the pitch range of vocal sound-making gradually narrows.

Wilson[64] provides very helpful mean speaking fundamental frequency (MSFF) charts for males and females, aged 1 to 18 years based on averages of compiled research from 1940 to 1985. His charts reveal 1–2-year-old infants at about 400 Hz/G4 in both sexes. The averages gradually decreased for each year, and they matched until ages 9 to 12 years, when the males began to average 5 to 10 Hz lower than females. During pubertal voice mutation, the females continued to lower by 5 to 10 Hz, but the males progressively lowered between 50 and 80 Hz below female averages. Andrews[65] reported a comparison of habitual MSFF and basal frequencies in 740 Australian children aged 5 to 13 years. She noted that significant differences between boys and girls began to appear at age 9.5 years, and the significance of the difference increased through puberty. Cooksey et al[66] followed 86 boys over 3 years, from ages 13 to 15, and found a progressive lowering of MSFF from a pubertal onset average of 226 Hz/Bb3 to a postpubertal average of 120 Hz/B2 (see Table 16–2).

Although no research has established practical scientific measurements for neuromuscular efficiency in speech coordinations, the low-end pitches in Wilson's lists of "acceptable limits" may indicate some degree of laryngeal hyperfunction. Clinical videolaryngoscopic views of healthy larynges reveal a hyperfunctional sphinctering of the laryngopharynx in people who habitually speak in the lower pitch areas of their voices.[67]

Young people who use their voices extensively and vigorously (daily talking, cheerleading) and who are involved in situations in which skilled speaking is required (public speaking, acting) will benefit from ongoing voice training. Increased speaking skill, when taught and learned well, results in physical and acoustic efficiency in the entire biomechanical act of speaking.[68] As that occurs, the expressive effectiveness of speech increases and a degree of voice protection is built in. Unfortunately, much of the training received by public speakers and actors includes very little useful, self-protective voice training.

Singing Skills

The ability to arrange the vocal folds so that the frequency of mucosal waving almost exactly matches and then sustains an aurally perceived or remembered vibrational frequency is a rather sophisticated ear–brain–voice coordination. To arrange the folds seven

Table 16–2 Comparison of Low Terminal Pitch With Mean Speaking Fundamental Frequency During Six Voice Mutation Stages*

STAGE	LOW TERMINAL PITCH	MSFF
Premutational	218 Hz A3	259 Hz C4
Early mutation	206 Hz Ab3	226 Hz Bb3
High mutation	174 Hz F3	210 Hz Ab3
Mutation climax	148 Hz D3	186 Hz F#3
Post-mutation stabilization	125 Hz B2	151 Hz D3
Post-mutation settling or development	95 Hz G2	120 Hz B2

*Data from Cooksey et al.[66]

different ways in 1 second to match seven remembered (audiated) vibrational frequencies with seven different word syllables, and then repeat the task later but one octave higher, is rather remarkable. The muscles of the larynx are capable of operating at very high speeds. Twitch contraction times for laryngeal muscles are among the fastest in the whole body.[69]

Most of the research on the development of children's singing abilities has been carried out in the field of music education. It has been descriptive of pitch accuracy and range when children of various ages are asked to sing songs. Many of the researchers were not informed in detail about the structure and function of voices, and the validity of some of the conclusions suffers as a result.

Prenate, Infancy, and Childhood

The ability to perform singing skills begins with auditory input of both spoken language and sung music. Auditory input of instrumental and vocal music can begin prenatally and continue through early childhood if parents are aware of the benefits to their children and have the inclination to provide them.[70–74]

Ries[62] found that 95% of all sustained "singing-like" sounds made by 7–19-month-old infants and children ranged between 233 Hz/A#3 and 494 Hz/B4. Kessen[75] found that 23 of 24 infants 3 to 6 months of age learned to match three different pitches reliably: 294 Hz/D4, 356 Hz/F4, and 440 Hz/A4. An experimental protocol involved mothers using pitch pipes as a pitch reference when presenting stimulus pitches with their own voices.

Very few studies have compared the pitch range and pitch accuracy findings of children who have experienced minimal prenatal and early childhood singing experiences with children who have had frequent prenatal, infancy, and early childhood family singing experiences. Kelley and Sutton-Smith[76] reported longitudinal observations of three children in differing socioeconomic and family settings. One female child who shared considerable prenatal and infancy singing experiences with mother and grandmother began singing whole songs by age 12 months and had learned a repertoire of songs by 24 months. Her singing pitch range at 24 months was assessed as 210 Hz/G#3 to 540 Hz/C#5.

Following a review of considerable research in the field of music education on the singing ability of school-age children, Welch[57,58] proposed a five-stage developmental continuum.

1.   The words of the song appear to be the initial center of interest rather than the melody. Often there is little variation in sung pitch, perhaps because some children find it impossible to attend to more than one parameter of the song at any one time, and the words are, for them, the dominant feature. In response to a pitch stimulus, the brain appears to engage in "target practice" and chooses a pitch that is within a "familiar" vocal pitch range (speech). There is some evidence, however, that attempted pitches are frequently in proximity to the pitch target.

2.   There is some variation in sung pitches that may occasionally coincide with the target melody. There is a growing awareness that vocal pitch production can be a conscious process and that the ability to change vocal pitch to match aurally perceived targets can be mastered.

3.   A more "active" attempt is made to master vocal pitch production by "jumping" pitch intervals toward targets. Pitch production follows the directional contours of a target melody, and more pitches within melodies are accurate. Vocal pitch range continues to increase.

4. "Fine tuning" of pitch production coordinations can be observed. The melodic contour and most of the pitches are accurate. Some children will change the tonal center of melodies during the song, however, after a breath. For instance, they may change the "key" or tonality of a song from C major to A major but maintain melodic pitch and interval accuracy in both keys.

5. No major pitch, melodic, or tonality errors occur; there is a high level of pitch accuracy. Vocal pitch range is both higher and lower than at an earlier stage of "target practice."

Welch and colleagues[77,78] have developed computer hardware and software for "practice," feedback, and documentation of the continuum in children's singing skill development. He proposed general applicability of these stages to anyone of any age who has had limited or restricted experience with singing coordinations.

Adolescence

Several renowned voice experts[79–83] have stated that pubertal adolescents, especially boys, should not sing at all because of special vulnerabilities in laryngeal tissues and dangers to their vocal future. Recent research questions that assertion and recommends singing under appropriate conditions.

Boys. In 1965, Naidr et al[84] published the results of a 5 year study of voice mutation onset and rate of mutation in 100 boarding school boys in Czechoslovakia, aged 12 through 15 years. They grouped the boys into three categories: (1) beginning of the change (12–13 years), (2) high point or crux of the change (13–14 years), and (3) end of change (14–15 years). Changes in speaking and singing capabilities were correlated with the development of primary and secondary sexual characteristics and with body height, weight, and laryngeal size. Average duration of mutation was 13 months. Principal voice mutation occurred in the first half of pubertal growth, paralleling the most extensive increases in body height. These changes preceded increases in larynx size. Naidr et al[84] observed that voice change first appeared as a lowering of the upper limits of singing pitch range. As pubertal changes proceeded, singing pitch range gradually lowered. During the high point of mutation, the extent of singing pitch range narrowed, but was followed by an expansion of pitch range.

Over a period of 10 years, Frank and Sparber[85,86] used sonographic analysis to study changes in the singing pitch ranges of 5,000 Austrian children, aged 7 through 14 years. They also found three stages of mutation, which they labeled *premutationsstimme* (premutation voice), *mutationsstimme* (mutation voice), and *postmutationsstimme* (postmutation voice). Their stages overlapped but extended the stages identified by Naidr et al.[84] They also used sonographic analysis to identify a lower register; an upper register; the emergence of male falsetto register; and an extremely high "whistle" range from about C6 to C7 that was present only during high mutation.

Cooksey[91] comprehensively surveyed the research on voice mutation and the methods of adolescent male voice classification that were then used in the field of music education.[87–90] Based on that survey and his years of experience in classifying changing boys' voices, assigning them to vocal parts in choirs, and teaching them voice skills, Cooksey[92,93] proposed six stages of mutation with concomitant voice classifications for use by vocal music educators (see Table 16–3).

Cooksey then allied with Beckett and Wiseman[66] to test his theory in a 3 year study of 86 vocally untrained boys beginning in their seventh grade year. Data were collected monthly during school months from October 1977 through June 1980. Over 6,500 sonograms were computer analyzed to detect patterns of change. The following variables were studied:

1. Physiologic: Sitting and standing height, weight, chest size, waist size, percent body fat, vital capacity and phonation time
2. Acoustic: Speaking fundamental frequency; gross and singing sound volume ranges; sonographic analysis of sustained lower, upper, and falsetto register tones to determine formant frequency regions, number of formants, "spread" between the first two formants, harmonics-to-noise ratios within lower and upper partial ranges (80 to 4,100 Hz and 4,100 to 8,000 Hz)
3. Vocal: Pitch range, tessitura (pitch range in which acoustic spectra showed clearest partials), voice quality, voice register development.

Some of the prominent findings can be summarized as follows:

1. Voice mutation proceeded at various rates in different individuals, but proceeded through a predictable, sequential pattern of stages over about a 14 to 24 month period. There was no sudden, "overnight" voice change, although some circumstances may lead casual observers to such a belief.

2. Onset of voice mutation occurred at different ages among individuals. Presumably, onset was genetically determined. The most common time of onset was age 12 to 13 years, but it may begin as early as 10 to 11 years.

3. The most active phase of mutation occurred between ages 12.5 and 14.0 years, but there were exceptions.

4. The mean number of months the boys were in Cooksey's Midvoice I classification was 4.76; in Midvoice II, 12.92; in Midvoice IIA, 5.24; and New Baritone, 5.04. The mean age of boys in the high point or crux of mutation (Midvoice IIA) was 13.6 years. After the high point, there was a tapering in the degree of mutational change through the New Baritone and Settling Baritone stages. According to Cooksey, an extended period of development then ensues at least through ages 20 to 21 years, as young male voices develop toward adult norms of laryngeal and vocal tract dimension and function.

5. Mean pitch range narrowed from 20.6 semitones during the premutational stage to 16.6 semitones in the early mutation stage, remained at 15.5 semitones through the other stages, and reexpanded to 19.2 semitones in the postmutation development stage.

6. One sequential pattern that recurred in all of the mutational stages was the initial appearance of instability in upper pitch range capability, followed by a lowering of the low terminal pitch.

7. Vital capacity increased steadily and consistently as the subjects passed through each of the maturational stages.

8. The pubertal stages of somatic and sexual development closely paralleled the stages of voice mutation.

In 1984, Cooksey[94] completed a short follow-up study. One finding indicated that experienced, trained observers can reliably determine the voice classifications and that acoustic measures will support those perceptual judgments. Other studies have substantiated the Cooksey Index of Voice Classification.[95–97] Further Cooksey, Beckett, and Wiseman findings are summarized briefly in Table 16–3.

The Cooksey voice classification guidelines and assessment procedures can be used to select solo and choral music that is within the vocally "comfortable" pitch range capabilities of pubertal males in the various stages of growth. When use of his guidelines is coupled with approaches to voice care and to physically and acoustically efficient voice skill development, pubertal males can learn to sing with expressive skill, confidence, and vocal safety.[98] Training in such methodology is not common among vocal music educators. The Cooksey guidelines are not universally known and are rarely used in music that is published for adolescent singers in the school system.

Girls. A major physical landmark of female puberty is the onset of menarche, but it follows breast budding, development of pubic hair, and usually the peak of the growth spurt in height.[44,45] According to Tanner,[44] menarcheal onset has been occurring earlier in recent decades. In the 1930s the average age of onset was 14 years. In the early 1970s it was shortly before the 13th birthday.

Voice change is one of several signs of female puberty. Voice change appears to begin before menarcheal onset and to continue through it. A landmark of voice change onset is increased breathiness in voice quality compared with the relative clarity of prepubertal voice quality. The breathiness is due in part to incomplete vocal fold adduction. During voicing, the membranous portion of the vocal folds adduct, but the cartilaginous portion does not achieve complete closure, forming a posterior glottal opening that is called a *mutational* or *glottal chink*.[79] Mutational chink is thought to result from insufficient contraction of the interarytenoid muscles.[99] Appropriate vocal training can result in reduction and/or elimination of the glottal chink, with vocal safety, after the most active phase of voice mutation.[100] Female voice change can be characterized by:

1. Lowering of mean speaking fundamental frequency by about three to four semitones
2. Increased breathiness, huskiness, hoarseness
3. Voice "cracking" during speech
4. Noticeable register "breaks" during singing
5. Decreased and inconsistent pitch range capabilities
6. Singing that feels more effortful, delay in phonation onset
7. Breathy, "heavier," "rougher" voice qualities.

To date, no longitudinal research into female voice change related to singing has been published. Huff-Gackle[100] (Gackle[101,102]) combined research findings in anatomic and functional voice mutation with empirical observations to develop a list of perceptual voice change characteristics, pitch range guidelines and voice training methods for pubertal females who sing. She theorized three stages of mutation based on a review of literature and on years of personal experience in teaching singing to young females (see Table 16–4).

Singing in a "Belted Way"

The term *belting* or *belt voice* was coined in the musical theatre of the United States and was popularized primarily by the singing of Ethel Merman in the 1940s and 1950s. That style of singing is a staple of musical theatre in Western civilization.

For thousands of years, children and adults of nearly all the world's cultures have sung their folk/popular music in a strong, belted way. That way of singing the music is integral

**Table 16–3   Cooksey Maturational Stages of Male Voice Change
Related to Singing; Voice Classification Labels;
Mean Pitch Ranges (Whole Notes); Tessitura Ranges
(Bracketed Quarter Notes); and Brief Descriptions***

MATURATIONAL STAGE	VOICE CLASSIFICATION/DESCRIPTION
I: Premutation	Unchanged: Displays full spectrum amplitude in partials throughout pitch range; largest premutational vocal tract dimensions result in a "rich boy soprano" voice quality
714 Hz / 462 Hz / 274 Hz / 218 Hz	
II: Early mutation	Midvoice I: Amplitudes of upper partials are not as pronounced; increased noise (breathiness) and internal and external laryngeal muscle effort when singing above C5; slightly fuller voice quality
535 Hz / 401 Hz / 251 Hz / 206 Hz	
III: High mutation	Midvoice II: First appearance of falsetto register and "whistle" range; increased loss of amplitude in all spectral partials with increased noise in the upper partial range (4,100–8,000 Hz); voice quality is "thicker," "huskier"
426 Hz / 341 Hz / 214 Hz / 174 Hz	
IV: Mutation climax	Midvoice IIA: Continued loss of amplitude in spectral partials with significant increase of noise in entire partial range regardless of fundamental frequency; laryngeal muscle control significantly reduced; breathier; hyperfunction is commonly used to "make voice stronger"
365 Hz / 299 Hz / 186 Hz / 148 Hz	

(Continued)

Table 16–3 (*Continued*)

MATURATIONAL STAGE	VOICE CLASSIFICATION/DESCRIPTION
V: Postmutation stabilization 308 Hz 239 Hz 155 Hz 125 Hz	New baritone: Little change in amplitude of upper/lower partials, slightly more noise; formant regions moving toward adult norms; falsetto register stabilizes; quality can be firm/clear but lacks full-bodied adult richness; pitch gaps can occur as motor control adjusts to new laryngeal and vocal tract dimensions
VI: Postmutation development 287 Hz 206 Hz 127 Hz 95 Hz	Settling or developing baritone: Noise increases in lower *pitch* range, decreases in upper; number of upper formants increase, first two formants are lower; laryngeal coordination becomes normalized in upper pitch range; pitch gaps can still occur; quality clearer, not yet adult full-bodied richness

*Data from Cooksey.[98] Used by permission of Dr. John Cooksey.

to its expressive style. Western civilization's popular and religious musical styles preponderantly use the belted way of singing, including those styles that have roots in the African-American experience (spiritual, blues, jazz, gospel, rock, hip hop, rap, and so forth).

The populations of many Western countries have become cultural mixtures. A current trend in music and choral education is the singing of music from many cultures, including African-American styles. Stylistic accuracy demands that the belted sound quality be performed.

Voice care professionals, singing teachers, and vocally informed music educators traditionally have opposed belted singing, believing it to be injurious to voices, especially the voices of children and adolescents. Clinical experience appears to support the belief. Voice scientists have not discovered all of the details about the physical and acoustic processes that produce "belting" voice quality,[103] but enough information has been discovered to permit very informed descriptions and the initiation of voice education methods.

There are inefficient, overly strenuous ways to produce belting quality, and there are efficient and strenuous ways, according to Estill.[104–107] When producing this quality efficiently, singers remark how easy it seems, yet how powerful it sounds. First time "belters" sometimes comment on the cathartic quality of the experience. Compared with the coordinations used for operatic singing, general physiologic characteristics of belting appear to involve:

1. Comparatively intense postural stabilization of the torso and back of neck
2. Comparatively intense contraction of abdominal wall and costal muscles during phonation, with strong checking force from inhalation muscles—primarily the diaphragm muscle

**Table 16–4   Gackle Maturational Stages of Female Voice Change
Related to Singing; Estimated Pitch Ranges (Whole Notes);
Tessitura Ranges (Bracketed Quarter Notes); and Brief Descriptions***

MATURATIONAL STAGE	DESCRIPTION
I: Prepubertal 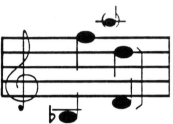	Common ages 8–10/11; voice quality not as full as males of same age due to slightly smaller larynx and vocal tract, no apparent register "breaks;" agile laryngeal motor control for singing wider, faster pitch intervals
IIA: Pubescence; premenarcheal 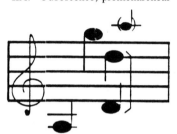	Common ages 11–12/13; correlates with first pubertal signs—breast budding, pubic hair, height increase; voice quality becomes breathy as "mutational chink" occurs, especially in "flutey" upper pitch range, less breathy in fuller quality of lower range; register "break" often appears between G4 and B4, and some girls find lower register is difficult to produce; previous volume levels are reduced; singing becomes more effortful and/or "uncomfortable"
IIB: Puberty; postmenarcheal 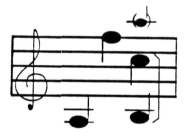	Common ages 13–14/15; peak of voice mutation and greatest instability in vocal coordinations; pitch range diminishes, especially "easy" range; breathy/husky quality still prominent in speaking and singing along with increased fullness; register "breaks" can appear at G4/B4 *and* at D5/F#5 (adult norm); lower pitch range may be temporarily easier for some girls to produce, yielding *illusion* of adult "alto" quality; singing in lower range may be helpful *temporarily*, but exclusive use of lower range will impose limitations on the capabilities of young voices due to tendency to sing with excessive laryngeal effort and vocal fold collision forces; singing continues to be more effortful and "uncomfortable" compared with prepubertal singing
III: Young adult; postmenarcheal 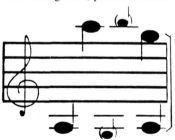	Common ages 14–15/16; pitch range capability increases and breathy voice quality decreases, especially with increased laryngeal conditioning, voice training, and experience; voice quality is clearer, more firm, fuller, and more rich and adultlike; sound volume, vocal "ease," and laryngeal agility resume; register transitions become more consistent and adultlike; vibrato may occur

*Data from Gackle.[102] Used by permission of Dr. Lynne Gackle.

3. Comparatively intense vocal fold adduction with a long closed phase and a short open phase during each vibratory cycle, with a comparatively intense vibratory collision force
4. Comparatively intense simultaneous contraction of both thyroarytenoid and cricothyroid muscles with adjustments that alter with changes in fundamental frequency
5. Comparatively intense stabilization of the larynx in a location that is above "at rest" location
6. Comparatively narrow lower vocal tract, particularly the laryngeal vestibule, with a rather open mouth/jaw
7. Comparatively intense stabilization of the soft palate in an arched upward location
8. Comparatively higher and more forward tongue on all vowels, particularly the normally tongue-back vowels.

General acoustic characteristics of belting appear to involve:

1. High amplitude (loud) sound wave
2. Comparatively greater upper partial/formant amplification than is present in classical "upper" or "head" register.

Singers who belt regularly and *in*efficiently can develop chronic vocal fold swelling, voice fatigue syndrome, and other more serious vocal abnormalities. These consequences, however, are not inevitable. When teaching, learning, and using the belt coordinations, great care can be exercised to protect vocal health.

Voice management skills that belt singers need to prevent voice disorders, and their consequent limits to singing capabilities, are:

1. Development and maintenance of all fundamental vocal skills
2. Development and maintenance of a well-conditioned upper or head register and a "falsetto" register (for men), and flute register (for women)—vital to vocal longevity and health
3. Continual maintenance of laryngeal lubrication and tissue compliance—drink five to seven 8 oz glasses of water per day (child-sized bodies), or seven to ten 8 oz glasses (adult-sized bodies)
4. Warm-up laryngeal muscles before extended singing
5. Balance of voice use time and voice restoration time (silence) based on monitoring of laryngeal sensations and vocal capabilities (swelling detector pitch patterns)
6. Continuous maintenance of general body conditioning and, *most importantly*, laryngeal muscle conditioning
7. Balance of personal energy expenditure with energy restoration—manage distressful circumstances.

Is belting appropriate for youngsters whose vocal anatomy is still developing and may be more vulnerable to the effects of intense collision forces? Even in childhood, the laryngeal muscles and tissues exhibit a strong degree of resilience and strength. Even though that is true, there are limits to the number of forceful collisions that the vocal folds can take before they will react to protect themselves; and there are limits to the amount of strenuous head and neck muscle use before some symptoms of vocal fatigue syndrome begin to appear.

After gathering considerable information about the physical and acoustic realities of belting; after directly experiencing efficient belting and teaching the skills for several years (or observing them being taught); after observing and teaching prepubertal children these skills; after considering health and ethical factors, we believe we can support the following beliefs:

1.   Preventing belted singing by children and adolescents will happen on the day playground yelling is prevented. Both are forms of strong, cathartic self-expression.

2.   Prepubertal children can learn to belt effectively and safely when their parents and vocal music teachers are thoroughly educated about its use.

3.   Belting by pubertal youngsters is a more delicate matter. We believe it can be done safely *if* there is precedent voice education and if the amount of time spent belting is moderated even more than for children, particularly during the climactic time of voice mutation.

4.   Singing teachers can learn one-to-one methods of teaching efficient belting, but current, deep-background training in voice and voice care is requisite. Singing teachers can learn to distinguish the voice qualities aurally that represent inefficient belting and efficient belting, exactly which parts of the vocal mechanism contribute to those qualities, and methods for remediating the inefficient coordinations.

5.   General music educators and choral conductors can learn methods of teaching efficient belting in group settings. Learning fundamental vocal skills—particularly laryngeal and vocal tract coordinations—and methods of voice care and protection is foundational. These methods are not tricks or gimmicks for producing a short-term musical effect. Using these methods well involves long-term goals, persistence, and patience.

A BRIEF PSYCHOSOCIAL CONTEXT FOR YOUNG-VOICE TREATMENT AND EDUCATION TEAMS

Aronson[108,109] has urged voice professionals to recognize that psychosocial history is a significant contributor to the development of voice disorders. "Psyche" and "personality" are thought to result from the confluence of genetic predispositions and the internal processing of unique psychosocial experiences. The processing of some psychosocial experiences involves conscious awareness, but most elements of personal experience are processed outside of conscious awareness.

Other-than-conscious learning capabilities of preborns, newborns, and infants appear to be rather sophisticated, as the process of language acquisition attests. As normal brain morphology continues (hardware development) and as sensory input and pattern detection continue with time, neurochemical networks or "programs" are elaborated and interfaced (software development).[110,111] These programs are commonly called "patterns of behavior," "patterns of thinking," and "emotional patterns." Other-than-conscious learning takes place, for instance, when youngsters observe the behavior of other people—such as parents; characters in cartoons, films and television programs; teachers; and peers and people who are admired such as pop culture stars. Other-than-conscious learning by observing the behavior of others is a lifelong reality.

Over time, youngsters become more adept in both other-than-conscious and conscious learning and communications. With the elaboration of conscious learning abilities comes increased sense-making and mastery (conscious awareness, analysis, categorization, symbol use, and precision and range of neuromuscular coordinations). *Lifelong learning* can be a synonym for all *psychosocial processing*.

The development of personhood or self-concept involves a blend of two well-known complex psychosocial processes: (1) self-identity, or the differentiation of self from other "selves," and (2) social integration. A prime influence on the development of self-identity is the extent to which children first bond with, and then differentiate themselves from, parents and develop "independent" mastery of self and "their world." A prime influence on social integration is the nature of parent–child bonding or disbonding. Relationships with other adults and peers throughout childhood and adolescence can be significant influences.

Genetic predispositions and psychosocial experiences tend to produce proportions of protective and constructive orientations to the people, places, and things of "the world." Protective orientations in young people reflect a psychosocial history in which a prominent number of experiences have been emotionally threatening. Behaviors that reflect a protective orientation can be described on a continuum from more withdrawn, hesitant, and dependent; to controlled and tense; to defensive and belligerent. Constructive orientations reflect a psychosocial history in which a prominent number of experiences have been emotionally safe and rewarding. Young people with a constructive orientation can be described briefly as more independent, productive, cooperative, confident, expressive, and creative.

During puberty, a surge of physical and biochemical changes erupts in young people.[44] Self-identity and social integration processes are richly affected by the changes. Changes in height, weight, and physiognomy are emotionally threatening to some youngsters and rewarding to others. The incidence of anorexia nervosa and bulimia in female teenagers has risen significantly in recent years.

The intensity of biochemically mediated emotional reactions dramatically increases with puberty. At the same time, there is increased cognitive capacity that enables increased conscious awareness of self in the social world, and of "the world as it is" versus "the world as it could be." These growing, but as yet unwieldy capacities increase the probability of heightened sensitivity to criticism and to conflict with parents, siblings, adult authority figures, and peers.

Over the past few generations, the cultural milieu in which young people grow up has dramatically changed. The intensity of stress reaction has generally increased,[112] and general health can be adversely affected.[113] Reactions to family relationship problems such as sexual, physical, or emotional abuse; alcoholism; divorce; and single parent families, two working parents, and less adult guidance result in more reliance on peers and pop culture idols as behavioral models. Those factors and the stresses of psychosexual growth and new social relationships can produce, in some youngsters, a threatening social milieu and protective behavioral orientations, including "feelings of inferiority," depression, anxiety, and overt rejection of "the world as it is." Various legal and illegal drugs are easily available to "blunt" emotional discomfort chemically. In the current psychosocial climate, teen pregnancy and suicide rates have been surging.

In preadolescence and adolescence, the clothing, lifestyle behaviors, and conscious and other-than-conscious expressions of admired pop culture stars influence the process of evolving sense-making, self-identity, and social integration.[114] In varying ways, all young-sters in this age group are "experimenting" with self-identities that are unique and distinct from their parents and other adults. They are exploring the integration of personal self-identities with those of their peers. The more the adults in their lives have attempted coercive controls on behavior, the greater the tendency to be "rebellious" or to conceal or even suppress expressions of self-identity. A form of alienation can occur that is a bar-rier to truly open, comfortable communication with some adults.

Many entertainers and popular art forms express rejection of "the world as it is" and reinforce the rejection of it. They also express the psychogenic-induced consequences of suppressed self-identity processes and a cathartic "release" of same. They do so by choosing clothing, lifestyle behaviors, and forms of expression that are opposite to the preferences of adult "controllers."

Parents, schools, and units of government often rely on coercive forms of threat to accomplish learning and behavior regulation. Nearly all behavioral rules are prohibi-tions with some form of punishment as consequences. School studies often are framed with similar coercive, punitive, and accusative prohibitions. These circumstances greatly diminish forms of intrinsic motivation by which the innate capacities of sense-making and self-mastery flourish.[115] Whether or not parents and other adult authority figures adapt to the changing psychosocial realities of young people will significantly influence the ex-tent to which a prominently protective orientation or a prominently constructive one will develop.

A consideration of "young voices" cannot be divorced from these psychosocial contexts. As young human beings grow up, their vocal behavior is intimately integrated with the processes of sense-making, self-identity, and social integration. Voice is a prominent component of the self-expression that occurs during the evolution of personhood.

The vocal characteristics of children and adolescents who are involved in these growing up processes are varied. Protective-withdrawn youngsters may show depression and have hypofunctional voices that are mildly breathy, soft, and underconditioned. Protective-controlled youngsters may present observable laryngeal, vocal tract, and articu-lator muscle tension with a history of hyperfunction and a pressed-breathy or pressed-edgy voice quality. Protective-defensive or belligerent youngsters may speak loudly, with pressed quality and general hyperfunction. Constructively oriented children are more at risk for developing voice abnormalities from extensive and hyperfunctional voice use if they are highly extroverted and involved in many activities that require voicing.

Parents are the most influential voice educators of all. How they coordinate their own voices while speaking or singing represents the predominant auditory input for other-than-conscious learning of respiratory, laryngeal, and vocal tract coordinations by their children. Other immediate family members also may become models. Family vocal communication patterns involving pitch, volume, timing, and quality usually are learned outside conscious awareness.

Admired peers and nonfamily adults in a child's community can contribute to the elaboration of behavioral patterns for speaking and singing. If electronic entertainment media are heard frequently during childhood, they may provide significant models for experimentation with and learning of voice coordinations. Cartoon characters, story characters, puppets, and costumed animal characters sometimes present voice coordina-tions that are rather hyperfunctional and abrasive to vocal fold tissue. Sometimes child entertainers who sing for children present voice qualities that are hyperfunctional. Voice models for speaking and singing in the entertainment media appear to increase their influence during adolescence.[114] Many youngsters may sing with popular music on radio or recordings surprisingly often and for surprising amounts of time.

According to Mehrabian,[116] about 7% of spoken communication may be delivered and received in conscious awareness—the "text" or denotative meanings of words. That means that 93% of spoken communication may be delivered and received outside of conscious awareness as "context." Fifty-five percent is presented in physical postures and gestures and are perceived visually. Thirty-eight percent of other-than-conscious communication is presented by voice and is received aurally, so that 45% of total spoken communications involves voice. Variables in other-than-conscious vocal communications include:

1. The connotative interpretations of the words presented (generated from the unique experience-feeling memories of each communicant)
2. The varied contextual ways that pitch, volume, quality ("tone of voice"), and speech timing are used.

If Mehrabian's statistics are even close to accurate, might programs that couple treatment for voice disorders with general student voice education be relevant to getting a job, earning a livelihood, and social success?

There is no universally consistent resource for meaningful voice education for all students in all schools, and yet the impact of dysfunctional voice on educational sense-making and self identity is known.[117] Pre-service training of school staff usually does not include efficient, effective use of their own voices, including school speech pathologists, music educators, choral directors, and theatre directors. The learning and use of effective methods for teaching physically and acoustically efficient voice skills— integrated speaking and singing skills—is often inadequate and inconsistent. Effective, constructive psychosocial methods for accomplishing such goals have been developed.[118–121]

An accessible resource now exists for vocal music educators, choral conductors, singing teachers, and school speech pathologists to experience current, science-based voice information and psychosocially constructive methodology that integrates efficient speaking and singing skills. The VoiceCare Network[121] is a nonprofit educational organization that is affiliated with the National Center for Voice and Speech (NCVS). NCVS, funded by the National Institute of Deafness and Other Communication Disorders, is a nationwide consortium of institutions that provide advanced training for voice professionals, research opportunities, and information dissemination programs. The Network's role is to disseminate research-based information about voice and to present teaching methodologies that are age-appropriate, psychosocially constructive, and oriented to voice health and care through courses titled "Lifespan Voice Education in the Real World." The Network is an auxiliary of the Music Educators National Conference, and its programs are endorsed by the National Association of Teachers of Singing.

OVERVIEW OF VOICE TREATMENT AND EDUCATION PROCESSES FOR YOUNG VOCAL PERFORMERS WITH DYSFUNCTIONING VOICES

Young vocal performers may be actors, public speakers, and/or singers in school, community nonprofit, religious, or professional organizations; and they may be leaders in school, religious, or community organizations; extroverted or hyperactive children; or involved in any number of activities that require extensive and/or vigorous voicing such as cheerleading or yelling at sports events.

Treatment of Voice Disorders in Young Vocal Performers

To provide the most effective care possible, five elements of voice disorder treatment may be used:

1. Focus all communications by team members on comfortable, cooperative learning and optimum resolution of the young patient-client's disorder
2. Diagnose the disorder and contributing factors through health history and videostroboscopic examination by ear-nose-throat physician
3. Evaluate and assess patient-client voice function (speaking/singing) through comprehensive, in-depth voice health and lifestyle history, assessment tasks, and videostroboscopic observation
4. Design a program of voice treatment and education that is tailored to the unique needs of each patient-client
5. Guide the patient-client through the treatment and education program by providing feedback, answering questions, reviewing tasks, and monitoring progress.

Communications Orientation

Two categories of communication may be interesting to examine: (1) communication that may affect motivation to resolve voice disorders and (2) communication that helps youngsters change their vocal behaviors in the direction of optimum voice.

On the first visit, the immediate psychological orientation of young patients-clients will fall into three broad categories (young vocal arts performers fall into the first category): (1) those who are distressed and anxious because their voice dysfunction is threatening the accomplishment of goals that are very important to them, (2) those who are not aware that their voice dysfunction limits their ability to communicate well with others, and (3) those who have not chosen to have their voices examined and are present only because an adult in authority has directed them. Treatment team members need to communicate four "messages" during the first and all subsequent visits.

Message 1.   "You are safe here." It may seem elementary to some, but, upon meeting a young vocal arts performer, a smile of welcome, a meeting of eyes, a firm handshake, and asking *them* to describe their circumstances will communicate safety and begin the next message.

During the first visit, when providing reaction to past vocal use, or during subsequent visits when providing feedback for task attempts and treatment progress, adopt a "language of accepting assessment" rather than a "language of punitive or accusative judgment." For example, instead of "You really did hammer your dried-out vocal cords, all right," say, "None of us can do what we don't know to do, right?" or "I heard more ease in those sounds; how did they feel to you?" instead of "I think you're still constricting your voice some, but it's better."

When setting treatment goals, adopt a "language of exploration and self-discovery" rather than a "language of coercion." For instance, say, "If you drink six to nine 8 oz glasses of water every day, that will help your voice operate more easily," rather than, "I want you to drink six to nine 8 oz glasses of water every day."

Message 2. "You are highly regarded here and your competence is respected." Overly solicitous communication will interfere with mutual respect.

Message 3. "We will tell you the truth about your voice as we see it and what can be done to restore optimum function. What you do with that information is up to you."

Message 4. "Your out-of-health voice can be resolved into a reliable, optimum voice, a voice that you will like and will be effective and accepted and admired by others. The process will take time, and you will have to summon your own strong determination to see it through." Some vocal conditions cannot be resolved to "normal" voice, of course. Language is then used to assist psychosocial adjustment to these circumstances so that constructive self-identity and social integration are optimized.

Comments. Young people who are not vocal arts performers will tend to fall into categories two and three above. The same four messages are needed, of course. The laryngologic diagnostic examination should proceed normally, but the speech–voice pathologist faces other communication challenges with youngsters in category two. The challenge is to design an experience in which *they* will discover how their ability to communicate effectively is limited and how the limitations might have occurred. The youngsters, then, may independently choose to initiate therapy or not.

When faced with youngsters in category three, a conference is needed that includes the parents–guardians and the adult who referred them. The same kind of direct learning as provided for category two youngsters can be helpful, while the parents–guardians and/or other adult observes. Guide the experience so that the decision on whether to initiate and continue therapy rests with the youngster. Young people who are coerced into therapy tend to evade doing the tasks that are necessary for restoration of optimum voice.

The younger the performers, the less they are capable of comprehending a technical–analytic mode of communication—a common mode of voice professionals. The language used, therefore, can be modified so that it is appropriate to age and experience.

Language labels can enhance or limit perception, understanding, and effective action. For instance, the terms *speaking voice* and *singing voice* are common labels among voice professionals. To young people who are still making sense of the world, the two terms communicate (other-than-consciously) the existence of two separate vocal entities. Young children may believe that they have two voices—one for speaking and another for singing—and that they operate independently of each other like their two arms.

That pattern of perception can have consequences into adulthood. Choral conductors may help young singers use their voices very efficiently and expressively when singing, but if a musical composition under rehearsal includes a speaking section, the singers may suddenly reveal esthetically "painful" voice qualities from hyperfunctional speech coordinations. If a patient is a singer, some otolaryngologists may not attend sufficiently to the contribution of the "speaking voice" to a voice disorder, because "singing voice" has captured their attention. In singers, the coordinations used to produce speech usually contribute more to development and maintenance of voice disorders than the singing coordinations.

A more accurate way to help young people is to help them appreciate that they have one voice, and it is used in a "speaking way," a "sound-making way," a "shouting way," and a "singing way." We may use such alternative phrases as, "When you use your voice for speaking" (or singing); "Your singing (speaking) coordinations are working your voice box muscles so hard and so much that they are hurting."

Physician Diagnosis of the Disorder

Adult vocal performers require special diagnostic consideration because their voices are an integral part of earning their livelihood. Some young vocal performers also may be earning a livelihood, but most are developing vocal skills that may either facilitate their future careers or inhibit them to some degree. Additional reasons for special diagnostic consideration for young vocal performers is that their anatomy and physiology are still forming and they are more vulnerable to vocal and emotional distress.

Use of a rigid fiberoptic videostrobolaryngoscope is valuable and may be essential for diagnosis of laryngeal tissue disorders. The degree of visual clarity and magnification of finer architectural detail provided by the rigid scope overrides the advantages of the flexible scope. In some cases, a video that includes both types of scope may be helpful. An adequate view may not be possible with smaller children, and some of them will not be able to tolerate either of the scopes. Videotaping of selected vocal tasks provides a clear record of organic state. Diagnosis of some disorders is aided by repeated viewing. When the laryngologist and the speech–voice therapist are both present, the patient–client can be asked to perform vocal tasks that serve both medical diagnosis and assessment of vocal coordinations.

Some young performers are so distressed by their "failing" voice and by the anticipation of "something stuck down my throat" or "through my nose" that they become physically very tense. Their laryngeal and vocal tract muscles may so narrow and shorten the vocal tract that a complete view of the vocal folds is denied. The "You are safe here" messages of the laryngologist and speech–voice pathologist can contribute to a moderation of adverse reaction. Advance talk that acknowledges their anxiety and suggests safety and relaxation can be very helpful. "Just about everybody who has never been "scoped" before feels a little anxious beforehand—just like you. I know I was. And yes, it may feel uncomfortable. I wish it didn't, but it may. And after they've finished and seen their own voices for the first time, nearly everyone who has done this says, 'You know, that wasn't so bad. I thought it was going to be awful, but it wasn't!' " An explanation of the viewing process using plastic models, followed by a brief practice session, may help. Taking time to "communicate safety" and to establish personal trust can benefit diagnostic accuracy and completeness, and is a foundation for successful therapy.

Before introducing the scope, ask the patient to wiggle the jaw left to right gently, then release the shoulders down, then breathe in two or three full breaths. Just as the scope begins to move in, have the patient-client begin sustaining the /ee/ vowel in order to direct their conscious awareness toward sustaining the pitch and away from worrying about the unpleasantness of gagging or nasal discomfort. If sustaining one pitch is insufficient to distract, ask them to sing a repeated pattern of two or three scale-wise pitches or the pitches of one phrase of a familiar song like "Happy Birthday."

When telling young performers about the diagnosis, use of the video is valuable. Orient them to the anatomic features that they are about to see with a plastic model of the larynx or a half head and neck. Then show a brief video of healthy vocal folds that show normal configuration, movement (adduction/abduction and shortening/lengthening), and a "slow motion" mucosal wave. Then show their video. Explain the diagnosis and give some indication of how the tissue changes happened. Choose words that communicate messages three and four above, focusing on reassurance of eventual resolution if the patient chooses to create the conditions that enable the body to resume optimum voice.

Address diagnostic findings primarily to the young patient-client. Including the speech–voice pathologist and/or accompanying adult by asking for information and opinions will communicate a "team" message. These matters may be of great emotional significance to young performers. If physician time cannot be devoted to all the elements of this process, a brief conference with the speech–voice pathologist about diagnostic observations—away from the young patient-client—can enable the spoken delivery of the diagnosis by the speech–voice pathologist.

The process described above provides the following advantages:

1.   The vocal constraints of emotional distress are diminished, and motivation to complete voice therapy is optimized.

2.   A more accurate and complete view of the vocal folds may be obtained due to reduction of some of the hyperfunction that results from anxiety.

3.   The disorder becomes a physical reality to the patients—not a fantasy—and they tend to react more like they do when they see a physical abnormality on the outer surface of the body. Motivation to do what is necessary to remove the tissue change is much greater than when only a verbal description is provided.

Assessment and Evaluation of Vocal Function

Evaluation and assessment of vocal function in young performers is intended to document reductions in vocal ability and to evaluate their relationship to any organic or functional abnormalities that may be present. A voice treatment and education program is based on the findings. Assessment and evaluation must include:

1.   Written general health history and written health and lifestyle history related specifically to voice
2.   Voice health interview
3.   Speaking assessment
4.   Singing assessment
5.   Videostroboscopic review
6.   Presentation of evaluation to client and parent–guardian.

Younger children sometimes prefer to have an accompanying adult in the room. Older children may not, and adolescents commonly do not.

History.   Reviewing a written general health history of young vocal performers and a written in-depth health and lifestyle history related to voice will be necessary for core members of a young-voice team. The voice history form should include information about all the circumstances in which voices are used, the extent and vigor of voice use, voice use occasions, voice communications patterns, and voice-related lifestyle patterns. Ask whether they sing with a radio or recorded music, and, if so, ask for an estimate of how many days and how much time each day. Parents–guardians and young performers can cooperate to provide complete information, and auxiliary team members may contribute, such as school teachers, singing teachers and theatre directors.

Voice Health Interview.   Following completion of a written history, a face-to-face interview can include a description by clients of when they first noticed reduced vocal function. Follow-up questions to their narrative and to their voice history will be necessary.

The information gained will identify factors which contributed to the disorder and will assist in developing a voice treatment and education plan. Some of the answers can be audiorecorded as a sample of habitual conversational speech.

Speaking Assessment.   When clients are speaking performers, a sample of how they speak conversationally and how they speak when they perform will be necessary. Other common voice assessments also will be helpful. A videotape of actual performance may be asked for and viewed, if appropriate, or a live performance may be attended. The actual performance situation often "triggers" vocal patterns that are different from the ones used in a clinic setting.

The following assessments will reveal basic functional information. The means of assessment will vary depending on the type of equipment available and its sophistication. See Chapter 8 for additional approaches.

1.   Audio record a sample of ordinary conversation during the voice health interview. The sample becomes a part of the client assessment record and can be used to assess MSFF. Informal, noninstrumental assessment of habitual average "anchor" pitch area can be determined by carefully listening to the client's speech and very softly "matching" several briefly sustained spoken pitches with one's own voice. The pausing expression "uhhh" may be used, for instance. Several very short, very soft "matches" during ongoing speech can help adjust an initial impression. The pitch can be verified on an electric piano keyboard. This assessment can be done during interviews if it is done in a way that does not disrupt the flow of the client conversation and shows that you maintain interest in what is being said. Use of the piano should be done during a convenient pause in the interview. Advance practice with colleagues is very helpful.

2.   In the absence of appropriate equipment to measure respiratory functions and capacities vis à vis adductory sufficiency, ask clients to breathe fully and sustain a sound as long as they can. A brief model on an /ah/ vowel will be helpful and sometimes necessary for youngsters. Perform the task two to four times. Record the time of the longest trial as maximum phonation time. An audiorecording of two or three of these trials may be made for subsequent acoustic analysis.

3.   Ask the young client to imitate the sound of a dripping faucet and model the task by making a series of rapid unvoiced "glottal pops" with an /uh/ vowel formation. Ask them to repeat the sounds with as little effort as possible and still do it. A clear "pop" indicates complete vocal fold adduction. Thickened mucus on the vocal folds and vocal fold swelling will prevent "pop" clarity. Instead, a brief breathy flow of air will occur.

4.   Next, ask clients to imitate a series of somewhat soft-voiced glottal "pops" after a provided model. This task assesses the combination of vocal fold adduction and mucosal wave onset.

5.   For additional assessment of MSFF and record-keeping, a computer-based instrument may be used.

6.   Available speaking pitch range may be assessed by using voice glides. Ask young clients to imagine that they have been cast in the lead role of a play that will be presented by a professional theatre company. They will be paid "big bucks." They play the role of the Wise Owl. In a key scene, the Wise Owl individually asks all the birds and animals of the forest a particular question. Because the Wise Owl is wise, he says the question differently for each creature in order to hear the truest answer possible. The speech–voice pathologist plays the role of director of the play and models a variety of ways to say "Who are you?" Begin in lower pitch range, speak slowly and softly, toward the mellow-breathy side of

quality, with a mysterious, distant, even "ghostly" inflection and an appropriate facial expression. Succeeding repeats of the question should include variable speech rates and intensity–volume variation. Expand the range of pitch inflection several times but remain within the lower half of speaking pitch range.

For upper speaking pitch range, suggest that clients also have been cast in a minor role in the play. In that human character's one scene, a group of friends are across the stage and just about to exit, and the script says that the client's character makes a particular vocal sound to get their attention so they stop for more dialogue. "Yoo hoo, yoo hoo!" is rehearsed twice in upper pitch range and register. "I wonder what your voice would do if you started in the 'yoo hoo' part of your voice and you slid it down to join the Wise Owl part like this: 'Yoo hoo—(descending voice glide)—are you?' " Then afterward: "Can you do another voice glide that begins in the Wise Owl part of your voice and slides up to join the yoo hoo part like this: 'Who are you—(ascending voice glide)—hoo?' "

7. Loudness capability and incidence of glottal attack in speech may be assessed by asking clients to imagine that they are on one side of a four-lane highway with no traffic, and they ask a stranger on the other side, "Am I the only aardvark in our area?" It has to be loud enough for the stranger to hear clearly. Then ask the question as though the highway was full of noisy cars and trucks.

8. The Bastian-Kaidar-Verdolini swelling test,[122] using the first phrase of "Happy Birthday," can be used to assess reliably the effects of swelling and other tissue abnormalities on vocal ability. Youngsters who cannot yet sing pitches accurately can imagine playing the role of a little newborn puppy who has been separated from its mother and is making a series of short "puppy crying sounds." Those sounds then can be converted into a small "sound siren" and "spiraled" up as high as it can go, several times.

9. The previous tasks can point the laryngologist and speech–voice pathologist toward the tasks that need documenting in videostroboscopy.

Singing Assessment.   If singing is one of the skills used by young performers—even though they may not presently be involved in a singing situation—then a singing assessment is necessary. The following assessments will reveal basic functional information. The means of assessment may vary. See Chapter 9 for additional approaches.

1. The "Wise Owl" and "yoo hoo" experiences described above provide baseline information about the ability to "match" the pitches of speech and vocal sounds. It also introduces a measure of comfort and an "atmosphere" of imaginative play into the assessment setting.

2. The same experience provides baseline information about the laryngeal coordinations that produce lower and upper vocal registers and whether the transition between the two is "blended" or produces an abrupt "break" in sound quality. Basic differences of register "strength" can be assessed. The most common imbalance between the two would be a stronger lower register coordination (the register coordination used in speech and most singing) but a weaker upper register coordination that produces a softer, breathy quality. If a voice disorder is not present, the "weakness" is due to lack of neuromuscular skill and conditioning. The "puppy cry" described above is a method of assessing baseline information about falsetto register for all males who are in or have passed the Cooksey Midvoice II classification (including adult males) and flute register for females.

3. Assessing low and then high terminal pitches can give a basic indication of present singing ability and an appropriate singing range for adolescent singers whose voices are changing. Low terminal pitch may be assessed by asking young clients to sing a series of

descending musical scales, each beginning on the fifth scale step of a major scale and ending on the first: 5, 4, 3, 2, 1. The beginning pitch of each scale lowers by one semitone. (A semitone is one musical half-step interval; adjacent keys on a piano keyboard are arranged in half-steps.) Eventually, the lowest pitch will "turn to breath." The lowest clear pitch is the low terminal pitch. The beginning pitch for the first five-note scale can be selected by first selecting a pitch from the habitual "anchor pitch area" in speech. Then, begin the first five-note scale on the fifth major scale note above the anchor pitch. The anchor pitch, then, will be the lowest pitch of the first five-note scale.

High terminal pitch may be assessed by asking the clients to sing a continuously ascending major scale (into the next octave), breathing when necessary, and then resuming the scale. Amount of training and experience, severity of voice disorder, or effects of adolescent voice mutation can be indicated by this task. Begin the scale in the habitual anchor pitch area of speech. To obtain the most successful results, less trained and experienced youngsters may be helped by asking them to open their mouths gradually wider as they ascend in pitch. That will help them to avoid some acoustic "loading" of the vocal folds and an unnecessary limitation on upper range ability.[123]

Males aged 11 to 15 years are most likely to be in some stage of voice mutation. Comparing their range compass to the ranges of the Cooksey Index (see Table 16–3) will provide an indication of mutational stage and the safe outer limits of pitch range in sung music. If the pitches are within the range compass but most of the pitches cluster in either the upper half or the bottom few notes of the range, then singing the music is likely to "teach" the boy to sing hyperfunctionally and produce a faster rate of laryngeal muscle fatigue through increased collision forces. The bracketed quarter notes indicate the pitch range (tessitura) in which most boys can sing with the greatest physical ease. The boys in Midvoice IIA, the high point of mutation, appear to be the most vulnerable to voice use disorders.

Females aged 11 to 15 years also are most likely to be in some stage of voice mutation. Comparing their range compass to the ranges proposed by Gackle (see Table 16–4) will provide an indication of mutational stage and the safe outer limits of pitch range in sung music. The girls in postmenarcheal stage IIB, the high point of mutation, appear to be least capable of singing easily in upper register range and more capable of singing in a loud belted way in their lower pitch range. They also appear to be the most vulnerable to voice use disorders. Softer singing and conversational speech tend to display a typically "husky" quality.

4.   Further information about register strength and transitions can be obtained when singing the pitch patterns described in the previous two tasks. Information related to voice quality and efficiency/inefficiency of overall vocal coordinations also may be obtained.

5.   The next task for assessing the voices of young clients is to have them sing four phrases or the chorus of a song of their choosing. It can be "Happy Birthday," a song from school, a song they have performed before, or one they are currently performing or rehearsing. The extent and strength of voice register use, extent of skill in performing register transitions, general hypo- or hyperfunctional voice use, and efficiency/inefficiency in the use of belting coordinations can be observed. The key tone of the songs can be raised or lowered to assess the limits of current register skills.

6.   While singing the song, *voice quality* observations can be made. General voice quality characteristics are produced by physical coordinations in two areas of the vocal mechanism—the larynx and the vocal tract. Word labels in common use for perceived voice

quality are almost entirely metaphoric, and many singing teachers confusingly use several terms and expressions to refer to perceived voice quality phenomena that emanate from both parts of the vocal mechanism.

The words we use to describe voice qualities are attached to documented phenomena within the larynx and vocal tract. The *larynx* contributes the following continuum of voice quality characteristics:

a. "Breathy" qualities are produced by incompletely adducted vocal folds or by vocal folds whose mucosal tissues have been changed from an optimum state and produce varying degrees of air-turbulence noise

b. "Pressed," "strident," "edgy," or "harsh" qualities are produced by intensely compressed vocal folds that in turn produce areas of chaotic vibration that produce the high-frequency spectral noise components that generated the above descriptors

c. "Firm-clear-mellow-warm" qualities are produced by a "balanced seal" of the vocal folds over the trachea that produces no perceivable noise.

Wide variation in perceived sound volume can be produced in each category. There is a subset continuum in the firm-clear-mellow-warm category:

i. "Lighter-softer," "thinner sounding" qualities that are produced by complete but lower-intensity adduction of the vocal folds, producing fewer upper spectral partials and upper formant regions; most partial amplitudes are "weaker."

ii. "Heavier-louder," "thicker sounding" or more "full-bodied" sounding qualities that are produced by higher intensity adduction of the vocal folds, producing more upper spectral partials and formant regions; most partial amplitudes are noticeably "stronger."

The *vocal tract* contributes the following continuum of voice quality characteristics:

a. Considerably "dark," "soblike," and "woofy" qualities are produced by a vocal tract that is hyperfunctionally longer and larger; that configuration amplifies the lower spectral partials and formant regions while attenuating the higher partials and formant regions. "Throaty" and "bottled up" qualities are produced by constricted tongue muscles, "shapes," usually with a back and downwardly depressed tongue base.

b. Noticeably "squeezed," "narrow," "pinched," and "shrill" qualities are produced by a vocal tract that is hyperfunctionally shorter and smaller; that configuration amplifies the higher spectral partials and formant regions while attenuating the lower partials and formant regions.

c. "Balanced resonance" qualities are produced by a vocal tract that is configured with neuromuscular economy (physical efficiency) for whatever expressive task is at hand and allows a relatively balanced amplitude in the lower and upper spectral partials and formant regions to emerge from the lips. Within this voice quality category is a subset continuum that ranges between "fuller" qualities and "brighter" qualities that emerge when the physically efficient singer is other-than-consciously expressing more somber or more celebratory emotional states.

7.   Singing the song with various amplitude and volume levels provides an opportunity to assess effects of a voice disorder on this singing ability.

8.   Singing the song provides the opportunity to observe habitual breathing coordinations and assess whether they provide appropriate breath-flow energy to support physically efficient phonation.

9.   Singing the song provides the opportunity to observe how young clients arrange their skeletons when seated, standing, and walking and to assess whether their habitual arrangements enable physical and acoustic efficiency or interfere with it.

10.   Singing the song provides the opportunity to observe excessive or appropriately minimal use of glottal attacks.

11.   Singing pitch patterns that require *laryngeal tissue flexibility and muscle agility*— wider pitch intervals and faster pitch changes—provides the opportunity to observe the extent to which mucosal stiffness, muscle tension dysphonia, or other abnormalities may have affected this important factor in singing ability.

Videostroboscopic Review.   The voice assessment findings should corroborate what is seen in the videostroboscopic views.

Evaluation Presentation.   Following a diagnostic examination and the gathering of all history and assessment information, the team members can now evaluate "the big picture" and design the voice treatment and education program. The status of the voice and a plan for regaining optimum voice then may be described to the young client and any family members, teachers, and directors who may be present.

Explaining the status of the voice provides an opportunity for voice education and "setting the stage" for intrinsic motivation to accomplish treatment goals. Common basic education at this time, using everyday vocabulary, will involve very basic anatomy, function, and tissue response to voice use. Refer frequently to the deficits in vocal ability that were described by the client at the beginning of the voice health interview. Plastic anatomic models, photo slides, and the videotape of the young client's own vocal folds can be used to increase the impact of the education on behavior. All youngsters need active participation or "doing" activities during the education. Adolescents have greater capacity to process more abstract, verbally delivered concepts. Some suggestions are described later, in the section on guiding clients through a treatment and education program.

Initial voice education will include informative experiences about how voices are made and operated and how they respond to use:

1.   How the sound of the voice is created by breath air flowing through closed vocal cords and how the flowing air makes ripple-waves happen in the outer layers of the vocal cords

2.   How the number of ripple-waves made produces the voice pitch and how the vocal cords make higher and lower pitches

3.   How the ripple-waves of the two closed vocal cords collide and rub into each other when vocal sound is made

4.   The high numbers of ripple-waves that happen when people talk and sing (see the section on guiding clients through a treatment and education plan for helpful information)

5.   How the impact force of the collisions is greater when voices are louder, just like hand-clapping is louder when people clap harder

6.   How the number of collisions and greater collision forces can cause the vocal cords to try to defend themselves by swelling up (or using other "defenses") to make a "padding" for protection against the collisions
7.   How the greater stiffness and larger size of swollen vocal cords affect pitch range, voice quality, and vocal agility
8.   How the muscles of the "voice box" sometimes work long hours
9.   That when the muscles work harder to make high, low, and loud sounds, they "tire" more.

During delivery of the information in items one through five above, the young client can be asked, "Does that make sense to you?" During delivery of the information in items five through nine above, the young client can be asked, "Does that help you understand what has happened to your voice?" Allowing young clients to use their pattern-detecting capabilities helps them to remain engaged and to appreciate the relationship between the voice education experiences and the current limitations on their speaking and/or singing ability.

Here is a sample of an "active-doing" educational experience that can be "put in your own words." It assumes that the client understands the information in items one through five above.

"Just for the fun of it, use the fingers of one hand to tap lightly on the back of your other hand. (Model it with the client.) Just keep on doing that while I talk. Now, what do you suppose that hand would feel like if you were to keep on doing that, oh, say, one thousand times? (Change pitch inflections and volume to convey changes in the numbers.) What about 50,000 times? 100,000 times? A million times? Keep on tapping your hand. Singing the pitch called middle C for one second means about 260 collisions have happened. (Play it on a piano keyboard or pitch pipe and ask the client to hum it with you for 1 second.) How many collisions would take place if we sustained it for 4 seconds? (About 1,040.) Just singing a song for three minutes may mean 50,000 to 90,000 collisions of your vocal cords. How many might there be when you rehearse your performance? How many in a whole day?

"How many times do you suppose we've tapped that hand? How does your hand feel? (Hurts?) Now, hit your hand almost as hard as you can about 15 times. (Do it together.) How does that feel? Take a look at that hand you hit. See a color that is different than your skin? (Red or dark.) Why do you suppose it is red? Why not green or some other color? (Blood.) Do you suppose that might happen to our vocal cords when we collide them real hard several hundred thousand times?

"Something else besides 'hurt' is happening on our hands, but we haven't hit our hands hard enough and long enough to be able to see it. When any part of us has taken hard hits or a lot of hits, our body tries to protect that part by sending extra water there to puff it up and form a padding, and more blood is sent there to begin healing work. Do you know what that padding is usually called? (Swelling.) (Further extrapolations of this scenario can address the formation of nodules, polyps, hemorrhage, and so forth.)

"Now I want to make one thing perfectly clear. Your vocal cords are very strong and resilient. They were 'built' to withstand millions of collisions a day *if* only some of the collisions are really hard, and *if* they have enough time to recover before the next millions happen, and *if* your voice allows your breathflow to do most of the work, rather than using a lot of unnecessary muscles to 'gang up' on your voice to make a lot of hard collisions and tire your voice out."

Designing a Voice Treatment and Education Program

Laryngologists.   For young performers, conservative treatment is the bedrock of voice recovery. When the extent and vigor of voice use have contributed to the disorder, timely therapy is the standard practice, followed by continuing voice skill education with a voice education team member in whom you have great confidence. Introduce the benefits of hydration and "voice recovery time" when indicated. Suggesting absolute voice rest for extended periods of time is never indicated. Absolute voice rest should never be extended more than 72 hours, and then only in very special circumstances. Reinforcing the competence of the speech–voice pathologist and voice education team members in such matters will be very helpful.

Surgical intervention in the treatment of any voice disorder in any young person should be an absolute last resort and only in the most extreme circumstances. The consequences of even the finest surgical technique to emerging anatomy and physiology are not known at this time. During the pubertal time, the tissues may be particularly sensitive to surgical disturbance. At no time should the possibility of surgery be used as a threat or consequence of not doing well in therapy.

Should surgery be required, therapy should begin well before the procedure is performed, just as it would with adults. Presurgical therapy begins the process of changing habitual hyperfunctional voice use patterns. When postsurgical talking begins with tissues that are still healing, the new vocal coordinations are already well on the road to change. This principle is particularly true for young singers, and the reconditioning of their laryngeal muscles and mucosal tissues must be supervised by someone who is knowledgeable and experienced in reconditioning processes for singing.

Speech–Voice Pathologists and Voice Educators.   The following elements of a therapy treatment and voice education plan for young vocal performers may be considered:

1. Itemize voice health and protection behaviors that are of immediate importance to young clients and those that are helpful for longer-term use
2. Design a regulated voice use regimen that enhances the restoration of laryngeal tissues to normal dimension, configuration, and function
3. Schedule a psychosocial interview to determine if referral for psychological assistance or family counseling may be appropriate and/or to introduce stress management experiences
4. Schedule sessions to begin learning fundamental voice skills for speaking and singing that are physically and acoustically efficient. Skills are regarded as fundamental if they apply to both speaking and singing
5. Determine the extent to which laryngeal muscle conditioning or reconditioning may be necessary after laryngeal tissues have resumed optimum function
6. Lay the foundation for educating young clients about the short- and long-term advantages of using voice protection methods and learning extended voice skills (beyond the fundamentals).

Guiding Young Patients-Clients Through a Voice Treatment and
Education Program

Interwoven into all of the elements of a voice treatment and education program are aspects of voice education that include (1) some basics of how voices are "made and played"; (2) some basics about how voice dysfunctions can occur and be prolonged; and (3) life-long methods of voice care and protection. In most cases, the education comes first because it points toward what has happened and what to do about it and provides intrinsic motivation for accomplishing program goals.

Voice Health and Protection Behaviors. A "tips list," given to the client and/or parent-guardian, can provide a beginning point for discovery of more detailed information about the benefits of new preventive and protective behaviors. Discuss the most essential behavioral changes during the evaluation—hydration, for instance—and include others in subsequent sessions.

Regulated Voice Use Regimen. When there is a need for "recovery time," then specific recommendations can be made. During 3 minutes of continual quiet conversation, females could experience from 30,000 to 45,000 vocal fold collisions and changed-voice males from 15,000 to 22,500 collisions. In songs with very average ranges, females singing in their higher pitch range (soprano, for instance) may experience from 80,000 to 90,000 collisions. Higher range adult males (tenors, for instance) may experience 40,000 to 50,000 collisions. Females singing lower range songs (such as alto) may experience from 55,000 to 65,000 collisions. Lower range adult males may experience 30,000 to 40,000 collisions.

There are a variety of standard practices that facilitate recovery time. Co-plan the specifics with young clients by asking such questions as, "During your day, when do you think you use your voice the most and the loudest?" and "How do you think you could give your voice more recovery time?" When young clients are involved in the planning, there may be more "ownership" of the task. Intrinsic motivation to carry out the tasks is greater when the therapy experience enables them to use their sense-making and self-identity (self-mastery) capacities. Introduce an element of fun or a game, when possible, with few extrinsic rewards such as stars or candy.

Psychosocial Interview. Psychosocial interviews are personal and may be emotionally delicate. They are best conducted after young clients have had time to get to know and feel comfortable with the speech/voice therapist. Aronson[108,109] suggests pleasant, relaxed surroundings for the interview, perhaps with a snack and beverage. Younger clients usually want a parental presence while adolescents usually prefer that adults wait outside.

Many organic voice disorders have psychogenic roots, and Aronson suggests that voice professionals "assume that all non-organic voice disorders are psychogenic until proven otherwise. . . ." He suggests that deteriorated relationships at home, school, or work may produce guilt, anger, and depression and that those physiochemical states can produce functional changes in voice. Suppressed and unexpressed emotional conflict is the common culprit, and denial of the conflict is a common first reaction.

The following questions are adapted from questions suggested by Aronson for psychosocial interviews: "Think back to when your voice trouble started. Was anything happening at that time that might have upset you? Is there anyone at home or at school (or at work) whom you have been having problems with (such as mother, father, brother[s], sister[s], best friend, boyfriend, girlfriend, other friends, other students at school, teacher, employer, co-workers)? Have you not been able to express your feelings to those people so far? Have you been concerned about your health or the health of someone in your family, or a friend's? Have you been concerned about your school work? How do you feel just before speaking, acting, or singing in front of other people? Does speaking, acting, or singing in front of other people ever make you feel scared or upset?"

Learning Fundamental Voice Skills. A helpful metaphor for learning and behavioral change is "The brain takes target practice." Brains can develop relatively new neurochemical networks (brain programs or patterns of behavior), or elaborate "old" ones, if they have some conscious "sense" of "where the bull's eye is" and "where the outside borders of the target are." When learners are taking target practice, many parents and educators have labeled bull's eye "misses" as "mistakes" or tell the learners that they "didn't do it right" or that they did something "wrong," "bad," "incorrect," or "improper." Such occasions, then, become "emotional ouches or hits" that can impact the development of protective versus constructive behavioral orientations.

When changing one or two parts of a complex habitual brain program like voicing, the new goals (bull's eyes) that are in conscious awareness will interfere with the automatic, other-than-conscious habitual program. Confusion will then occur, and under those conditions "confusion is the first sign of progress." Desirable but temporary confusion should be complimented and celebrated. Undesirable confusion can result from attempting conscious awareness of two or more activities at once. Conscious processes can handle only one "bull's eye" at a time.

Fundamental voice skills are applicable to both speaking and singing. Physical and acoustic efficiency in speech and song is a prime principle of establishing optimum voice. Learning to speak and sing more by sensation than by sound is an important direction for fundamental skill development. The kinesthetic sense is a more important source of feedback for skilled speakers and singers than the auditory sense.

Physical efficiency means coming as close as humanly possible to learning what it feels like to (1) use only the muscles that are necessary for voicing, thus releasing the interfering "unnecessaries"; and (2) use the necessary muscles with only the amount of contraction energy that is necessary for the vocal task at hand. Acoustic efficiency means learning what it "feels like" when the throat part and the mouth part of the "voice tube" (vocal tract) are appropriately "shaped" to enable the supraglottic sound waves to pass through and out of the vocal tract relatively unimpeded. Fundamental voice skills are:

1. *Enabling, flexible arrangement of the skeleton and general body movement*, as recommended in Alexander Technique and Feldenkrais Movement.[124–127]

2. *Efficient creation of airflow through the vocal folds*. "Midsection breathing" involves a visible (but not exaggerated) expansion of the abdominal wall and lower rib cage during inhalation and primary use of the abdominal muscles to create comfortably an appropriate breathflow energy for "athletic" speaking and singing. The shoulders and upper rib cage are "quiet."

3. *"Breaking up" and releasing of unnecessary muscular tensions or "holdings" in the postural arrangement of skeleton and in the head and neck areas*. Self-massage tasks for face, neck, and upper shoulders and motion tasks for temporomandibular joints, lips, and tongue can begin the goal of reducing unnecessary work in head and neck muscles during speaking and singing. Appropriate stretching, shaking, and slapping of legs, torso, and arms will bring mental–emotional "energizing" and "freeing" of the muscles that can restrict muscle movements that are necessary for phonation and pitch change. After

massage and motion tasks, the conscious attention of young clients can be focused on comparing posttask bodily sensations with pretask sensations and describing same.

4. *Efficient initiation and continuation of phonation.* There are three ways to initiate vocal sound: (1) aspirate, or air-then-sound, as in the /h/ consonant; (2) "glottal attack," or strong-closure-then-force-air-through; and (3) balanced initiation or near-simultaneous-closure-and-breathflow. A priority in voice therapy is elimination of glottal attack and nonlanguage aspirate initiations of sound in both speaking and singing—unless they convey special expressive impact for words that begin with vowels.

A major priority of voice therapy and voice education is "balancing" the coordination of the following two muscle groups: (1) those that primarily produce adduction and adductory force and (2) those that primarily produce the shortening, lengthening, stiffening, and thickening–thinning of the vocal fold mucosa that result in pitch changes and voice registers. These muscles can produce a continuum of voice qualities that range from breathy-airy to firm-clear-mellow-warm to pressed-edgy-harsh.

To establish what the outside borders of this target are, clients can be asked to "play Rich Little Time and make the sounds I make back to me." Say, "Hello there, how are you?" with a very breathy quality. (They respond.) Next model the same words in a loud, very pressed-edgy quality. (They respond.) Ask, "Did you notice a different feeling in your throat when you did that one compared with the first one?" (They respond.) "Now, we'll do those two again and add a third sound. On that one, make it just as loud as the second one, but make it *almost* breathy at the same time." Model the same words in those three ways followed by a response each time. Improvise target practice until relative mastery occurs. For singers, these qualities can be sung on a 5–4–3–2–1 scale in easy range.

The bull's eye is to learn ways to make quieter and louder sounds with a firm-clear-mellow-warm quality. A visually perceived horizontal line, with "B" for breathy on the left side and "P–E–H" for pressed-edgy-harsh on the right side can be presented to youngsters to further their target practice voice exploration. The bull's eye middle can be labelled "F–C–M–W" for firm-clear-mellow-warm.

5. *Efficient "shaping" of the vocal tract for optimum "release" of supraglottic vocal sound waves and formation of basic vowel qualities.* At the level of fundamental skills, the principle to follow is that the higher the spoken or sung pitch, and the greater the sound volume regardless of the pitch, the more both parts of the vocal tract must incrementally open to accommodate the changing nature of the acoustic sound waves. When performing higher pitches and louder volumes, the more either part of the vocal tract is inappropriately narrowed, the more the sound pressure waves will be deflected onto the waving vocal folds. The vocal folds are then impacted from below by the subglottic sound pressure waves and from above by deflected supraglottic sound waves (acoustic loading).[123] The greater the intensity of the "double impact," the greater will be the interference with the waving.[128] If the executive command of the brain is to sustain vocal sound-making, then an adjustment will take place in the relative tension of the laryngeal muscles to adapt to the acoustic loading. Laryngeal muscle tension will either increase to hyperfunctional levels or decrease to hypofunctional levels. In the former case, squeezed-pressed-edgy voice quality will begin, and in the latter case sudden breathiness or an abrupt register-quality change or "voice crack" will be heard. In either case, the effectiveness of vocal self-expression can be affected.

To establish what the outside borders of this target are, young clients can be asked to observe what the inside of their throats feel like when they are silent. Then, playing Rich

Little Time again, they can respond to the speech–voice therapist modeling a ten-foot tall giant saying, "Ho, ho, ho, how are you?" with maximum yawn-like forced-open throat. (They respond.) Ask, "How did the back of your throat feel to you compared with when you were silent?" (They respond. Several trials may be helpful.) Explain that the brighter parts of vocal sound are stifled when people make vocal sound that way, and that is why it sounds so "low and big, bottled-up and dark."

Next, ask them to make a Bugs Bunny sound on, "Eeaah, what's up doc?" (They respond.) Ask how that feels compared with the ten-foot giant. (They respond.) Explain that the fuller parts of vocal sound are stifled when people squeeze their voice tubes so much, and that is why Bugs Bunny sounds so "pinched and piercing."

To establish the bull's eye of this target, ask them to pretend that their flatted hand is a glass windowpane that they want to fog up with their breath air to clean it. First, model a sharp, loud whisper sound, and after they respond, ask if the feel of that was more like the ten-foot giant or Bugs Bunny. Most youngsters will respond with "Bugs Bunny," but some will not. Accept their description and say, "Some people squeeze their voice tube when they do that loud sharp whisper, and to them it feels like Bugs Bunny. Now, can you make a noiseless, silent, slow-air window fog?" (They respond.) "Compared to doing nothing, did you notice anything move in the back of your throat? Did it feel more like Bugs Bunny or the ten-foot giant? (They respond.) Was it as big and open as the ten-foot giant? (They respond.) Could it be described as a 'gentle, easy, released open feeling in the back of your throat?' " Then take target practice on quite a few toward-the-breathy-side, downward sigh-glides using the "window-fogger" feel. Eventually, add language sounds to the sigh-glides. Thus the throat part of the voice tube can learn appropriate openness for speaking and singing with an appropriately open pharyngeal cavity and an *appropriately* "full" voice quality.

A visually perceived horizontal line, with "TFG" for the ten-foot giant on the left side and "BB" for Bugs Bunny on the right side, can be presented to youngsters to further their target practice voice exploration. The middle is labeled "WFF" for windowfogger feel.

6.   *Equalization of the strength of upper and lower register coordinations and "blending" of the transition between the two registers.*[128–131] Conversational speech involves laryngeal coordinations in which the vocalis portion of the thyroarytenoid muscle is prominently involved in pitch inflections. That is a prominent feature of the laryngeal coordinations that produce lower pitch range and modal register voice quality ("chest" register to many singing teachers). Some people have evolved ear–brain–voice coordinations for speech that do not include upper pitch inflections for speech. In other words, their brains do not have a program for "easing" of vocalis contraction so that cricothyroid lengthening of the vocal folds can occur. That is a prominent feature of the laryngeal coordinations that produce upper pitch range and loft register voice quality ("head" or "falsetto" register to many singing teachers). This coordination produces higher pitched speaking inflections and singing pitch range with slightly lighter voice quality.

In many speakers and singers, the coordinations that produce upper register pitches are at underdeveloped levels on a continuum of ability development and neuromuscular strength. Upper pitch range inflection in expressive speaking and upper pitch range in singing will be enhanced by developing the fundamental skill of equalized upper and lower register skill and strength. The most helpful beginning point in developing this skill is to use downward sigh-glides and pitch patterns that start in the upper register coordination, somewhat softly at first, and move downward in pitch to "blend" or "melt" into the lower register coordination. Ask clients to invite the "yoo hoo" part of their voice to go lower and lower until "yoo hoo" melts into the "Wise Owl" part of their voices.

Conditioning or Reconditioning Laryngeal Muscles and Tissues. Young people who are newly involved in extensive and vigorous vocal performance may experience laryngeal discomfort or even pain. Vocal performers who have undergone a period of reduced voice use following upper respiratory infection or a course of voice therapy may experience similar symptoms after they return to "athletic" vocal performance. Prior to a resumption of athletic vocal use, these performers need a warm-up routine and a period of laryngeal reconditioning.

Laryngeal muscles respond to use and disuse similarly to other musculature. During relative disuse atrophy occurs, and during relatively vigorous use over time trophy occurs. Four factors that change in the laryngeal muscles under these conditions are (1) strength (intensity of contraction), (2) endurance (sustained intense contraction over time before fatigue begins), (3) bulk (margins of the vocal folds are moved slightly closer to or further away from adductory midline due to changes in thyroarytenoid muscle bulk), and (4) precision, speed and "smoothness" of neuromuscular coordinations. During relative disuse, atrophy involves a reduction in the above characteristics. During increased use, trophy involves an increase in them.

Although we are not aware of studies that verify this conclusion, we believe that vocal fold mucosal tissues also experience forms of atrophy and trophy. Well-conditioned vocal fold mucosa may evidence increased elasticity and resilience in response to increased waving frequencies, collision forces, and relative epithelial abrasion.

A program of conditioning or reconditioning involves two factors: (1) relative vigor or strenuousness of laryngeal use—louder volumes, higher pitches, lower pitches, and faster, more precise but fluid movements; and (2) gradual increases of time spent using voice vigorously after an appropriate warm-up period.

Recent voice use history will provide the basis for estimating the current trophic state. Very atrophic larynges may begin reconditioning with soft, breathy-side, downward sighglides in easy middle pitch range for 3 minutes five times per day. Eventually, an audiotape of sound patterns and/or pitch patterns may be made for the youngster to "perform with" several times per day. Sound making, speech making, and singing can be used as appropriate. Time and voice vigor increase as strength and endurance increase. When young performers have learned to observe vocal sensations more than sounds, they will be able to detect if and when their larynges begin to fatigue, feel irritated or sore, or to sound slightly "fuzzy." Should these signs occur, they should stop voicing and wait until the next time they are to "exercise" their voices. The speech–voice pathologist or voice educator will need to provide clear voice use time and strenuousness goals and to monitor progress.

Laying a Foundation for Lifelong Voice Protection and Learning Extended Vocal Self-Expression Skills. Experiencing diminished vocal ability because of a disorder can be frightening to young people who are interested in the vocal performing arts. A therapeutic process not only can restore optimum voice function, but also boost the sense-making, self-mastery, self-confidence, self-identity, and social integration processes of growing up. Effective therapy for a voice disorder underlines the advantages of learning extended voice skills. Deepening the vocal skills of conversational talking, performance speaking, and singing during youth with an experienced voice educator can provide many advantages to people in almost any chosen career.

Table 16–5   Voice Care Checklist

POSSIBLE CHILD/ADOLESCENT TERMINOLOGY	ADULT TERMINOLOGY
Easy voice; open feeling when speaking or singing; midsection breathing	Efficiency
Always having firm, strong, in-shape voice muscles	Conditioning
Stretching arm, leg, and face muscles; gently moving head, neck and throat muscles before strong singing and speaking	Warming up
Resting tired and used throat muscles and vocal cords so they can recover	Recovery time
Drink lots of refreshing water, at least five to seven drinking glasses each day; helps with your easy voice	Hydration, lubrication, tissue flexibility
How is my throat feeling? How does my voice sound?	Self-monitoring
Am I having fun? Am I happy? Do I laugh?	Managing, modifying stress reactions
Am I feeling OK, or do I stay home a lot because I'm sick?	Maintenance of general health

If young-voice teams do their voice treatment and education jobs well, and if young vocal arts performers respond well, young people will be able independently to care for their voices and avoid vocal "disasters" in the future. Near the end of the therapeutic process, a Voice Care Checklist can be provided (see Table 16–5) and discussed for future reference. Using age-appropriate language will be important.

Two sources that provide more detailed treatment of voice evaluation and assessment, and the design and guidance of voice therapy for children and adolescents, are *Voice Problems of Children* by Wilson[1] and *Voice Therapy for Adolescents* by Andrews and Summers.[132]

REFERENCES

1. Wilson DK: *Voice Problems of Children*, 3rd ed. Baltimore, Williams & Wilkins, 1987, p 323.
2. Pont C: Hoarseness in children. *Western Michigan Univ J Speech Ther* 2:6–8, 1965.
3. Baynes RA: An incidence study of chronic hoarseness among children. *J Speech Hear Disord* 31:172–176, 1966.
4. James HP, Cooper EB: Accuracy of teacher referrals of speech handicapped children. *Except Child* 33:29–32, 1966.
5. Senturia BH, Wilson FB: Otorhinolaryngologic findings in children with voice deviations. *Ann Otol Rhinol Laryngol* 77:1027–1041, 1968.
6. Silverman EM, Zimmer CH: Incidence of chronic hoarseness among school-age children. *J Speech Hear Disord* 40:211–245, 1975.
7. von Leden H: Vocal nodules in children. *Ear Nose Throat J* 64:473–480, 1985.
8. Hirano M, Kurita S, Nasashima T: The structure of the vocal folds, in Hirano M (ed): *Vocal Fold Physiology*. Tokyo, University of Tokyo Press, 1981.
9. Hately BW, Evison G, Samuel E: The pattern of ossification in the laryngeal cartilages: A radiological study. *Br J Radiol* 38:585–591, 1965.
10. Kahane JC: Postnatal development and aging of the human larynx. *Semin Speech Language* 4:189–203, 1983.
11. Eisenberg RB: Development of hearing in children, in Romand R (ed): *Development of Auditory and Vestibular Systems*. New York, Academic Press, 1983.
12. Purpura DP: Normal and aberrant development in the cerebral cortex of the human fetus and young infant, in Buchwald NA, Brazier MA (eds): *Brain Mechanisms in Mental Retardation*. New York, Academic Press, 1975.

13. Kolata G: Studying learning in the womb. *Science* 225:302–303, 1984.
14. Birnholtz JC, Benacerraf BR: The development of human fetal hearing. *Science* 222:517–519, 1983.
15. Grimwade J, Walker D, Bartlett M, et al. Human fetal heartrate change in response to sound and vibration. *Am J Obstet Gynecol* 122:86–90, 1971.
16. Querleu D, Renard K: Les perceptions auditives du foetus humain. *Med Hyg* 39:2102–2110, 1981.
17. Querleu D, Renard K, Crepin G: Perception auditive et reactivite foetale aux stimulations sonores. *J Gynecol Obstet Biol Reprod* 10:307–314, 1981.
18. DeCasper A, Fifer W: Of human bonding: Newborns prefer their mothers' voices. *Science* 208:1174–1176, 1980.
19. DeCasper A, Spence M: Prenatal maternal speech influences human newborns' perception of speech sounds. *Inf Behav Dev* 9:133–150, 1986.
20. Jansen AH, Chernick V: Development of respiratory control. *Physiol Rev* 63:437–483, 1983.
21. Eichorn DH: Physiological development, in Mussen PH (ed): *Carmichael's Manual of Child Psychology*, 3rd ed, vol 1. New York, John Wiley & Sons, 1970.
22. Bouhuys A: *The Physiology of Breathing*. New York, Grune & Stratton, 1977.
23. Cotes JE: *Lung Function*, 4th ed. Oxford, England, Blackwell Scientific, 1979.
24. Dunnhil MS: Postnatal growth of the lung. *Thorax* 17:329–333, 1962.
25. Peiper S: Cerebral function in infancy and childhood, in Wortis J (ed): *International Behavioral Science Series*. New York, Consultants Bureau, 1963.
26. Mitchell RA, Berger AJ: Neural regulation of respiration, in Hornbein TF (ed): *Regulation of Breathing*. New York, Marcel Dekker, 1981.
27. Laitman J, Crelin ES: Postnatal development of the basicranium and vocal tract in man, in Bosma JF (ed): *Symposium on Development of the Basicranium*. Washington, DC, Department of Health, Education and Welfare, 1976.
28. Laitman J, Crelin ES: Developmental change in the upper respiratory system of human infants. *Perinatol Neonatol* 4:15, 1980.
29. Wilder CN: *Respiratory Patterns in Infants: Birth to Eight Months of Age*. Unpublished Ph.D. dissertation, Columbia University, 1972.
30. Hollien H: Developmental aspects of neonatal vocalizations, in Murry T, Murry J: *Infant Communication: Cry and Early Speech*. New York, College Hill Press, 1980.
31. Fleming P: Development of respiratory patterns: Implications for control, in *17th Annual Intra-Science Symposium, International Symposium on Sudden Infant Death Syndrome*. Santa Monica, California, February 1984.
32. Laufer MZ: Temporal regularity in prespeech, in Murry T, Murry J: *Infant Communication: Cry and Early Speech*. New York, College Hill Press, 1980.
33. Lieberman P: *The Biology and Evolution of Language*. Cambridge, Harvard University Press, 1984.
34. Murry T, Murry J: *Infant Communication: Cry and Early Speech*. New York, College Hill Press, 1980.
35. Hixon TJ: *Respiratory Function in Speech and Song*. Boston, College Hill Press, 1987.
36. Bosma JF: Anatomic and physiologic development of the speech apparatus, in Tower DB (ed): *The Nervous System: Human Communication and Its Disorders*, vol 3. New York, Raven Press, 1975.
37. Ballenger JJ (ed): *Diseases of the Nose, Throat and Ear*. Philadelphia, Lea & Febiger, 1969.
38. Ogura JH, Mallen RW: Developmental anatomy of the larynx, in Ballenger JJ (ed): *Diseases of the Nose, Throat and Ear*, 12th ed. Philadelphia, Lea & Febiger, 1977.
39. Hirano M, Kurita S, Nasashima T: Growth, development and aging of human vocal folds, in Bless DM, Abbs JH (eds): *Vocal Fold Physiology: Contemporary Research and Clinical Issues*. San Diego, College Hill Press, 1981.
40. Kahane JC: Weight measurements of infant and adult intrinsic laryngeal muscles. *Folia Phoniatr* 36:129–133, 1984.
41. von Leden H: The mechanism of phonation: A search for a rational theory. *Arch Otolaryngol* 74:72–87, 1961.
42. Klock LE: *The Growth and Development of the Human Larynx From Birth to Adolescence*. Unpublished M.S. thesis, University of Washington School of Medicine, 1968.
43. Timeras PS: *Developmental Physiology and Aging*. New York, Macmillan, 1972.
44. Tanner JM: Sequencing, tempo and individual variation in growth and development of boys and girls aged twelve to sixteen, in Kagen J, Coles R (eds): *Twelve to Sixteen: Early Adolescence*. New York, W.W. Norton, 1972.
45. Lee PA: Normal ages of pubertal events among American males and females. *J Adolescence Health Care* 1:26–29, 1980.
46. Kahane JC: A morphological study of the human prepubertal and pubertal larynx. *Am J Anat* 151:1:11–19, 1978.
47. Kahane JC: Growth of the human prepubertal and pubertal larynx. *J Speech Hear* 25:446–455, 1982.
48. Maue WM: *Cartilages, Ligaments and Articulations of the Adult Human Larynx*. Unpublished Ph.D. dissertation, University of Pittsburgh, 1971.

49. Tossi O, Postan D, Bianculli C: Longitudinal study of children's voice at puberty, in *Proceedings: XVIth International Congress of Logopedics and Phoniatrics*. 1976, pp 486–490.
50. Allen TH, Anderson EC, Lagham WH: Total body potassium and gross body composition in relation to age. *J Gerontol* 15:348–357, 1960.
51. Kahane JC: Anatomy and physiology of the organs of the peripheral speech mechanism, in Lass NJ, McReynolds LV, Northern JL, Yoder DE (eds): *Handbook of Speech–Language Pathology and Audiology*. Philadelphia, B.C. Decker, 1988.
52. Sundberg J: *The Science of the Singing Voice*. DeKalb, IL, Northern Illinois University Press, 1987, p 102.
53. Wind J: *On the Phylogeny and the Ontogeny of the Human Larynx*. Groningen, Sweden, Wolters Noordhoff Publishing, 1970.
54. Kalmus H, Fry DB: On tune deafness (dysmelodia): Frequency, development, genetics and musical background. *Ann Hum Genet* 43:369–382, 1980.
55. Welch GF: A schema theory of how children learn to sing in-tune. *Psychol Music* 1:3–18, 1985.
56. Welch GF: Variability of practice and knowledge of results as factors in learning to sing in-tune. *Bull Council Res Music Educ* 85:238–247, 1985.
57. Welch GF: Children's singing: A developmental continuum of ability. *J Res Singing* 2:49–56, 1986.
58. Welch GF: The developing voice, in Thurman L, Welch GF (eds): *Bodymind and Voice: Foundations of Voice Education*. Minneapolis, The VoiceCare Network, 1992.
59. Condon WS, Sandor LW: Neonate movement is synchronized with adult speech: Interactional participation and language acquisition. *Science* 183:99–101, 1974.
60. Rosenthal MK: Vocal dialogues in the neonatal period. *Dev Psychol* 18:1:17–21, 1982.
61. Eimas PD: The perception of speech in early infancy. *Sci Am* 252:1:34–40, 1985.
62. Ries N: An analysis of the characteristics of infant-child singing expressions: Replication report. *Can J Res Music Educ* 29:1:5–20, 1987.
63. Keating P, Buhr R: Fundamental frequency in the speech of infants and children. *J Acoust Soc Am* 63:567–571, 1978.
64. Wilson DK: *Voice Problems of Children*, 3rd ed. Baltimore, Williams & Wilkins, 1987, pp 116–124.
65. Andrews ML: *Frequency Characteristics of the Voices of 740 Australian School Children*. Unpublished manuscript, Bloomington, Indiana University, 1982.
66. Cooksey JM, Beckett RL, Wiseman R: A longitudinal investigation of selected vocal, physiological, and acoustical factors associated with voice maturation in the junior high school male adolescent, in Runfola EM (ed): *Proceedings: Research Symposium on the Male Adolescent Voice*. Buffalo, State University of New York Press, 1984.
67. Lawrence VL: Habitual pitch of speaking voice and the singer. *Natl Assoc Teachers Singing J* 44:1:25–26,44, 1987.
68. Raphael BN: Loudness and projection as related to public speaking and acting, in Lawrence VL (ed): *Transcripts of the Thirteenth Symposium: Care of the Professional Voice*. New York, The Voice Foundation, 1985.
69. Mårtensson A, Skoglund CR: Contraction properties of intrinsic laryngeal muscles. *Acta Physiol Scand* 60:318–336, 1964.
70. DeCasper A, Fifer W: Of human bonding: Newborns prefer their mothers' voices. *Science* 208:1174–1176, 1980.
71. DeCasper A, Spence M: Prenatal maternal speech influences human newborns' perception of speech sounds. *Inf Behav Dev* 9:133–150, 1986.
72. Panneton RK: *Prenatal Auditory Experience With Melodies: Effects on Postnatal Auditory Preferences in Human Newborns*. Unpublished Ph.D. dissertation, Greensboro, University of North Carolina, 1985.
73. Shetler DJ: The inquiry into prenatal musical experience: A report of the Eastman project 1980–1987. *Pre-Peri-Natal Psychol J* 3:3:171–189, 1989.
74. Thurman L: Parental singing during pregnancy and infancy can assist in cultivating positive bonding and later development, in Fedor-Freybergh PG, Vogel MLV (eds): *Prenatal and Perinatal Psychology and Medicine: Encounter With the Unborn*. Park Ridge, NJ, Parthenon Publishing, 1988.
75. Kessen W: The imitation of pitch in infants. *Inf Behav Dev* 2:93–99, 1979.
76. Kelley L, Sutton-Smith B: A study of infant musical productivity, in Peery JC, Peery IW, Draper TW (eds): *Music and Child Development*. New York, Springer-Verlag, 1987.
77. Welch GF, Howard D, Rush C: Real-time visual feedback in the development of vocal pitch accuracy in singing. *Psychol Music* 17:2:146–157, 1989.
78. Welch GF, Rush C, Howard D: A developmental continuum of singing ability: Evidence from a study of five-year-old developing singers. *Early Child Dev Care* 69:107–119, 1991.
79. Weiss DA: The pubertal change of the human voice. *Folia Phoniatr* 2:3:126–159, 1950.
80. Luchsinger R: Physiology and pathology of respiration and phonation, in Luchsinger R, Arnold GE (eds): *Voice–Speech–Language. Clinical Communicology: Its Physiology and Pathology*. Belmont, CA, Wadsworth, 1965.

81. Fritzell B: Singing and the health of the voice, in *Research Aspects on Singing: Autoperception, Computer Synthesis, Emotion, Health, Voice Source*. Stockholm, Sweden, Royal Academy of Music, ADEBE Reklam & Tryckservice AB, 1981.

82. Sataloff RT: Professional singers: The science and art of clinical care. *Am J Otolaryngol* 2:251–266, 1981.

83. Brodnitz FS: On the changing voice. *Natl Assoc Teachers Singing Bull* 40:2:24–26, 1983.

84. Naidr J, Zbořil M, Ševčík K: Die pubertalen veranderungen der stimme bei jungen im verlauf von 5 jahren. *Folia Phoniatr* 17:1–18, 1965.

85. Frank F, Sparber M: Stimmumfluge bei Kindern aus neuer sicht. *Folia Phoniatr* 22:397–402, 1970.

86. Frank F, Sparber M: Die premutationsstimme die mutationsstimme und die postmutationsstimme in sonagramm. *Folia Phoniatr* 22:425–433, 1970.

87. McKenzie D: *Training the Boy's Changing Voice*. London, Bradford and Dickens, Drayton House, 1956.

88. Cooper IO, Kuersteiner KO: *Teaching Junior High School Music*, 2nd ed. Conway, AR, Cambiata Press, 1973.

89. Swanson FJ: *The Male Singing Voice Ages Eight to Eighteen*. Cedar Rapids, IA, Ingram Press, 1977.

90. Cooksey JM: The development of a continuing, eclectic theory for the training and cultivation of the junior high school male changing voice. Part I: Existing theories. *Choral J* 18:2:5–13, 1977.

91. Cooksey JM: The development of a continuing, eclectic theory for the training and cultivation of the junior high school male changing voice. Part II: Scientific and empirical findings: Some tentative solutions. *Choral J* 18:3:5–16, 1977.

92. Cooksey JM: The development of a continuing, eclectic theory for the training and cultivation of the junior high school male changing voice. Part III: Developing an integrated approach to the care and training of the junior high school male changing voice. *Choral J* 18:4:5–15, 1977.

93. Cooksey JM: The development of a continuing, eclectic theory for the training and cultivation of the junior high school male changing voice. Part IV: Selecting music for the junior high school male changing voice. *Choral J* 18:5:5–17, 1978.

94. Cooksey JM: Vocal–acoustical measures of prototypical patterns related to voice maturation in the adolescent male, in Lawrence VL (ed): *Transcripts of the Thirteenth Symposium: Care of the Professional Voice*. New York, The Voice Foundation, 1985.

95. Groom M: *A Descriptive Analysis of Development in Adolescent Male Voices During the Summer Time Period*. Unpublished Ph.D. dissertation, Florida State University, 1979.

96. Rutkowski J: The junior high school male changing voice: Testing and grouping voices for successful singing experiences. *Choral J* 22:4:11–15, 1981.

97. Barresi AL, Bless DM: The relation of selected aerodynamic variables to the perception of tessitura pitches in the adolescent changing voice, in Runfola EM (ed): *Proceedings: Research Symposium on the Male Adolescent Voice*. Buffalo, State University of New York Press, 1984.

98. Cooksey JM: Adolescent male changing voices, in Thurman L, Welch GF (eds): *Bodymind and Voice: Foundations of Voice Education*. Minneapolis, The VoiceCare Network, 1992.

99. Vennard W: *Singing: The Mechanism and Technique*. New York, Carl Fischer, Inc., 1967.

100. Huff-Gackle ML: *The Effect of Selected Vocal Techniques for Breath Management, Resonation, and Vowel Unification on Tone Production in the Junior High School Female Voice*. Unpublished Ph.D. thesis, University of Miami, 1987.

101. Gackle L: The adolescent female voice: The characteristics of change and stages of development. *Choral J* 31:8:17–25, 1991.

102. Gackle L: Understanding adolescent female changing voices, in Thurman L, Welch GF (eds): *Bodymind and Voice: Foundations of Voice Education*. Minneapolis, The VoiceCare Network, 1992.

103. Miles B, Hollien H: Whither belting? *J Voice* 4:64–70, 1990.

104. Estill J: Observations about the quality called "belting," in Lawrence VL (ed): *Transcripts of the Ninth Symposium, Care of the Professional Voice*. New York, The Voice Foundation, 1980.

105. Estill J: The control of voice quality, in Lawrence VL (ed): *Transcripts of the Eleventh Symposium, Care of the Professional Voice*. New York, The Voice Foundation, 1982.

106. Estill J, Baer T, Honda K, Harris KS: The control of pitch and voice quality: An EMG study of supralaryngeal muscles, in Lawrence VL (ed): *Transcripts of the Twelfth Symposium, Care of the Professional Voice*. New York, The Voice Foundation, 1983.

107. Estill J: Belting and classic voice quality: Some physiological differences. *Med Prob Perf Artists* 2:3:37–43, 1988.

108. Aronson AE: Importance of the psychosocial interview in the diagnosis and treatment of "functional" voice disorders. *J Voice* 4:287–289, 1990.

109. Aronson AE: *Clinical Voice Disorders: An Interdisciplinary Approach*, 2nd ed. New York, Brian C. Decker, 1985.

110. Churchland PS, Sejnowski TJ: *The Computational Brain*. Cambridge, MA, The MIT Press, 1992.

111. Pert C: The wisdom of the receptors: Neuropeptides, the emotions and bodymind. *Advances* 3:8–16, 1986.

112. Lipsett LP: Stress in infancy: Toward understanding the origins of coping behavior, in Garmezy N, Rutter M (eds): *Stress, Coping, and Development in Children*. New York, McGraw-Hill, 1983.

113. Odent M: *Primal Health*. London, Century Hutchinson Ltd., 1986.
114. Brown EF, Hendee WR: Adolescents and their music: Insights into the health of adolescents. *J Am Med Assoc* 262:1659–1663, 1989.
115. Deci EL, Ryan RM: *Intrinsic Motivation and Self-Determination in Human Behavior*. New York, Plenum Press, 1985.
116. Mehrabian A: *Nonverbal Communication*. Englewood Cliffs, NJ, Prentice-Hall, 1972, pp 186, 187.
117. Bless DM: The educational impact of voice disorders, in *Voice and Voice Disorders Newsletter*. Rockville, MD, American Speech–Language–Hearing Association, 1991, pp 6, 7.
118. Thurman L: Voice education in school music education, in Lawrence VL (ed): *Transcripts of the Thirteenth Symposium: Care of the Professional Voice*. New York, The Voice Foundation, 1985.
119. Lamb D: Teaching voice skills to children: The Orff-Schulwerk approach, in Lawrence VL (ed): *Transcripts of the Thirteenth Symposium: Care of the Professional Voice*. New York, The Voice Foundation, 1985.
120. Langness AP: Developing children's voices, in Thurman L, Welch GF (eds): *Bodymind and Voice: Foundations of Voice Education*, 4th ed. Minneapolis, The VoiceCare Network, 1992.
121. Thurman L, Welch GF (eds): *Bodymind and Voice: Foundations of Voice Education*. Minneapolis, The VoiceCare Network, 1992.
122. Bastian RW, Keidar A, Verdolini-Marston K: Simple vocal tasks for detecting vocal swelling. *J Voice* 4:172–183, 1990.
123. Rothenberg M: The voice source in singing, in *Research Aspects on Singing*. Stockholm, Sweden, Royal Academy of Music, 1981.
124. Alexander FM: *Use of the Self*. Long Beach, CA, Centerline Press, 1984.
125. Feldenkrais M: *Awareness Through Movement*. New York, Harper & Row, 1972.
126. Rickover RM: *Fitness Without Stress: A Guide to the Alexander Technique*. Portland, OR, Metamorphous Press, 1988.
127. Pryor A: The Alexander technique, in Thurman L, Welch GF (eds): *Bodymind and Voice: Foundations of Voice Education*. Minneapolis, The VoiceCare Network, 1992.
128. Titze I: A framework for the study of vocal registers. *J Voice* 2:183–194, 1988.
129. Hollien H (ed): *Report on Vocal Registers*. New York, Collegium Medicorum Theatri, 1982.
130. Hollien H, Schoenhard C: A review of vocal registers, in Lawrence VL (ed): *Transcripts of the Twelfth Symposium: Care of the Professional Voice*. New York, The Voice Foundation, 1983.
131. Thurman L: Vocal registers: A summary, in Thurman L, Welch GF (eds): *Bodymind and Voice: Foundations of Voice Education*. Minneapolis, The VoiceCare Network, 1992.
132. Andrews M, Summers A: *Voice Therapy for Adolescents*. Boston, College Hill Press, 1988.
133. Thurman L: Human compatible learning and human antagonistic learning, in Thurman L, Welch GF: *Bodymind and Voice: Foundations of Voice Education*. Minneapolis, The VoiceCare Network 1992.

17

The Aging Voice

HANS VON LEDEN, MD
DAVID M. ALESSI, MD

As we approach the 21st century, life expectancy in the United States continues to climb. This well-documented trend has led to an increase in the geriatric population[1] and a higher incidence of age-related voice problems.[2] The gradual senescence is compounded by an increase in the birth rates during the years after World War II. Whereas individuals over 65 years of age comprise 11% of the population in 1980, this figure is projected to be 13% in the year 2000 and 21% in the year 2030. Currently, the fastest growing segment of the population consists of individuals above 75 years of age.[3] Advancing years place their toll upon the vocal system; it has been estimated that 12% of elderly individuals have some type of vocal dysfunction.[4]

HISTORICAL OVERVIEW

Although the effects of age on the human voice have been recognized since time immemorial, a scientific study of these phenomena had to await the development of modern technology. Unfortunately, there has been considerable disagreement in the findings of various authors.

Early observations on the ossification of the laryngeal cartilages date back to the late 19th and early 20th centuries: Chievitz[5] in 1882, Scheier[6] in 1902, and Fraenkel[7] in 1908. However, the Austrian otolaryngologist Imhofer[8] was apparently the first scientist to conduct detailed histologic studies of the aged larynx. In 1912 he reported an increase in the lipoid pigment in the sarcolemma with advancing years. Two years later he described involutionary changes in the elastic tissue.[9] By 1923, Max Nodoleczny[10] in Munich had released his fundamental studies on tremor.

In 1931, Kofler[11] of Vienna published his extensive histologic studies on the aged larynx; he observed calcification and ossification of the cartilages, atrophy of the soft tissues, reduction and interruption of the elastic fibers, and deposition of fatty material. The changes in the laryngeal epithelium were similar to those encountered in the skin of the elderly. During the following year, 1932, another Viennese physician, H. Stern,[12] published his observations on the relation of audible changes in the singing voice to the underlying organic changes in the aging larynx. Stern stressed the importance of general hygienic measures for the preservation of the voice—vox sana in corpore sano!

A series of Italian authors, Amprino and Bairati,[13] Malan,[14] Segre,[15] and Carnevale-Ricci,[16] reported their observations during the same decade. Segre's article is of particular

269

interest because the author discusses both the anatomic and the physiologic aspects of the aging voice.

In the United States in 1941, Bach and his associates[17] presented the first major article on the aging voice. These authors confirmed definite degenerative changes in the laryngeal muscles of old persons that they attributed to vascular disturbances by insufficient nourishment. In 1949, Terracol and Azemar[18] called attention to vocal function in relation to the biologic aspects of aging in their comprehensive publication "La Senescence de la Voix." They described both anatomic and biologic factors of aging and their effects on the voice: reduction in pulmonary ventilation, reduced endocrine function and water metabolism, decreased collagenous connective tissue, flaccidity of the cervical muscles, decreased vitamin C metabolism, and so forth.

Interest in the aging voice increased after 1950. In 1959, Mysak[19] discovered that adult males voices aged 80 to 92 years are characterized by significantly higher measures of average fundamental pitch levels than males aged 65 to 79 years. In both groups the pitch demonstrated a central upward trend and greater flexibility. In 1963, McGlone and Hollien[20] examined two similar groups of older women and found no corresponding changes in their pitch levels.

In 1965, Luchsinger and Arnold[21] published their monumental book on human voice and speech. In that volume Luchsinger and Arnold discussed a wide variety of changes in the aging voice. They stressed that senility of the voice in both sexes reflects the general process of aging in body and mind. In general, vocal involution in the male begins after age 60 years, while in the female the aging of the voice is closely related to menopause. With advancing age, the vocal range becomes smaller through loss of the high tones. Vocal intensity becomes reduced, and vocal quality may become husky and muffled, or thin and sharp. The overall sound of the voice may become rough and tremulous.

Also in 1965, Appaix and associates[22] described spectrographic studies of the spoken voice, and during the following year Sedlackova and colleagues[23] reported their sonographic measurements of aging voices. Also in 1966, Ptacek and associates[24] measured younger adults and geriatric subjects in diverse vocal tasks—maximum pitch range, maximum vocal intensity, maximum vowel duration, and so forth. On all of these tasks, the geriatric subjects showed reduced scores.

In Eastern Germany, Böhme[25] described a series of experiments with the aging voice in successive years, 1968 and 1969. In 1971, Segre,[26] by then in Argentina, summarized his experiences with the symptoms, findings, and treatment of the senile voice. In 1972, Hommerich[27] presented an excellent review of the morphologic aspects of the aging voice.

In the same year, Habermann[28] summarized the functional aspects of the aging voice as follows:

Deterioration of the voice with age is an extremely complex process, involving degeneration in the lungs, larynx and pharynx. Endocrine factors especially in women are important. Decline of voice does not coincide with actual age. There are far more old people than "old" voices. The various single factors involved are rarely found in one and the same person.

Indication of change of voice properties in respect to aging are loss of the chest register; rapid change of pitch and timbre; decrease in vocal depth; reduction of resonance; change in quality especially timbre; reduced ability of voice regulation together with difficulty in intonation; and voice tremor. There is also reduction in vocal range and lastly one finds phonasthenia. Whilst most people hardly notice the aging of their voices it is of importance to artists, especially concert singers, although actors normally find usefulness in the noticeable change of their voice.

Also in 1972, Ryan[29] described his acoustic studies of the aging voice in 80 normal male subjects. He noted a significant increase in the mean vocal intensity for reading and speaking and a significant decrease in the overall reading rate and mean sentence reading rate. In the same year, Hollien and Shipp[30] investigated a large population of male talkers ranging in age from 20 to 89 years. They confirmed a rise in the fundamental frequency level from age 60 years through the 80s.

Finally, in 1977, von Leden[31] stressed the interrelations of communication disorders in advanced years, particularly the relation between the voice and impaired hearing. He also stressed the importance of the biologic rather than the calendar age and discussed newer aspects of rehabilitation.

A vast amount of additional information has been produced in the 1980s. Extensive bibliographic data for this period may be found on the subsequent pages and in the inaugural issue of the *Journal of Voice*.[32]

THE AGING BODY

An exact description of an "old" voice is a complex undertaking. Not every elderly person has a cranky "granny-like" voice. In fact, young lay people judging the age of a single unseen speaker exhibit considerable error.[30] This difficulty in evaluation decreases with the judges' age and experience.

With the normal aging process, changes are exhibited in the hormonal, circulatory, skeletal, and neuromuscular systems. For example, decreases in sex hormones and in the basal metabolic rate are seen after late middle age.[33,34] With advancing years, the cardiac output decreases, and arterial intimal thickening occurs with atherosclerosis.[35,36] Moreover, loss of bone and muscle mass, a "dying-back" neuropathy,[37] and a progressive decrease in central nervous system function occur with age.[38,39] These changes have a significant impact on the function of the larynx.

To understand the clinical findings in the aging voice, we should start with a discussion of the normal anatomic and physiologic changes that occur within the larynx over this period. However, it is important to note that many aspects of the aging voice are not well-documented or have inherent problems. For example, there are few well-controlled studies on hormonal influence. Most studies have been on men to avoid confusing data on age with data influenced by hormonal changes. Also, there may exist an elderly dialect, which may produce changes in the articulatory variables in speech production. This could have a subtle effect on the analysis of speech samples. A dialectic variation might exist with vowels, thereby also affecting the analysis of sustained vowels.[36]

As stated, the literature on the effects of hormonal changes on the voice is sparse, but some data are known. The slow decrease in thyroid function seen with aging can affect voice quality. Moreover, the menopausal effect on the voice has been reported by professional singers who experienced a loss of brilliance and power as well as decreased ability to reach high notes during and after their "change of life."[40]

ANATOMIC CHANGES

The anatomic structures that change with time and have an impact on voice formation include the laryngeal cartilages and joints, the intrinsic laryngeal musculature, the vocal fold epithelium and the laryngeal innervation. Structures surrounding the larynx also change with age.

Cartilage

Both elastic and hyaline cartilage are found within the larynx. The elastic cartilages (vocal process and apex of the arytenoid cartilage, corniculate, and epiglottis) do not ossify.[26,41] However, with aging the hyaline cartilages (thyroid, cricoid, and most of the arytenoid) ossify. Associated with this age-related calcification and ossification is a decrease in the cell density of chondrocytes and a fatty degeneration of chondrocytes.[42] Rother and Riodel[42] also noted the following changes with age in the hyaline portion of the arytenoid cartilages: "albuminoid" degeneration, partial loss of intercellular substance with exhibition of well visible collagen fibers, and a basophilic reaction of intercellular substance up to the fourth decennium, which later becomes more and more eosinophilic.[43] This ossification may have a role in voice production by the following mechanism. Normally, compression of the thyroid laminae by the inferior constrictor leads to increased cord adduction. This cord adduction may be hindered by stiffening of the thyroid cartilage.[43]

Joints

There is erosion of the joint surfaces with age.[26] In the cricoarytenoid joint, age-related changes can include thinning of articular surfaces, breakdown in collagen fiber organization in articular cartilage, and irregularities of the articular surfaces.[43] Kahn and Kahane[44] investigated age-related changes in the articular surfaces of human cricoarytenoid joints and found consistent patterns of orientation of collagen fibers in cricoarytenoid joint surfaces in young and old age groups. Older articular surfaces exhibited extensive fibrillation and ossification, suggesting that articular cartilage undergoes alteration in ground substance and/or fiber structure as a function of age. These joint changes may impact on voice production. Cricoarytenoid joint cartilage changes in older males may limit range of motion of arytenoid cartilages and reduce degree and extent of vocal fold closure. Additionally, the tight enarthrosic joint formed by the arytenoids and the cricoid shows the impact of aging through a loosening of the capsule and the erosion of the joint surfaces. As a result, the meticulous approximation of the arytenoids, which is indispensable for the emission of a given tone, is jeopardized.[26]

Muscles

In the laryngeal musculature, there are significant age-related changes. There is degeneration of muscle tissue[53]; as the number of myofibrils decreases, they are replaced by loose connective tissue.[26] In baboons, the thyroarytenoid muscle contracts more slowly and recovers less rapidly with advancing age. This phenomenon may be associated with age-related alterations in the biochemical properties of muscle, such as a decrease in the ATPase activity of myosin. However, the active tension of endolaryngeal musculature increases with age, suggesting an extramuscular (vascular or nervous) mechanism for age-related changes in the larynx.[45] In the thyroarytenoid muscle, there is a loss of type II muscle fibers and a compensatory hypertrophy of the remaining muscle fibers with age.[46] Studies on the thyroarytenoid muscle indicate that the number of neuromuscular junctions decreases with age, a finding consistent with the limited "dying-back" phenomenon seen in peripheral nerves.[47] The posterior cricoarytenoid muscle is unique in many ways and has a tendency to undergo significant early age-related changes. Interestingly, the number of neuromuscular junctions increases from young to old age, suggesting that the aging changes are intrinsic to the muscle and not the result of peripheral nerve changes.[48]

Nerves

Substantial age-related changes are seen in the recurrent laryngeal nerve and are probably a type of "dying-back" neuropathy found in peripheral nerves.[48–50] Fiber type grouping by selective type II muscle fiber denervation and reinnervation by type I motoneurons as seen commonly in limb muscles is not found in the thyroarytenoid muscle.[46] The type I fiber hypertrophy noted in the thyroarytenoid muscle is probably secondary to its high constant activity. Age-related changes are also seen in the superior laryngeal nerve. When compared with superior laryngeal nerve sections from young cadaver specimens, there is a decrease in myelinated fibers with small axonal diameters in the old age group.[51] Additionally, aging of superior and/or recurrent laryngeal nerve Schwann cells is shown by the reduced number of mitochondria and the presence of giant mitochondria.[49]

Age-associated central nervous system impairment can affect the fine neuromuscular control of the larynx. This is best seen with neurologic diseases that occur in the elderly and affect the voice. Essential tremor, Parkinson's disease, amyotrophic lateral sclerosis, and stroke can all result in a deterioration of the quality of the voice.[4]

Circulation

Many of the degenerative changes seen in the laryngeal musculature are related in part to the decreasing blood supply to the aging larynx.[52–54] Also, the elastic or myoepithelial cushions of the arteriolar intima in the thyroarytenoid are altered and reduced in number. This may decrease the control of blood flow into this metabolically active muscle.[26]

Circulatory support of the larynx is important in not only maintaining nourishment to the laryngeal structures but also in the physiology of phonation. Fundamental frequency and vocal intensity of sustained phonation vary with cardiac contractions. This phenomenon appears to be related to the increased stiffness of the vocal folds, which in turn is caused by engorgement of the vascular beds.[53] This normal laryngeal circulatory physiology is affected by age-related vascular changes leading to an alteration in vocal quality.

Vocal Ligament and Epithelium

In a study of excised cadaveric larynges, vocal fold atrophy, bowing, and sulcus vocalis were seen in 72%, 8%, and 64% of senile cadaver larynges, respectively (young controls measured 0%, 7%, and 7%).[55] Eighty-one percent of senile vocal cords were noted to have a yellowish or grayish discoloration, which was thought to be the sequel of fatty degeneration and keratosis.[55] Hirano et al[56] histologically studied 64 human cadaver larynges ranging in age from 70 to 104 years. He noted the following, albeit somewhat variable, age-related tendencies: (1) the membranous vocal fold shortens in males; (2) the mucous membrane thickens in females, probably secondary to postmenopausal endocrine changes[57]; (3) the epithelium of the vocal fold thickens in females; (4) edema develops in the superficial layer of the lamina propria in both sexes; (5) the intermediate layer of the lamina propria thins, with this deterioration greater in males; (6) elastic fibers in the intermediate layer become less dense and have a tendency to atrophy in males; (7) the deep layer of the lamina propria thickens in males; and (8) collagenous fibers in the deep layer become denser and fibrotic in males.[56] Kahane[43] has corroborated these findings.

As a result of the decrease in elastic fibers and increase in collagenous fibers in males, there are sex-related differences in the connective tissue composition of the vocal fold. The female vocal cord consists mainly of elastic fibers, and the male cord consists mainly of collagenous fibers. In old age the two kinds of fibers degenerate.[58,86] With age, the mesenchymal cells responsible for the normal turnover of connective tissue decrease in both number and function, thus influencing the type and amount of connective tissue present.[59] Atrophy of laryngeal epithelium is often seen in aged men. Also demonstrable are prolongation of mitotic cycles, an increasing tendency of cornification, and a decreasing formation of pegs in the range of the basilar membrane.[60]

The mucous glands become atrophic and reduced in number.[61] Thus there is a loss of lubrication in the senescent larynx.[62]

Supraglottic and subglottic mucosal changes also occur, and some of these changes may correlate with a higher incidence of airway tumor formation with advanced age. The thickness of the supraglottic mucosa increases with age.[63] The squamous epithelium seen subglottically[64] and in the ventricles[65] increases with age. Both of these changes are greater in smokers and may play a role in the further development of squamous metaplasia.[65]

Gradual loss of elasticity of the thyroarytenoid ligament causes imperfect approximation of the true vocal cords.[66] Since the thyroarytenoid muscle is one of the main protectors of the laryngeal airway, gradual diminution of this muscle's function may be associated with the increase in aspiration that accompanies aging.[67] This is compounded by diminished sensory innervation to the larynx as seen with the decrease in superior laryngeal nerve function.[51]

Lungs

The lungs undergo major age-related changes. The trachea softens and widens.[26] The peribronchial muscles atrophy, and the pulmonary alveoli and bronchioles dilate, with the resulting development of pulmonary emphysema and reduced elasticity of the thoracic cage, all of which produce a reduction in expiratory breath.[26] There is also an increase in alveolar thickness and capillary number, which can be associated with a decrease in oxygen diffusion.[68]

Pulmonary function decreases with age. As much as a 40% reduction in vital capacity occurs between the ages of 20 and 80 years, and the tensile strength and elasticity of the lungs deteriorates with age.[69] There is also a decrease in the forced expiratory volume and an increase in the residual volume.[68] These alterations result in a loss of breath support for voice production.

Articulators

The articulators, which form the voice into speech, also show age-related changes. The loss of teeth and presence of dentures create obvious articulation difficulties. These difficulties are aggravated by a chronically dry mouth. The elderly patient experiences a decrease in production of saliva caused by a loss of 25% of the secretory parenchymal volume, acinar hyalinization, and salivary duct adhesions.[70]

ACOUSTICS

A lower laryngeal position of the larynx in elderly females may contribute to a lowered vocal resonance.[57] However, the literature on the change in dimensions of the vocal tract itself with age is sparse. In phonated vowels, the first formant and the mean second formant values become progressively lower with advancing age. This finding would support an increase in vocal tract dimensions in elderly speakers. In whispered vowels, however, mean second formant values rise slightly with age.[57] In general, the size of the female larynx grows smaller with increasing age, but the effect on voice is not well understood.[65]

The stereotypic aged voice has an altered pitch, hoarseness, lack of intensity, and warble. Phonatory deviations with age are well documented. In a study of 175 males reading the Rainbow Passage, there was an initial decrease in the fundamental frequency to age 40 years, but a gradual increase from 60 to 80 years.[73] In a study of 60- to 80-year-old nonsmoking men, the fundamental frequency and acoustic variability increased.[53] In a study of 75 women, the stability and the frequency of the fundamental frequency decreased with age.[57] The stability was determined by the standard deviation of the fundamental frequency during a single sustained vowel phonation. Other authors have also found a decrease in fundamental frequency,[71] or a minimal change,[72,73] with age in females.[71] In males, a slow increase in speaking fundamental frequency is seen after age 40 years.[71,73] Hormonal changes play a role, as seen in fundamental frequency changes in post-menopausal women.[57]

Changes in the resonating chambers also may influence pitch. These alterations include the growth of the craniofacial structure from young adulthood to old age, the lowering of the larynx in the neck with age, and the dilation of the pharyngeal muscles as a result of the loss in tonus.[36]

Some authors feel that there is an increase in vocal loudness with age,[69] while others report a gradual loss of intensity with increasing age.[31,57] Segre[26] reports a loss of intensity with age, as the result of a reduction in the expiratory breath and the amplitude of vocal fold vibrations.

In aging, one sees a loss of fine control over the vocal folds,[36] as well as an increase in the roughness of the voice.[69] The vocal timbre may become muffled or thin and sharp. The overall sound of the voice may become monotonous and tremulous, leading occasionally to a peculiar and characteristic wobbling.[31]

The jitter also increases with age.[57,74] The increase in jitter value is greatest for certain vowels, /i/, for example.[74] The cycle to cycle frequency variability (mean percent jitter) and amplitude perturbation (shimmer) both increase with advancing age.[53,75] This variability was found to be even greater in patients with significant atherosclerotic disease or poor general condition.[75] The deterioration of hearing can also affect the fine control of voice.[31]

The senescent speaking voice often shows vocal fatigue, hoarseness, and the pitch changes described above.[26] A diminution in the vocal intensity is described by most authors, although acoustically measured sound pressure levels of intensity in male voices may increase with age.[61] "Senile tremolo" is often found, as is wobbling of the voice, and is attributed to irregular respirations.[61] According to Morrison and Gore-Hickman,[61] two types of voice are seen with aging. In one, phonation is in the lower part of the voice range with a husky or muffled timbre, as with a thickened, chronically edematous larynx. Atrophic changes predominate in the other type. These patients develop a squeaky voice from using the upper end of their range, and the vocal timbre is thin and reedy.[61] There is an increase in hyperfunctional dysphonia as the elderly patient tries to compensate for the changes in fundamental frequency noted above.[43]

CLINICAL FINDINGS

The changes associated with the senescent singing voice include weak, breathy glottal attack, shorter duration of sustained notes, lessened intensity, and a deterioration in the timbre and range.[26,31] On laryngoscopic examination of the aged larynx, Segre[26] found a yellowish discoloration of the mucous membrane, atrophy of the ventricular folds, loss of normal tension, flaccidity, and a fissure in the middle or anterior third of the glottis during phonation. Honjo and Isshiki[71] described yellowish or dark grayish discoloration of the vocal cords in 39% of men and 47% of women, edema of the vocal cords in 56% of men and 74% of women, vocal fold atrophy in 67% of men and 26% of women, a glottal gap in 67% of men and 58% of women, and a sulcus vocalis in 10% of both sexes.[71] Stroboscopic examination may reveal irregularities in symmetry, periodicity, amplitude, mucosal waves, and vibratory closure, which explain abnormalities in the aged voice in spite of a normal appearance on indirect laryngoscopy.[26,76]

Our personal observations have been performed with both fiberoptic laryngoscopy, stroboscopy, and phonatory function analysis. Most patients with laryngeal complaints are recorded videographically. The recorded image can then be played at very slow speeds for careful analysis. Besides the findings listed above, we observed that the sulcus vocalis is much more prevalent in the elderly. We have frequently found minor vocal cord movement abnormalities that were not appreciated until the tape review. Phonatory function shows a decrease in the maximum phonation time, the airflow rate, and the total volume. As part of any laryngeal examination, especially in the geriatric population, a measure of hearing is indicated.[31]

THERAPEUTICS

Probably the most important determinant of how rapidly a voice will age is genetics.[36] Anything that maintains the neurologic, circulatory, and muscular systems is beneficial. Therefore a certain level of fitness must be maintained. The type of exercise may be important. Some singing teachers feel that jogging causes a weakening of the voice. However, exercises that encourage deep breathing, such as swimming and walking alternating with sprinting, are beneficial.[36] Regular practice without long layoffs is important for the singer.[77]

Often, minor deficiencies in the voice and speech patterns of older persons can be corrected by expert therapy.[26,31] Selection of the appropriate speech or voice pathologist is critical. The therapist needs to have a good knowledge of voice disorders, approach the patient professionally, and treat the patient as an intelligent adult.

Vocal hygiene is the cornerstone for effective therapy. Intelligent conservation of the speaking and singing voice during and after the climacteric often prevents phonatory trauma. The avoidance of loud talking or singing in the presence of ambient noise is desirable. The elimination of smoking and other irritants and maintaining adequate humidification and copious hydration are also crucial.

Segre[26] recommends prostigmin and potassium salts and the use of androgens in men and corticosteroids in women for loss of tone in the vocal folds. The use of steroids is controversial and should be considered with caution.[31] Iodinated glycerol or high doses of guaifcncsin arc useful for control of secretions. Improved oral hygiene will prevent a chronically dry mouth. Vitamins A, B, and C supplements may also prove helpful.[26,31]

Laryngeal framework surgery as described by LeJeune et al,[66] Tucker,[78] and Isshiki et al[79–81] offers the opportunity to augment vocal fold tension in an attempt to strengthen the voice. LeJeune et al[66] described a type of laryngoplastic phonosurgery involving the advancement of the anterior commissure. He reported success in six patients, although the follow-up was inconsistent. At first LeJeune et al achieved their objective by bending forward the vertical strut of the thyroid cartilage containing the anterior commissure attachment. The strut remained attached inferiorly, and the superior portion was maintained in position by a horizontal graft placed between the free end of the vertical strut and the remaining thyroid cartilage.[66] Tucker[78] modified the procedure by using a superiorly based strut. He used this procedure in 10 patients exhibiting the breathiness and quavering voice typical of an "elderly" larynx, eight of whom have been followed for at least 6 months. After an initial good result in all patients, the voice regressed to the preoperative state in 3 to 7 months. Thus the procedure is of limited value in elderly patients because of eventual relaxation of tissues.[78] Subsequently LeJeune[82] described a procedure that completely separated the strut superiorly and inferiorly so that the entire vertical component is advanced. The strut was secured with two horizontal grafts above and below the anterior commissure. Koufman[83] further added the injection of a prosthetic substance bilaterally to enhance the closure of the glottis. Isshiki et al[80] performed the thyroplasty type III using the same principles and have obtained some initial favorable results. Tightening of the vocal fold can also be achieved with a thyroplasty type IV, a cricothyroid approximation.[81]

Bouchayer and Cornut[84] and Roch et al[85] used a microflap for senile larynges with a sulcus vocalis. Although this procedure is not performed widely in the United States, their results sound promising.[84]

The interaction of psychodynamics and the voice is well known. It is important to be able to differentiate normal aging from psychological abnormalities. For example, lowered and narrowed pitch variability has been linked to depression and sadness; hoarseness may be associated with similar moods, fatigue, or tension.[54] In the absence of mental instability, psychotherapy can still make an important contribution. In the initial stages of vocal involution, it can act as a stimulating factor for better vocal hygiene or, later, as a suggestive factor to obtain an attitude of calm adaptation to phenomena that are physiologic in origin and therefore shared by all singers.[26]

THE SINGER AND ACTOR

The voice of the vocal artist deserves special consideration, for both the preservation of the vocal system and the rehabilitation of early vocal changes. Since the vocal manifestations tend to parallel the biologic changes of the host, a general attention to the health of the organism is essential.

Almost 2,000 years ago Marcus Fabius Quintilianus, the first author on the art of public speaking, described his recommendations in the 12 volumes of his *Institutio Oratoria*. He stressed the need for:

1. A simple life
2. Sensible eating habits
3. Ample rest and sleep

While these basic instructions are not easy to follow, they form the core of a regimen for increased resistance to the many ills that aging flesh is heir to. A simple life presumes sufficient exercise to challenge the major organ systems; swimming and walking are especially recommended. Eating habits should be moderate, and irritants should be avoided. The prescription for sufficient rest includes, of course, careful use of the vocal organ.

The preservation of the voice begins during the first acting or singing lessons and lasts into advanced age. No less a singer than Caruso continued to see his voice coach regularly until his final illness. General ailments of the thoracic and the abdominal structures must be thoroughly treated, endocrine dysfunctions must be carefully eliminated, and the mental health of the entertainer requires special attention.

Fortunately, most seasoned entertainers make up in experience what they lose in vigor. They have learned the "tricks of the trade" and are able to dazzle their audiences with their expertise. In addition, skilled laryngologists, voice pathologists, and singing teachers are at their disposal to assist them with the maintenance and rehabilitation of their art.

When female entertainers reach menopause, estrogen replacement therapy may prove helpful in avoiding or diminishing the associated vocal changes. Thyroid dysfunction is often difficult to diagnose in the elderly; indicated thyroid therapy may help to restore significant changes in the vocal range and quality.

Vitamin C seems to be helpful for the sustained health of the mucous membranes lining the vocal tract. Vitamin A and vitamin B_{12} may also prove beneficial during advancing years. Ample fluids are essential to counteract the reduction in glandular secretions in the mouth and throat.

Above all, entertainers must keep their voices agile by constant exercises. Humming, vocaleases, and other warming-up exercises can not only retard vocal involution, but also reverse early age-related vocal changes. Wobbles, tremors, and similar findings frequently associated with senescence can often be eliminated by proper vocal training.

Many great actors like Hume Cronyn and Jessica Tandy have reached the zenith of their careers during their latter years. Tito Schipa, Benjamino Gigli, Ezio Pinza, Lauritz Melchior, Lily Lehmann, Amalia Materna, and Renate Peters have proved that singers can continue their art into their 60s or even 70s. With good vocal conditioning, sensible nutrition, proper medical supervision and appropriate medication, many singers should be able to emulate their example.

As Voltaire said so aptly, "Qui n'a pas l'esprit de son age, de son age a tout le malheur"—whoever does not understand the spirit of his age, receives only unhappiness from his age.

REFERENCES

1. Hurst PS: Geriatric dentistry. *Otolaryngol Clin North Am* 23:1097–1107, 1990.
2. Ward PH, Colton R, et al: Aging of the voice and swallowing. *Otol Head Neck Surg* 100:283–285, 1989.
3. Johns M, Brackmann DE, et al: Goals and mechanisms for training otolaryngologists in the area of geriatric medicine. *Otol Head Neck Surg* 100:262–265, 1989.

4. Shindo ML, Hanson DG: Geriatric voice and laryngeal dysfunction. *Otolaryngol Clin North Am* 23:1035–1044, 1990.
5. Chievitz: Untersuchungen über die Verknöcherung der Kehlkopfknorpel. *Arch Anat* 1882.
6. Scheier M: *Arch Mikr Anat* 59:220, 1902.
7. Fraenkel E: *Fortschr Röntgenstr* 12:151, 1908.
8. Imhofer F: Ueber das Abnutzungspigment in der Muskulatur der Stimmbänder. *Ztschr Laryngol Rhinol* 5: 389, 1912.
9. Imhofer F: Ueber das elastsiche Gewebe im Stimmband aepter Individuen. *Zentralbl Allg Pathol Pathol Anat* 25:337, 1914.
10. Nadoleczny M: *Untersuchungen füber den Kunstgesang*. Berlin, Julius Springer, 1923.
11. Kofler K: Der Alterskehlkopf. *Wiener Med Wochenschr* 48:1468–1472, 1931.
12. Stern H: Ueber einige Ursachen und Folgen der Alterserscheinungen. *Stimmgebung Mschr Ohrenheilk* 66: 1143–1149, 1932.
13. Amprino, Bairati: *Z Zellforsch Mikros Anat* Vol 20, 1933; Vol 20, 1934.
14. Malan: *Arch Biol* Vol 45, 1934.
15. Segre R: La Laringe senile. *Il Valsalva* Vol 15, 1936.
16. Carnevale-Ricci F: Osservazioni istopatologiche sulla laringe nella senescenza. *Arch Ital Otol* 49:1, 1937.
17. Bach A, et al: Senile changes in the laryngeal musculature. *Arch Otolaryngol* 34:47–56, 1941.
18. Terracol J, Azemar R: La senescence de la voix. *Largentiere* 1949.
19. Mysak ED: Pitch and duration characteristics of older males. *J Speech Hear Res* 2:46–54, 1959.
20. McGlone R, Hollien H: Vocal pitch characteristics of aged women. *J Speech Hear Res* 6:165–170, 1963.
21. Luchsinger R, Arnold GE: Vocal involutions or senescence of the voice, in *Voice Speech Language*. Belmont, CA, Wadsworth, 1949, pp 135–137.
22. Appaix A, et al: Etude spectrographique de la voix parlee en fonction de l'age. *Trans 13th Intl Congr Logop Phoniatr* 2:105–115, 1965.
23. Sedlackova E, et al: Das Altern der Stimme. *Trans 7th Int Congr Gerontol* 4:469–472, 1966.
24. Ptacek P, et al: Phonatory and related changes with advanced age. *J Speech Hear Res* 9:353–360, 1966.
25. Böhme G: *Stimm-, Sprech-, und Sprachstorungen*. Stuttgart, Gustav Fischer, pp 156–159, 1974.
26. Segre R: Senescence of the Voice. *EENT Monthly* 50:223–227, 1971.
27. Hommerich RW: Der alternde Larynx: Morphologische Aspekte. *HNO* (Berl) 20:115–120, 1972.
28. Habermann G: Der alternde Larynx: Funktronelle Aspekte. *HNO* (Berl) 20:121–124, 1972.
29. Ryan WJ: Acoustic aspects of the aging voice. *J Gerontol* 27:265–268, 1972.
30. Hollien H, Shipp T: Speaking fundamental frequency and chronologic age in males. *J Speech Hear Res* 15: 155–159, 1972.
31. von Leden H: Speech and hearing problems in the geriatric patient. *J Am Geriatr Soc* 25:422–426, 1977.
32. *Journal of Voice* 1:2–67, 1987.
33. Dequeker J: Bone and aging. *Ann Rheum Dis* 34:100, 1975.
34. Guyton AC: Energetics and metabolic rate, in Guyton AC (ed): *Medical Physiology*, 5th ed. Philadelphia, WB Saunders, 1976, pp 934–945.
35. Bierman EL, Ross R: Aging and atherosclerosis, in Paoletti R, Gotto AM (eds): *Atherosclerosis Reviews*. New York, Raven Press, 1977, pp 79–111.
36. Michel JF, Brown WS, Chodzko-Zaiko W, et al: Aging voice: panel 1. *J Voice* 1:53–61, 1987.
37. Krinke G: Spinal radiculopathy in aging rats: Demyelination secondary to neuronal dwindling? *Acta Neuropathol* (Berl) 59:63–69, 1983.
38. Corsellis JAN: Ageing and the dementias, in Blackwood W, Corsellis JAN (eds): *Greenfield's Neuropathology*. Chicago, Year Book Medical Publishers, 1976, pp 796–848.
39. Wang HS: Dementia in old age, in Wells CE (ed): *Dementia*. Philadelphia, FA Davis, 1978, pp 15–26.
40. Hollien H: "Old voices": What do we really know about them? *J Voice* 1:2–17, 1987.
41. Keen JA, Wainwright J: Ossification of the thyroid, cricoid and artyenoid cartilages. *S Am J Lab Clin Med* 4: 83–108, 1958.
42. Rother P, Riodel P: Stereological studies of aging changes in epiglottal cartilage cells. *Z Mikros Anat Forschung* 89:839–858, 1975.
43. Kahane JC: Connective tissue changes in the larynx and their effects on voice. *J Voice* 1:27–30, 1987.
44. Kahn AR, Kahane JC: India ink pinprick assessment of age-related changes in the cricoarytenoid joint (CAJ) articular surfaces. *J Speech Hear Res* 29:536–543, 1986.
45. Mardini IA, McCarter RJ, et al: Contractile properties of laryngeal muscles in young and old baboons. *Am J Otolaryngol* 8:85–90, 1987.
46. Krieger L, Malmgren LT, Gacek RR: Age-related muscle fiber change in the human thyroarytenoid muscle: A histochemical stereologic study. *Otolaryngol Head Neck Surg* 105:193–194, 1991.
47. Evangelisti PA, Malmgren LT, Williams EF: Age-related changes in the volume of the neuromuscular junctions of human thyroarytenoid muscle: A stereologic study. *Otolaryngol Head Neck Surg* 105:194, 1991.
48. Gambino DR, Malmgren LT, Gacek RR: Age-related changes in the neuromuscular junctions in the human posterior cricoarytenoid muscles: A quantitative study. *Laryngoscope* 100:262–268, 1990.

49. Choo D, Malmgren LT, Rosenberg SI: Age-related changes in Schwann cells of the internal branch of the rat superior laryngeal nerve. *Otolaryngol Head Neck Surg* 103:628–636, 1990.
50. Urich H: Diseases in peripheral nerves, in Blackwood W, Corsellis JAN (eds): *Greenfield's Neuropathology*. Chicago, Year Book Medical Publishers, 1976, pp 688–770.
51. Mortelliti AJ, Malmgren LT, Gacek RR: Ultrastructural changes with age in the human superior laryngeal nerve. *Arch Otolaryngol Head Neck Surg* 116:1062–1069, 1990.
52. Bach AC, Lederer RL, Dinolt R: Senile changes in the laryngeal musculature. *Arch Otolaryngol* 34:47–56, 1991.
53. Orlikoff RF: The atherosclerotic voice. *ENT J* 69:833–837, 1991.
54. Mueller PB, Sweeney RJ, Baribeau LJ: Acoustic and morphologic study of the senescent voice. *ENT J* 63:292–295, 1984.
55. Mueller PB, Sweeney RJ, Baribeau LJ: Senescence of the voice: Morphology of excised male larynges. *Folia Phoniatr* 37:134–138, 1985.
56. Hirano M, Kurita S, Sakaguchi S: Ageing of the vibratory tissue of human vocal folds. *Acta Oto-Laryngol* 107:428–433, 1989.
57. Linville SE, Fisher HB: Acoustic characteristics of women's voices with advancing age. *J Gerontol* 40:324–330, 1985.
58. Leutert G: Age dependence of functional systems, exemplified by the vocal cord and cricothyroid articulation. *Z Ges Innere Medizin Ihre Grenzgebiete* 41:131–133, 1986.
59. Grasedyck K, Krohn J, et al: New results on ageing of connective tissue. *Aktuelle Gerontol* 8:585–594, 1978.
60. Bentz W, Laue R: Aspects of healthy and pathologically changed laryngeal epithelium in a model. *Z Alternsforschung* 43:59–64, 1988.
61. Morrison MD, Gore-Hickman P: Voice disorders in the elderly. *J Otolaryngol* 15:231–234, 1986.
62. Pont NA: Lubrication of the vocal mechanism. *Folia Phoniatr* 26:287–288, 1974.
63. Hirabayashi H, Koshii K, Uno K, et al: Laryngeal epithelial changes on effects of smoking and drinking. *Auris Nasus Larynx* 17:105–114, 1990.
64. Stearns MP, Cummings CW: Age-related changes in the epithelium of the monkey larynx. *Ann Otol Rhinol Laryngol* 91:370–371, 1982.
65. Stell PM, Stell IM, Watt J: Age changes in the epithelial lining of the human larynx. *Gerontology* 28:208–214, 1982.
66. LeJeune FE, Guice CE, Samuels PM: Early experiences with vocal ligament tightening. *Ann Otol Rhinol Laryngol* 92:475–477, 1983.
67. Pontoppidan H, Beecher HK: Progressive loss of protective reflexes in the airway with the advance of age. *JAMA* 174:2209–2213, 1960.
68. Chodzko-Zajko WJ, Ringel RL: Physiological aspects of aging. *J Voice* 1:18–26, 1987.
69. Hollien H: Inferring laryngeal characteristics from phonatory output, in Cummings C, et al (eds): *Otolaryngology / Head and Neck Surgery*. Saint Louis, CV Mosby, 1986, pp 1828–1838.
70. Close LG, Woodson GE: Common upper airway disorders in the elderly and their management. *Geriatrics* 44: 67–72, 1989.
71. Honjo I, Isshiki N: Laryngoscopic and voice characteristics of aged persons. *Arch Otolaryngol* 106:149–150, 1980.
72. McGlone RE, Hollien H: Vocal pitch characteristics of aged women. *J Speech Hear Res* 6:164–170, 1963.
73. Hollien H, Shipp T: Speaking fundamental frequency and chronologic age in males. *J Speech Hear Res* 15:155–159, 1972.
74. Wilcox KA, Horii Y: Age and changes in vocal jitter. *J Gerontol* 35:194–198, 1980.
75. Ramig LA, Ringel RL: Effects of physiological aging on selected acoustic characteristics of voice. *J Speech Hear Res* 26:22–30, 1983.
76. Kitzing P: Stroboscopy—a pertinent laryngological examination. *J Otolaryngol* 14:151–157, 1985.
77. Michel JF, Coleman R, Guinn L, et al: Aging voice: panel 2. *J Voice* 1:62–67, 1987.
78. Tucker HM: Laryngeal framework surgery in the management of the aged larynx. *Ann Otol Rhinol Laryngol* 97:534–536, 1988.
79. Isshiki N, Morita H, et al: Thyroplasty as a new phonosurgical technique. *Acta Otolaryngol* 78:451–457, 1974.
80. Isshiki N, Taira T, Tanabe M: Recent advances in phonosurgery. *Folia Phoniatr* 32:119–154, 1980.
81. Isshiki N, Taira T, Tanabe M: Surgical alteration of the vocal pitch. *J Otolaryngol* 12:335–340, 1983.
82. LeJeune FE: Vocal ligametry, update. *Ann Otol Rhinol Laryngol* 96:597–600, 1987.
83. Koufman J: Surgical correction of dysphonia due to bowing of cords. *Ann Otol Rhinol Laryngol* 98:41–45, 1989.
84. Bouchayer M, Cornut G: Microsurgery for benign lesions of the vocal folds. *ENT J* 67:446–466, 1988.
85. Roch JB, Bouchayer M, Cornut G: Le sulcus glottidis. *Rev Laryngol* 102:332–346, 1981.
86. Engelmann G, Leutert G: The aging alterations of the arytenoid cartilage. *Z Mikrosk Anat Forschung* 103:597–619, 1989.

Performance Anxiety

ALLAN B. DEHORN, PhD

Oh, no.
Today's the day. I can't believe it got here so quickly.
I'm not ready. I'm going to make a fool of myself.
Why am I doing this?
Today I have to audition for the scholarship.
I don't think I can do it.
What if I blow it?
What if I get anxious again and my throat clogs up?
What if I can't swallow? I'll be so dry I'll sound like sandpaper.
This is terrible. See, I'm getting anxious already.
I just know I'm going to fail.
See, my throat's getting tight. I'll sound terrible.
I'm on after those two. Boy, they look great—so calm, so relaxed.
Look at me. I'm a basket case. Maybe I should go into accounting.
I can't do it. I just know I'm going to have a terrible anxiety attack.
Oh, no. I'm up next. What am I going to do? What if I pass out?
What if I can't remember the lyrics? I'll be the laughing stock of the audition.
I just know I will.

Sound familiar? This poor soul is in the process of initiating and suffering through performance anxiety. Is he going to make it? That depends largely upon whether he has learned and practiced various interventions that are available to him. We will check in on him later in the chapter.

There are several major theories about the nature of performance anxiety. This chapter focuses on the theory that is illustrated in the above scenario, although other theories will be examined as well. The rest of the chapter is devoted to examining various types of treatment or intervention available to those who suffer from performance anxiety.

DEFINITION AND DESCRIPTION

Performance anxiety, sometimes called *stage fright,* is a condition that has been experienced at one time or another by just about everyone who has had to give an important performance, whether in music, a sporting event, or even a business meeting. The performance anxiety can be rather mild and forgotten or can grow, unfortunately, to disabling proportions. Those whose livelihood does not depend on performing might say, "So what?" But those performing artists who suffer from performance anxiety, usually silently and in agony, know how debilitating it can be.

Even such luminaries as Arthur Rubenstein[1] and Pablo Casals[2] have suffered from performance anxiety. In fact, in a study of 2,212 classical musicians surveyed by the International Conference of Symphony and Opera Musicians in 1988,[3] 24% reported that performance anxiety was a problem and 16% indicated that the problem was severe. There are indications that performance anxiety is even more prevalent among amateur and student musicians.[4,5] It is a tragic event when a promising musical career is abandoned because of performance anxiety.

Anxiety is a physiologic response by the body to perceived threat. It was very adaptive when we roamed the forests and plains and were confronted by beasts with large teeth. It remains an adaptive response when we are confronted by beasts of a different type, perhaps on our own big city streets. It is not necessarily adaptive during a musical audition, even though the judges may seem bestial.

In the presence of threat, the body responds with a "fight or flight" reaction. To run or fight, the skeletal muscles become tense and over time may feel fatigued, "rubbery," trembling, tingling, and/or numb. The heart rate increases to provide greater blood flow to the muscles, and respiration increases to oxygenate the increased blood flow. The field of vision narrows, perhaps to focus better on the threat. Palms become sweaty; feet become sweaty or cold. The smooth muscle systems slow down. Nausea often results, or diarrhea, or urinary urgency. The mouth and throat become dry, and swallowing feels more difficult. Voice timbre and resonance diminish. Since concentration and attention are focused on the source of the threat, attention to other things, such as lyrics, can be affected. Lightheadedness and dizziness often result, perhaps because of the changes in breathing pattern.[6]

Anxiety is not always a detriment to performance. There is evidence to suggest that moderate anxiety can actually enhance performance.[4] Some who feel moderate anxiety might, because of previous anxiety experiences, interpret this as trouble and begin a disruptive, anxiety-evoking spiral, which can have devastating effects. Others might interpret the same moderate anxiety as a good sign—"Now I'm pumped; now I'm ready"—which is likely to enhance the performance.

A COGNITIVE–BEHAVIORAL MODEL

A useful model in the understanding and effective treatment of performance anxiety is one that combines behavioral and cognitive components. It is by no means the only model that precedes effective treatment, but it offers efficacy and utility.

Since almost everyone has some degree of performance anxiety, at some point or other, it is likely that on one or more occasions the anxiety grew to disruptive proportions. Perhaps it was because of being unprepared musically; perhaps it was because of being unprepared for the levels of tension evoked by a major performance. Perhaps it was because of a confluence of many factors that together elicited sufficient anxiety to disrupt a prior performance. Once that performance is disrupted, it frequently develops that the performer then anticipates trouble prior to the next performance. ("Oh, no. What if I blow it?")

Perhaps the next performance goes well and the performer gets thunderous applause;

then the troubled recital is quickly forgotten. Conversely, the anxiety might start to rise at the next recital with the anticipation of trouble, generally in the form of "what ifs." As in the scenario opening this chapter, "what if I get anxious again and my throat clogs up"; "what if I can't swallow"; "what if I can't remember the lyrics"; and "what if I pass out" are all good examples of catastrophic *spook thoughts*.

As the anxiety rises in the stage-frightened person, a second level of spook thought kicks in. This might be nicknamed the "body spook thoughts" or the intensive-care monitoring: "Oh, no. I can't feel my tongue. My throat's so dry a gallon of water won't help. My throat is getting tight. My heart is pounding so hard I think I'm having a heart attack. I just know I'm going to pass out and make a fool of myself." The effect of this second level of spook thought, or, in psychological parlance, cognitive anxiety-evoking cue, is to elicit greater levels of the anxiety.

The entire system is driven by the catastrophic thought that somehow the anxiety, if not controlled, will continue to rise until the sufferer is overwhelmed and probably dies, passes out, goes crazy, or somehow loses control. These catastrophes, of course, do not occur, but the sufferer does not wait long enough in the situation to discover this crucial fact.

Unfortunately, the anxious performer learns very quickly that escaping the anxiety situation while anxious or choosing to avoid the situation altogether readily offers anxiety relief. The effect of this avoidance can be devastating in the forms of missed auditions or even abandonment of career. If allowed to occur, the avoidance is likely to spread into more situations. The sufferer feels as if he has saved his life, mental health, or career by not entering into the performance situation in which he is anticipating overwhelming anxiety. The thought occurs in a new situation, such as at rehearsal, "What if the anxiety should happen here?" The anxiety starts to rise until the body spook thoughts kick in, and an anxiety attack occurs. In addition, each time the reluctant performer tries to challenge an anxiety situation, but escapes at the last minute, he is only adding to the strength of the belief that catastrophe undoubtedly would have occurred if he had stayed.

Sometimes one cannot escape the situation, but must perform. In this case the development of superstitious protection devices frequently results. As long as the performer has his lucky rabbit's foot, warms up in a certain routine, or carries his 5 year old tranquilizer, he feels he is protected from the overwhelming anxiety. The protective devices may work for awhile, giving the performer a sense that the anxiety is controlled and that the recital will go well. Problems arise, however, when the anxiety rises to what feels like scary proportions, and the so-called protective devices do not seem to hold the anxiety level anymore. The protections can become more elaborate and time consuming and not having or performing them at the time of recital can be the anxiety-evoking event even though all else was going well up to that point.

Anxiety is a natural, reactive event. In most instances it only takes a few seconds after the perceived threat is gone before the anxiety symptoms diminish. Most people who suffer from performance anxiety say to themselves, "Mine must be different. It doesn't go away within seconds. It just hangs on until I leave the recital." Their anxiety does react normally. However, the performers are still "spooking" themselves with catastrophic thinking (e.g., "I just know I'll do poorly. What if I screw up?"). The effect of the ongoing spook thinking is to continue to perceive threat and therefore to continue to trigger anxiety reactions. Once the performer stops spooking himself or herself, the anxiety diminishes as expected. Figure 18–1 illustrates the anxiety levels associated with performance and the various anxiety-evoking cognitive components in operation.

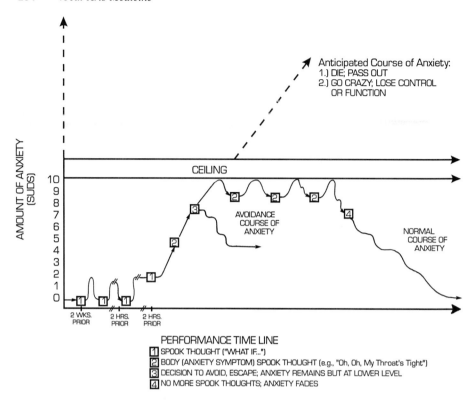

Figure 18–1.

COGNITIVE–BEHAVIORAL TREATMENTS

What can be garnered from the above discussion is that there are basically three components to the problem of performance anxiety: (1) anxiety symptoms, (2) avoidance or protection devices, and (3) the anticipation of catastrophe, or "spook thoughts." The good news is that there are effective cognitive and behavioral treatments available for each of these components.[4,6,7] We first consider the issue of biologic models of performance anxiety and then pharmacologic treatment.

The first component is the anxiety symptoms. Certainly they are scary; they can interfere with performance, and they make the performer feel miserable. However, they are not the major focus of effective treatment, since the anxiety system is merely reacting normally and as it should to perceived threat. ("Oh, no. What if I fail; what if I get overwhelming anxiety? I'll feel like such a fool.") Two very effective behavioral approaches for anxiety management are breathing techniques such as slow and rhythmic diaphragmatic breathing—which should not need to be explained to a group of vocal musicians, and several of the various relaxation techniques. Our clinic prefers to use the Jacobsen progressive deep-muscle relaxation technique because the proprioceptive sensations seem to help the participant focus. Our participants feel it is hard to concentrate on lovely beach images with a lot of anxiety chatter swirling in their heads.

We encourage the relaxation techniques to be used when the anxiety levels are still low before the "body spook thoughts" (see Fig. 18–1) trigger the second level of additional anxiety. It is difficult to begin relaxation exercises when one is experiencing an anxiety level of eight or nine on a subjective scale that goes to ten. These relaxation techniques should be practiced until confidence in them grows. Many people, unfortunately, do not practice them, wait until a key performance, and try the relaxation exercise just before going onstage, all the while saying to themselves, "This won't work. It's not working. I'm still anxious. What if. . . ." (Guess what happens?)

If the relaxation and/or breathing techniques can avert an emerging anxiety attack, it is encouraging, and it demonstrates that anxiety is not automatic and catastrophic. Early in treatment, however, it is much more likely that the spook thoughts and consequent anxiety will prevail.

The second component of performance anxiety is avoidance and protection, which can be very devastating. Very effective behavioral treatments exist for the avoidance and protection devices. These fall under the general category of exposure techniques. The basis for performance anxiety is the mistaken belief that anxiety will become overwhelming and catastrophe will occur. Performance anxiety is not overwhelming; it only seems so, on occasion. The fundamental tenet of *exposure therapy* is to face the fearful situation and see that catastrophe does not result. This can be done on a gradual basis, working up to the most fearful situation in a process called *systematic desensitization*. Alternatively, this can be done in a rapid manner, in a process called *flooding*.

To use an analogy, think of going to a scary movie. When the lightning and thunder occur as the young girl walks through the cemetery, and the cello music starts, we all begin to experience some anxiety. Then, when the monster jumps out, we all experience an anxiety attack. But, looking at the reality of the situation, we see a dark room, with only moderately comfortable seats, with patterns of light on the wall. In reality, what is there of which to be afraid? What is triggering the anxiety is our cognitive anticipation and evaluation, and yet the anxiety reaction is real. If we go to the same scary movie three times, we begin to respond with less anxiety. If we see the same movie ten times, we are likely to be bored; we have become desensitized to the movie cues and to the cognitions triggering anxiety.

The same phenomenon occurs during the exposure therapies. The participant encounters the fearful situation over and over until the anxiety dissipates, which it will, since no catastrophes do occur. Both the gradual, systematic approach and the flooding, or face-the-worst, approach are effective. In our clinic we offer both and let the participant choose. Treatment is complete not when the anxiety has been averted by breathing, relaxation, or avoidance, but rather when the performer has encountered the performance-anxiety beast face to face and has seen it dissipate on its own. When the performer comes to this realization experientially, not just intellectually, the performance anxiety is likely to fade rather dramatically ("Yes, but what if . . . ?").

The early exposure work was done in the therapist's office using the participant's imagination to recreate the fearful situations.[18] The recent literature on exposure therapies strongly suggests that actual, or in vivo, exposure to the fearful situation produces the best results.[6,9]

Music teachers have inherently known about exposure therapy for years. The early initiation of recitals in a musician's performance history and the need to practice repeatedly from informal to dress rehearsals are examples of using exposure techniques. One might question, "How can I use exposure techniques for my Carnegie Hall debut since I can't use the Hall for desensitization purposes?" Sometimes recreating fearful situations is more difficult since the fearful stimulus might be a particular judge or 3,000 people in the audience. Creative solutions or at least approximations can often be found to the problem of recreating fearful performance situations.

Again, the goal of exposure therapy, whether of a gradual or flooding nature, is to encounter the fearful situations and the anxiety and to stay in the situation until the anxiety lessens. No catastrophes will occur.

A problem that sometimes occurs when people try to use exposure therapies is that they stay in the fearful situation to a certain point but escape when they feel the anxiety is about to become overwhelming. Then they come in to the behavior therapist's office and say, "Your techniques don't work!" What has happened is that the person is, in fact, contributing to the performance anxiety by additional lessons of "anxiety is overwhelming," rather than staying in the situation until the anxiety diminishes. The latter is essential for effective treatment.

But sometimes more rehearsal or more recitals do not produce less performance anxiety. Sometimes the participant has not stayed in the situation long enough as above, but sometime performers do stay in the recital and do not feel their anxieties diminishing. What now, go to drugs?

Remember that the precipitants for performance anxiety are the spook thoughts. As long as these spook thoughts are allowed to run rampant, the effects of exposure are likely to be compromised. When exposure therapies work without the benefit of cognitive–behavioral interventions, it may be because, informally and luckily, the participant's cognitions about the fearful situation shifted to more positive and more realistic cognitions.[10,11] Why leave this to chance?

Cognitive behavior techniques are available to identify systematically and change the spook thought patterns and thereby change the anxiety experiences. Studies of performance anxiety and related cognitions do indicate that certain types of thinking are related to anxiety. The most common patterns significantly associated with performance anxiety are unrealistic appraisal, lack of confidence, worry about the effects of tension, and, especially, catastrophising—exaggerating in the imagination the consequences of a minor mishap and the fear of losing control.[4,10]

Cognitive–behavioral approaches that address these concerns have been shown to be very effective in the treatment of performance anxiety.[4,7,10,11] *Self-instructional training*[10] is a method in which the performer is taught to recognize the current negative thought patterns (e.g., the spook thoughts—"What if . . . ?") and to substitute not only positive, task-oriented statements but also more reality-based statements (e.g., "I can manage this. It's very similar to the other recital when I did very well.") rather than catastrophic extremes. One helpful tip is to continue to say the new statements even though they are not believed initially. The belief in them will come later.

Visualization as a technique can be a very effective cognitive intervention. Usually when anxious performers visualize, they reach a point in their fantasies in the pre-performance or performance activities at which the anxiety starts to intrude; they assume catastrophe awaits; and they cognitively escape the scene. If visualization is to be used successfully, the outcome needs to be positive, but not grandiose, and to be realistic, but not negative and overwhelming. The more vivid the scene, it seems, the more effective the visualization technique. Repetitive practice is an important element.

Any cognition that effectively challenges the spook thoughts is likely to be helpful. Simple *disputation* seems more effective than other techniques such as *thought-stopping* or *distraction*, since, as with the exposure techniques, one is challenging the cognitions directly rather than trying to shy away from them. Using disputations, if the spook thought says, "What if I collapse on stage?"[11] one replies, "I'm not going to collapse on stage. I'll be fine." Rather than memorize certain mantras, disputation allows the performer to react to the specific spook thoughts of the immediate situation, and it combines the important elements of positive and realistic appraisal.

Some performers with anxiety problems start to learn the cognitive–behavioral techniques before anything else. They are in their behavioral therapist's office working diligently on their cognitive patterns, and feeling great and feeling ready and feeling confident . . . until they get to the next recital when they let the spook thoughts reemerge and the anxiety results. In our clinic we feel it is important to approach both the behavioral and the cognitive components of the problem. As Meichenbaum[10] suggests, let the participant become a personal scientist, testing hypotheses in anxiety situations. Does the anxiety overwhelm?—let's test it out. Will I collapse or sound like a frog?—let's find out. The combination of a new, more positive and realistic set of cognitions generally encourages more behavioral exposures. When the catastrophe does not occur during the exposure, the performer realistically appraises this, which reinforces the new cognitions. More confidence in the cognitions; more confidence in the exposure techniques—Look out, Luciano! The two approaches working together can offer very effective treatment.[7]

BIOLOGIC APPROACHES

Any discussion of treatment for performance anxiety would be remiss if the use of medication were not included. In the study of 2,212 classical musicians of the ICSOM mentioned previously,[3] 27% of the entire group reported the use of propranolol (Inderal), a popular beta-blocker. Of that group, 19% used the propranolol daily by prescription; 11% used the propranolol occasionally by prescription; and the other 70% reported occasional use without a prescription. In addition, approximately 20% of the entire group were concerned about their alcohol use and their use of prescription and nonprescription drugs. Another study of 94 musicians with performance anxiety[11] showed that 20% had tried benzodiazepines, 26% had tried beta-blocker drugs, and 41% had tried alcohol as a method of reducing performance anxiety. Sixty-seven percent of the professional musicians in this study had tried beta-blockers, as did 37% of the part-time professionals. This study group is one of the few to include vocal musicians. Other studies of musicians have shown lower levels of drug use,[5] but the use of medications seems to be a popular intervention for performance anxiety among musicians.

Benzodiazepines (tranquilizers) and alcohol have been tried by performing artists, but do not seem as popular, probably because they cause sedation and impaired psychomotor functioning, which can affect performance.[12–14] In fact, one study[13] showed that even small doses (2 mg) of diazepam (Valium) caused deterioration of performance among musicians. Both the benzodiazepines and alcohol act directly on the central nervous system.

They can alter mood and thus leave the performer excited and confident after an inferior performance, and they can decrease normal dexterity and intellectual keenness.[5]

The beta-adrenergic blocking drugs, or beta-blockers, are not centrally acting and do not cause the same level of sedation. Instead, they block the action of the beta-receptors of the sympathetic nervous system and decrease the peripheral effects of anxiety, especially increased heart rate and motor tremor.[16] For these reasons, initially beta-blockers were proposed as a treatment for anxiety.

Despite the popularity of beta-blockers with performers and the enthusiastic endorsement by investigators,[13–15,17–19] reviews of controlled studies have concluded that beta-blockers only demonstrate an equivocal effect on performance anxiety.[12,20] Controlled studies are important because they can demonstrate whether a treatment effect is real or just enthusiasm, whether the treatment effect is greater than a placebo effect or even a no treatment control group experience. The best conclusions from the controlled studies are that beta-blockers can lower heart rate and tremor[13–15,18] but have almost no effect on anticipated or subjective anxiety.[13,15,18] This bodes fairly well for string musicians for whom improved bowing technique has been identified,[13,14] although no differences in technical performance quality or musicianship were found for keyboard musicians among those given propranolol (Inderal) or placebo.[14] Almost no controlled studies include vocal musicians, however, except those investigating cognitive and behavioral techniques.

It is curious that several of the controlled studies reporting some efficacy of beta-blockers also report a similar effect.[13,14,17] The first performance during each study seems to favor the beta-blocker over placebo, even significantly, but by the second or third performance the placebo group is doing just as well. This is very similar to controlled studies of other medications for anxiety that not only show the placebo group performances equalling those of the medication group but also show that the placebo group can do better during the long-term follow-up.[17] To a cognitive–behaviorist these observations only support the notion that the effective components of treatment are not the medication but rather (1) the repeated exposure to the fearful situation and (2) the developing belief that nothing catastrophic will happen, whether because of the assumption of protection by the pill or the realistic appraisal of the performance situation.

A concern about the unsupervised use of beta-blockers is that of side effects. Physicians are warned to use extreme caution in the use of beta-blockers with patients who suffer cardiac disease, particularly involving the conduction system, and those who suffer bronchial asthma.[16] Minor side effects may include fatigue, lightheadedness, nausea, and insomnia. Another unsubstantiated concern for vocal musicians may be that nonselective beta-blockers have a considerable effect on the bronchi and bronchioles and increase airways resistance.[16] While this can cause bronchospasms in asthmatics and is "not clinically important" in normal individuals, does this reaction affect the performing vocal musician? The answer is conjectural, and the question warrants a set of well-controlled studies. Another concern about unsupervised use of beta-blockers is long-term use, which is not recommended.[15,16] It is very important to see a physician if one wants to utilize beta-blockers to deal with performance anxiety.

What practical conclusions might be drawn from this discussion of biologic treatment of performance anxiety? The first is that alcohol and benzodiazepines are not effective for performance anxiety and may, even at low levels, have a detrimental effect on performance. The second conclusion is that, in the words of one of the proponents of beta-blockers, "Beta-blockers on their own are not the whole answer. . . ."[13] It appears that beta-blockers reduce heart rate and tremors. For the vocal musician with severe performance anxiety, this may give him a sufficient sense of control over the anxiety to proceed with performance exposure techniques. To put this in the cognitive–behavioral model presented earlier, the reduced somatic response may help the performer cognitively challenge the second level, body spook thoughts, and thus maintain only lower levels of anxiety during the performance. The third conclusion is that beta-blockers might be a useful component in a multimodal treatment approach, especially to help the sufferer of severe performance anxiety to initiate and maintain the behavioral and cognitive–behavioral components of treatment.

The lack of vocal musicians as subjects in these treatment studies severely restricts the conclusions that can be drawn. The next time your local, friendly researcher solicits your participation in a study of the effective treatments for performance anxiety perhaps you might volunteer yourself . . . or a friend.

Let's return to our performer at the audition and see how he is doing since he has been to his cognitive–behavioral therapist.

"What if I blow it? I'll just. . . .
Wait a minute. Why am I doing this to myself?
I'll be all right.
I'm not going to fail. I'm well-prepared.
I've warmed up. I know my music.
A little bit of anxiety can be helpful in performance enhancement—I'll use it rather
    than let it scare me.
I'm ready to go. Well, here goes.
Recitar! Mentre preso dal delirio. . . .

[applause]

REFERENCES

1. Sobel D: For stage fright, a remedy proposed. *New York Times.* November 20, 1979, C1.
2. Corredor J: *Conversations with Casals.* New York, EP Dutton, 1956.
3. Fishbein M, Middlestadt S, Ottati V, et al: Medical problems among ICSOM musicians: Overview of a national survey. *Med Probl Perf Art* 3:1–8, 1979.
4. Steptoe A, Fidler H: Stage fright in orchestral musicians: A study of cognitive and behavioral strategies in performance anxiety. *Br J Psychol* 78:241–249, 1987.
5. Wesner RB, Noyes R, Davis TL: The occurrence of performance anxiety among musicians. *J Affect Disord* 18:177–185, 1990.
6. Barlow D: *Anxiety and Its Disorders.* New York, Guilford Press, 1988.
7. Kendrick M, Craig K, Lawson D, Davidson P: Cognitive and behavioral therapy for musical performance anxiety. *J Consult Clin Psychol* 50:353–362, 1982.
8. Wolpe J: *The Practice of Behavior Therapy.* New York, Pergamon Press, 1973.
9. Emmelkamp PMG: *Phobic and Obsessive–compulsive Disorders: Theory, Research, and Practice.* New York, Plenum Press, 1982.
10. Meichenbaum D: *Cognitive Behavior Modification.* New York, Plenum Press, 1977.
11. Clark DB, Agras WS: The assessment and treatment of performance anxiety in musicians. *Am J Psychiatry* 148:598–605, 1991.
12. Clark DB: Performance-related medical and psychological disorders in instrumental musicians. *Ann Behav Med* 11:28–34, 1989.
13. James I, Savage I: Beneficial effect of nadolol on anxiety-induced disturbances of performance in musicians: A comparison with diazepam and placebo. *Am Heart J* 4:1150–1155, 1984.

14. James IM, Pearson RM, Griffith DNW, Newbury P: Effect of oxprenolol on stage fright in musicians. *Lancet* 2:952–954, 1977.

15. Brantigan CO, Brantigan TA, Joseph N: The effect of beta-blockage on stage fright: A controlled study. *Rocky Mountain Med J* 76:227–232, 1979.

16. Hayes PE, Schulz SC: Beta-blockers in anxiety disorders. *J Affect Disord* 13:119–130, 1987.

17. Meibach RC, Dunner D, Wilson LG, et al: Comparative efficacy of propranolol, chlordiazepoxide, and placebo in the treatment of anxiety: A double-blind trial. *J Clin Psychiatry* 48:355–358, 1987.

18. Neftel KA, Adler RH, Kappeli L, et al: Stage fright in musicians: A model illustrating the effect of beta-blockers. *Psychosom Med* 44:461–469, 1982.

19. Liden S, Gottfries C: Beta-blocking agents in the treatment of catecholamine-induced symptoms in musicians. *Lancet* 2:529, 1974.

20. Nies AS: Clinical pharmacology of beta-adrenergic blockers. *Med Probl Perf Art* 1:25–29, 1986.

19

The Speech–Language Pathologist's Role in the Management of the Professional Voice

R.E. STONE, JR, PhD

The professional voice user is no less susceptible to vocal foibles and laryngeal problems than are members of the general public. Along with the usual dysfunctions, however, professional voice users seem particularly susceptible to specific disorders and often require unique medical and nonmedical voice care. Differences between behavioral and medical/surgical treatment models serve as a point of departure for this chapter. Then, two different treatment endpoints are identified as varying according to conditions that alter the voice. Finally, considerations that may enter into management of the professional voice user are presented under the major headings of vocal care and reinstating voice use after voice rest. This may be the first literature focusing on commercial rather than classical singers. For completeness sake, some of the more common problems seen by the behavioralist in the voice clinic and their ICD code numbers are presented in Appendix A. To treat these difficulties, several intervention procedures are typically applied by speech–language pathologists and are identified in Appendix B of this chapter along with their CPT code numbers.

DIFFERENCES BETWEEN BEHAVIORAL AND MEDICAL–SURGICAL MODELS OF INTERVENTION

Several features related to patient and clinician involvement differentiate medical/surgical intervention from behavioral intervention. In the medical model, responsibility of etiology and responsibility for personal improvement is placed outside the realm of the person seeking help. The patient participates by giving consent and then passively receives that which is done to or for that person's benefit in the form of the specialist's observation, medication, or surgical activity. The active agent is the surgeon or physician, whose involvement with the patient is for relatively short periods. Cognitive skills and abilities for the most part come from the medical specialist, and little cerebral activity is required of the patient.

In a behavioral model great understanding and involvement is required of the patient, hereafter referred to as *client* to emphasize that the speech–language pathologist may wish to view the dysphonic's role as different than in a physician–patient relationship. The clinician is obligated to extensive time commitments for teaching—not just admonishing but instructing and helping in the learning process. The client learns to take better care of the voice. The client learns that redevelopment of voice involves altering belief systems. What at first seems impossible may, with proper instruction, become a realistic expectation. The individual must recognize both the undesirable and the desirable behaviors brought to the task of producing voice and must assume responsibility for using that desired or undesired behavior, as well as for the ensuing consequences of each. The client, not the clinician, is the important ingredient in the clinical recipe. Little is done to or for the person except that which the person does himself. Successful intervention hinges on the client's learning to carry out the suggestions of the clinician. This can only be done by making the behavioral management of voice problems a highly cognitive activity of the client. Admittedly, the clinician is a significant part of the intervention by guiding the client (1) to set realistic goals, (2) to design suitable learning activities, and (3) to learn responsibility for behaviors used. Yet the clinician has a less active role in assuming responsibility for the patient's betterment than does the medical specialist in a medical model. Often it is necessary for the clinician to teach these themes as well as teach the mechanics of improved voice production.

The Influence of Palliation and Correction Purposes on the Speech–Language Pathologist's Selection of Treatment Endpoints

Endpoints of intervention depend on the palliative or corrective purposes of treatment. Most texts involving the study and treatment of voice and its disorders (vocalogy, as Titze[1,2] and Gates[3] might call it) seem to encourage implementation of intervention strategies for nearly all vocal problems regardless of etiology. Yet the clinical literature fails to give the physician and speech–language pathologist guidelines for expecting varying degrees of success from behavioral management. Behavioral intervention that attempts full restoration of normal voice and normal vocal physiology for all clients regardless of etiology of dysphonia will be unsuccessful more times than not. Instead of trying to correct all dysphonias, at least two treatment expectations may be adopted by the speech–language pathologist. One is built on concepts of palliation and the other on correction. Selection between these two hinges on the etiology of the dysphonia and the associated pathophysiology. Figure 19–1 presents a few of the etiologies or conditions altering normal voice production categorized according to those that are compatible with palliative and with corrective expectations.

With palliation, the expected endpoint is voice produced different from that at the entry of treatment and closer to normal. The endpoint of correction is normal voice. An assumption underlying palliation is that the client does not have the potential for normal voice. In the case of papillomatosis, for example, the growth on the vocal folds alters mucous membrane properties such that the abnormal glottal duty cycle and glottal incompetence obviate normal vocal fold vibration. A change in this pathology is not

Assignment of Therapy Roles as a Function of Laryngeal Aberration

CONDITIONS	DIAGNOSES	
	CORRECTIVE	PALLIATIVE
Anatomic changes		Web, sulcus, scar, bowing
Pathologies*	Nodules, vocal polyps, contact ulcers	Polyps (hemorrhagic, pedunculated), non-TVF polyps, laryngitis, papillomas, keratosis, leukoplakia, Reinke's edema, foreign body reactions, cysts, asthmatic edema, neoplasms
Traumas*		Edemas, dislocations, scars, granulation tissue, hemorrhage
Systemic*	Functional sicca	Syndromes (Sjögren, Addison, scleroderma, hormonal disorders (myxedema, gonadal, menstrual)
Neuro/myologic disturbances†	Incipient dystonia, nerve paralyses (with expected regeneration)	Dystonia, tremor, nerve paralyses (with no expected regeneration)
Maladaptive laryngeal behavior†	Postexposure to irritants, mutational falsetto, functional (a)dysphonias, chronic vocal fry, speaker's throat, non-senile bowing	Paradoxical cord motion

*Vocal care (varp/lubrication/hygiene).
†Vocal reeducation.

Figure 19–1. Conditions and diagnoses altering voice that may best be associated with corrective and palliative treatment roles.

expected from only behavioral intervention even if vocal fold activity can be brought closer to normal. Likewise, only behavioral intervention in a case of an intubation granuloma may improve vocal function but probably will not end in normal voice or in elimination of the pathology. Often, however, there are associated undesired vocal dynamics that result from maladaptive compensation for such pathologies. If these dynamics can be ameliorated by behavioral change to make voice more effective at a lower cost/benefit ratio to the client, then a palliative intervention program may be justified even though voice will never be normal.

Assumptions underlying corrective intervention are (1) that normal voice is reasonably expected and (2) that misuse of the vocal apparatus is the sole etiology of dysphonia. *Vocal misuse* is defined as the application of wrong vocal physiology most often observed as excessive muscle activity (hyperkinetic) or inadequate airflow. Vocal misuse, identified by various terms, including *functional dysphonia* or *aphonia, conversion dysphonia,* and *hysterical dysphonia,* is best treated by vocal reeducation with a goal of complete restoration of voice.

Another suitable application of a corrective focus in intervention is indicated by polyps and nodules in association with a patient history of vocal abuse. Such history includes lesion location and characteristics that can be attributed to vocal abuse. *Vocal abuse,* as used here, is defined as normal vocal physiology carried out to an abnormal degree usually either in loudness or duration. Experimental evidence shows that elevated pitch may be deleterious as well.[4,5] Johnson[6] has pointed out that the use of even normal vocal loudness and duration in the presence of infectious processes also may constitute vocal abuse. He developed a vocal abuse reduction program for children that is effective in eliminating the pathology arising from the abuse and giving normal voice in 80% of the clients within 5 to 15 weeks of intervention. Presumably, modification of the program for adults would give a similar therapeutic endpoint and success rate. Because this program is adequately described by him it will not be reiterated here.

Many speech–language pathologists are taught to apply techniques to facilitate better voice production in instances of vocal abuse and vocal misuse (see, for example, Boone and McFarlane[7]). For the problems of abuse of professional voice users that this chapter addresses, such techniques could seem contraindicated. This author takes no exceptions to such activities in cases of misuse. In cases of abuse and in dysphonias resulting from vocal fold pathology, however, it seems wiser to pursue strategies that are designed to eliminate the abuse and pathology first. Then, when the mechanism is normal or as good as it can be, activities to optimize laryngeal function seem timely and appropriate. When facilitative techniques are applied before resolution of the pathology, the clinician risks teaching the client to compensate for the pathology. Physiology of compensation presumably would be different from physiology that is possible with normal anatomy. Thus the clinician applying facilitative techniques risks teaching abnormal physiology.

Applying such techniques to cases of abuse before addressing issues discussed by Johnson[6] often focuses clinical activities on other than elimination of the abuse. Such intervention therefore is misdirected and often has been found in our facilities to be counterproductive.

Consequently, discussion of facilitative techniques in the management of professional voice users has been omitted because such professionals usually present with problems that contraindicate such approaches. When they can be justified, facilitative techniques are a useful armamentaria. The reader is encouraged to refer to the excellent presentation of facilitative techniques by Boone and McFarlane.[7] Other considerations in ameliorating vocal abuse specifically in professional users, however, are presented here.

Whereas speech–language pathologists generally expect full correction of laryngeal pathology arising from abuse, with the professional voice user one sometimes must settle for palliation. Gates[3] writes that in their enthusiasm for care, therapists must be sure that "the treatment is not worse than the disease." He continues this line of thinking by posing that prolonged therapy (to teach proper vocal hygiene, providing information about amplification and noise reduction in the work place, instructing the person in stress management, and keeping this person in therapy until the dysphonia resolves) may be more costly than suggesting a job change, particularly if the person wanted in the first place to escape from undesirable employment. On the other hand, learning proper vocal hygiene and techniques would possibly solve some professionals' problems, but to implement these would require unwanted change in job or vocal style. But, doing these *in so far as possible* and retaining their entertainment jobs changes the procedures from correction to palliation—helping professionals cope with their limitations and still work. Thus suggestions necessarily are to be applied in some instances with a palliative endpoint in mind because the professional cannot usually follow the instructions to a degree that is sufficient for full correction.

VOCAL CARE FOR THE PROFESSIONAL

Ensuring proper laryngeal lubrication, abstaining temporarily from voice use, limiting voice use, initiating voice training and reestablishing voice use following voice rest or surgery often help to eliminate and sometimes prevent voice problems.

Laryngeal Lubrication

Undesirable physical characteristics of laryngeal mucus, the chief complaints of the patient, and patient response to questions about diet and personal habits may indicate the need for a lubrication regime. Increased production and viscosity of mucus are the most frequently observed laryngoscopic signs of inadequate vocal fold lubrication. Potential signs of poor lubrication include thickening of laryngeal mucus. Roping and stranding of mucus from one cord to the other probably represents the greatest viscosity of mucus. The location of the stranding may indicate the site of previous vocal fold injury or may foretell the site of impending injury. Whitish pooling of mucus on the upper lip of the folds or on their superior surfaces also can be viewed as an indication of increased viscosity but of a lesser degree than that seen in stranding. Yet whitish pooling of mucus would seem to suggest viscosity that is greater than that associated with pooling of colorless mucus. An ordinal scale of viscosity from lesser to greater may therefore be considered: increased amount of mucus, clear pooling, whitish pooling, stranding (see Fig. 19–2). Although such a scale of viscosity

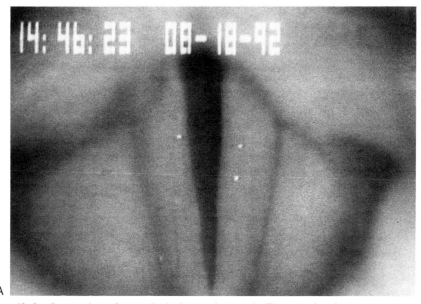

A

Figure 19–2. Presentations of mucus in the larynx: **A**, normal. (Figure continued on next page)

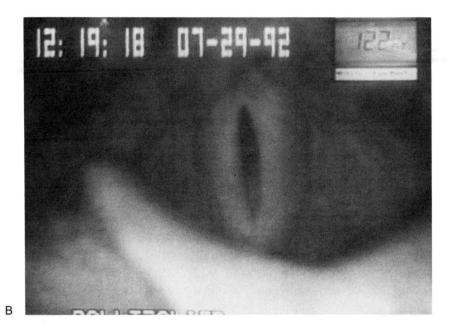

Figure 19–2, cont.   B, Decreased amount contributing to lack of light reflections. **C**, Clear pooling. (Figure continued on next page)

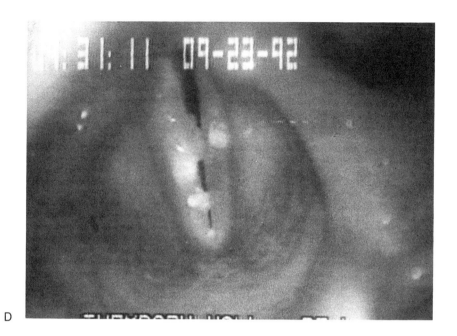

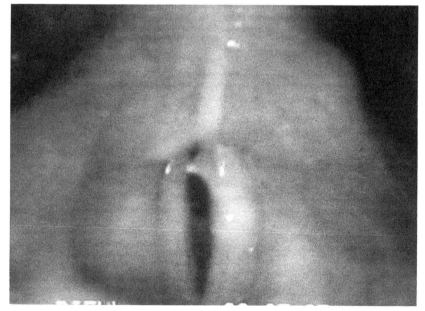

Figure 19–2, cont. **D**, White pooling. **E**, Stranding.

needs validation, these laryngeal signs can signify a need for clinical attention to modification of mucus consistency. These signs are often associated with various symptoms of which the patient complains, including sensation of dryness of the nose, mouth and throat; frequent throat clearing; momentary arrest in voice usually released by a cough or throat clearing; sudden changes in voice quality; mouth breathing; and decreased durability and range of the voice with pitch breaks. When asked, patients often admit to the use of milk products; caffeine; decreased liquid intake; smoking and marijuana use; ethanol consumption; antihistamine (ab)use; use of birth control pills and diuretics; and spending increased time in low humidity environments.

Improving lubrication of the larynx involves the elimination of certain undesirable behaviors and the implementation of desirable behaviors. The clinician who is attuned to the problem of thickened mucus or dryness (sicca) may first suggest that the individual avoid or at least limit dehydrating factors. This would include primary smoking, which probably dries the larynx because of the heat associated with the burning tobacco, be it cigarettes, cigars, in pipes, or marijuana. Additionally, irritants in the smoke may cause an outpouring from the mucous glands to a point that they cannot keep up with the amount of liquid necessary for proper viscosity and then produce mucus that is too thick. One also must consider the possibility of the irritating effects of passive smoking on the speaker's larynx and consider ways of reducing it. For example, a singer on stage may place a slow-moving fan behind the bandstand to blow the smoke back out in front of the singer into the audience.

The clinician may guide the client to avoid various sources of caffeine, which is a dehydrating agent. Caffeine can be found, of course, in most coffees and teas, cola-based drinks, chocolate products, and some medicines. An article in *U.S. News & World Report*, May 22, 1988, has ranked certain popular beverages by caffeine content (see Table 19–1).

Voice clients may also benefit from encouragement to avoid alcohol. Alcohol is a drying agent and therefore increases the viscosity of mucus. Milk products also are substances known by performers to create thick mucus; therefore, they fervently avoid milk products several hours prior to performance. The substance in milk that forms thickened mucus is not known, but the effect nonetheless is significant.

Table 19–1 Caffeine Content of Common Beverages

BEVERAGE	CAFFEINE (MG)	BEVERAGE	CAFFEINE (MG)
Coffee (5 oz.)		Soft drinks (12 oz.)	
Brewed, drip	116	Jolt Cola	71
Brewed, perc.	80	Mountain Dew	54
Instant	65	RC Cola	48
Decaf. brewed	3	TAB	47
Tea (5 oz.)		Coca-Cola	46
Brewed, U.S.	40	Dr. Pepper	41
Brewed, Imp.	60	Sugar-Free Dr. Pepper	41
Instant	30	Pepsi-Cola	41
Iced (12 oz.)	70	Diet Pepsi	38
		Pepsi Light	36
		Canada Dry D/C	2
		Diet Rite	0

A "thou shalt not . . ." approach may be balanced by more positive approaches, and the clinician may recommend various things on a "do more of . . ." basis. Included in this category would be to hydrate the body adequately. Some clinicians will recommend that patients drink approximately 6 to 10 glasses of water per day. In dry environments, such as in an airplane, one might drink a glass of water or juice every 40 minutes. Another guideline as to how much liquid to take might be suggested by a phrase posed by the late otolaryngologist Van Lawrence: "drink until you sing wet—pee pale."

Individuals may benefit from mucolytic agents. The oldest substance in existence may be lemon wedges. Individuals divide a lemon into six wedges and take one six times a day, chewing the pulp and discarding the peel—one wedge after breakfast, one at midmorning, one after lunchtime, one at midafternoon, one after supper, and one before going to bed. Done on a short-term basis, this probably will not cause significant erosion of the enamel of the teeth. It is not recommended on a long-term basis. Some otolaryngologists will recommend supersaturated potassium iodide (SSKI). Guaifenesin is another mucolytic agent that may be prescribed by a physician.

One of the most common causes of laryngeal dehydration involves mouth breathing. Singing and speaking are nearly synonymous with mouth breathing. When these activities are done in dry environments, found in nearly every air-conditioned or heated room, drying of the airways is unavoidable. Voice professionals must establish ways to modify breathing characteristics and/or the atmospheric environment to effect a more physiologic and hygienic condition of the larynx. A clinician is ill-advised to recommend nasal breathing only. It is too slow, looks too awkward, and does not allow for air intake of sufficient volume during speech and song. Open mouth breathing seems to be the posture of choice for most performers. The drying effect, however, can be decreased by having the client use tongue-tip-up breathing. The clinician can instruct and practice the patient to place the tip of the tongue on the upper alveolar ridge and draw air around the sides of the tongue. This has a tendency to warm and moisten the air before it hits the oropharynx and the larynx. It is a procedure that can be efficiently and unobtrusively employed so that a listener is unaware that the speaker is an "upper" instead of a "downer." Additionally, the clinician may consider the possibility of increased nasal airways resistance that could be relieved by beclomethasone dipropionate, monohydrate nasal spray, or surgical alteration of nasal anatomy. Testing the efficacy of topical nasal medications or of mucolytic agents in improving vocal performance has not been reported abundantly in the experimental literature. This may represent potential horizons for clinical trials.

Voice Rest

Management of vocal problems may involve temporary elimination of vocal fold vibration or decreasing amount of potentially abusive vocal fold contact. Brodnitz[8] has advised voice rest to promote undisturbed, quick healing. Voice rest that essentially makes the individual mute may not be met with full compliance by patients except in the most motivated individuals. A case in point might be postoperative patients who want to avoid repeated procedures or in other cases, individuals whose continued or potentially recurring vocal disability means great financial loss. The following case illustrates the benefits of voice rest and gradual removal from rest.

CASE **1**

A singer with several gold records executed her next to last note in the last song of her last performance on a 2 week tour of England. The last note would have been her highest of the concert and the
next to last was the second highest and second loudest. The next to last note became her last in Europe.

She reported "something strange happened in my throat and I just couldn't even try to sing the
last note. I knew something had gone wrong. I was hoarse ever since the concert but now I'm
somewhat better but still can't sing through the break in my voice."

Videoendoscopy with stroboscopy (see Fig. 19–3) showed evidence of a left true vocal fold
hemorrhage in the form of a polyp on the laterosuperior surface. Questionable puffiness of the cord
was appreciated and judged to be the source of present vocal limitations.

Also, two varices were evident on stroboscopy. One was just anterior to the rubylike polyp. The
other was on the medial surface of the same vocal fold and could be seen only by varying the phase
of illumination so that the upper lip of the fold was seen to be lateral to the lower lip. These
observations were made just before a planned week-long series of public relations meetings and
appointments and 2 months before opening the year's touring season.

Due to schedule demands, there was a need to restore the larynx and voice as much as possible as
quickly as possible. Experience inclined us to anticipate incomplete resolution of the polyp. Vocally,
this was acceptable because its lateral location appeared not to alter vocal fold dynamics to a
substantial degree. The varices were of greater concern. A vascular leak of the aneurysm on the glottic
margin would surely disable her and require surgical removal followed by a rehabilitation period that
essentially would not allow her to perform for the rest of the season. Economically and professionally,
she might never recoup the losses from such an event.

The potential for devastation of her career necessitated dramatic intervention and absolute voice
rest to allow healing of the varices. This was implemented for 3 weeks with weekly interval
stroboscopic examinations. The laryngeal picture never changed during this time frame except for
resolution of the slight puffiness of the cords. During voice rest, she maintained P.R. commitments and
other face-to-face communication via the use of a notebook computer. For talking with groups, the
notebook was connected to a larger monitor so all could read her messages.

First, by humming, she came out of the 3 weeks of voice rest and quickly established voicing in
sentences. She progressed gradually from one-to-one conversation limited to just a few sentences
the first day, to quiet radio interviews by the end of the second week, to limited vocalizations the third
week, to rehearsals with the band the sixth week. She sang a 45 minute concert during the seventh
week. By 3 months she embarked on her previously arranged tour itinerary and did not miss a concert.
Seven months later, the medial varix had disappeared, the polyp was reduced minimally in size, and
the second varix near the polyp was unchanged. Throughout the touring season interval laryngeal
examinations, on-tour consultations, and follow-up clinic visits to learn vocal care and wise management of the voice were provided.

Most patients will not follow elimination of vocal fold vibration as well as this patient.
A modified voice rest approach may enjoy greater receptivity. Here, *modified voice rest*
means the use of a soft, easily produced whisper. It is not stage whisper that is associated
with increased laryngeal tension and a high flow rate. Musicians often are the most insistent
that whispered speech is vocally damaging to the larynx. Yet, when the facts are
investigated with videoendoscopic techniques, one finds that a soft, easy whisper does not
involve vibration of the vocal folds, but merely the flow of air through a narrowed glottal
aperture. Therefore, when cessation of the vocal cord vibration is desired to promote
healing or to avoid the risks of injury associated with voice production, it seems that a
whispered speech may be reasonable. One need not worry about atrophy of the vocal cord
because the arytenoids are not immobilized and the vocal cords abduct and adduct and are
tensed during respiration, lifting, and so forth. All that is desired under this type of voice
rest is cessation of vibratory action. Even teachers are able to conduct their classroom

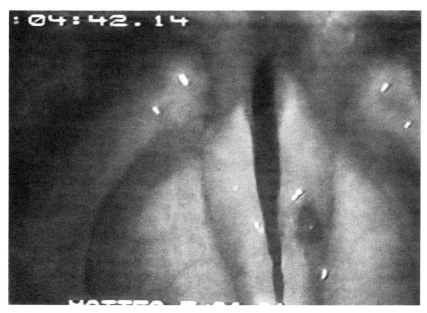

Figure 19–3. Hemorrhagic polyp on the left vocal fold with ipsilateral varices, one on the glottal surface and the other on the superior surface anterior to the polyp.

activities using this desirable type of whispered speech, particularly when it is supplemented with amplification.

Decreasing amount and/or force of vocal cord vibration may serve as an alternative when cessation of vibration or whisper is not a recommendation of choice. Working substantially with professional voice users, one finds that the advice of either strict voice rest or "whisper only" is often not a viable alternative unless the expected benefits offset the consequences of being put "on ice." This sometimes involves the expense of $2,000 to $85,000 per engagement, depending on the "star" status of the performer. Consequently, we have found ourselves in the position of allowing the client to engage in limited professional use of the voice. The limitation may merely be in regard to duration, using voice only when people are paying to hear that voice. This decreases vocalizations for most performers to a substantial degree. Such advice is recommended in cases in which there is vocal fold edema and/or vocal fold nodules/polyps related to suspected vocal abuse. Limiting voice also may be in terms of intensity and fundamental frequency. Accordingly, advice may be offered to give less than a 100% vocal effort and transpose songs to another, more comfortable pitch range. This allows the individual to meet scheduled venues even though the person may have to settle for something less than his or her best performance. Most audience members wish to hear and see a performer rather than to hear a particular high note or specific intensity level. Modified voice rest is represented by case 2.

CASE **2**

Two days before the opera, a singer arrived in Tennessee from Germany. In less than 24 hours she was expected to do a blocking rehearsal, then an informal and finally a dress rehearsal. She came to the clinic to investigate possible causes of mild changes in technique necessary to perform in her midrange. Although she could hear voice quality differences from what was normal, she admitted that probably these differences would not be noticed by others (a fact borne out by critics' raves over her performances on subsequent days).

Laryngeal videoendostroboscopic examination revealed moderately large immature bilateral vocal nodules (polyps) at the junction of the anterior and middle thirds of the vocal folds (Fig. 19–4). Retrospectively, she attributed their onset to having sung while experiencing a cold 2 weeks previously.

The only feasible intervention was to suggest elimination of all unnecessary vocal use (eg, attend no cast parties) and use minimum conversation (only to order food, etc). Transposition of music to a lower key was not an option, and she had to sing as required by the score. By arrangement with the conductor, however, she was able to reduce the dynamic markings of her solo parts.

Such modifications were employed for the 3 days of her performance. This was followed by 2 weeks of using reduced vocal intensity in required communication and the avoidance of unnecessary voicing. She experienced resolution of the pathology and she resumed an active operatic singing schedule in her opera house back in Germany without problems.

For necessary voice use such as in noncancelable radio or television interviews, patients are advised to use reduced intensity by suggesting they talk no louder than if the interviewer and listening audience were only 3 feet away.

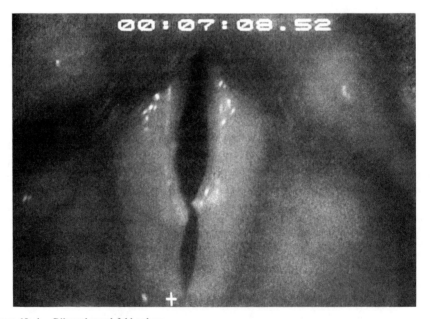

Figure 19–4.   Bilateral vocal fold polyps.

Reduction of potential abuse in voice production judged by the client to be necessary, such as throat clearing, needs further consideration. In the professional, throat clearing is one of the more common abuses. Although most clinicians seem inclined to admonish the performer not to clear the throat, the admonitions are "hollow words" when, while performing, a person finds difficulty because of mucus collected in the larynx. Proper laryngeal lubrication as outlined earlier may be of help, along with alternative behaviors to throat clearing when possible. One such activity is "laryngeal squeezes." The individual engages in a valsalva-like activity (such as in bearing-down or lifting heavy weights), relying on the constriction of the larynx to move the collection of mucus from one sensitive area of the larynx that stimulates throat clearing to an area that does not bother the performer. If such squeezes of the larynx do not work, then one may try swallowing. During the swallowing act the laryngeal space is compromised by muscle contractions that may move mucus to a nontroublesome part of the larynx. If this does not help, the clinician may ask the individual to engage in producing a high flow rate of air through the larynx without vocalization; this would auditorially result in the production of a loud whispered /ha/. Throat clearing may be necessary when all other alternatives fail, beginning with a soft easy throat clearing and then repeating it more vigorously on successive trials until relief is obtained.

Inventory of all voice use and elimination of that which is unnecessary should receive the greatest amount of attention from both the clinician and the client. Such behaviors might be easily recognized by asking the person to consider use of voice in which vocal intensity is elevated. Examples of such unnecessary abusive behaviors include:

1. Giving commands during set-up of the band and during sound checks
2. Talking immediately after a performance, when the adrenaline rush is still flowing
3. Giving "rebel yells" during vocal performance or during attempts to liven up a crowd
4. Talking while in flight on airplanes, particularly when seated near engines (where intensity levels may reach 85 dB)
5. Talking between sets while visiting audience members at their tables in the cocktail lounges
6. Vocalizing at "after hours" parties
7. Conversation with friends during performance by other groups on the venue.

Sometimes client insight is best developed by "on tour consultations" when the clinician can witness and point out in real-time such abuses. Elimination of the behavior begins with identification and then with instructions that inform the client of the laryngeal physiology associated with loud voice productions. Instruction should develop the theses that (1) greater loudness is associated with stronger adductive forces of the vocal cords; (2) increased subglottal pressure increases the amplitude of excursion of the vocal cords; and (3) greater excursions lead to greater colliding forces during vocal cord vibration. Frank yelling and rebel yelling probably are associated with vertical as well as horizontal movement of the vocal cord and potentially produces a rubbing effect, setting up the vocal cords for increased likelihood of injury. The client in case 3 frequently produced high intensity vocalizations as well as extensive amounts of voice.

CASE **3**

After 7 years of performing 6 hours per night 6 days a week in small "dives," this performer of honky-tonk music found himself now with a regular band, a tour bus, a high-powered manager, and 4 months into a year-long tour schedule. His most popular cut on his first album was number eight on the charts. A unilateral full-cord hemorrhage was also something new and caused his first-time dysphonia (except for frequent post-performance hoarseness of a transient nature). His chief complaints were gradual worsening of hoarseness over a 2 week period, inability to sustain notes, difficulty staying on key, and presence of large, uncontrollable pitch breaks.

Following vocal care consultation and follow-up evaluation of the effectiveness of modified voice rest for 9 weeks, he felt compelled to return to touring because "buyers" were cancelling their commitments. On the first time out, his clinician accompanied him for 3 days and performed stroboscopic examinations before and after each concert to study laryngeal response to entry back into performance. This also provided the opportunity to inventory vocal use and provide timely voice management suggestions.

The schedule of activities revealed previously unappreciated demands for vocalizations, partly because the artist had to serve also as his own road manager.

Day 1:
Arrive in town at 3 PM; check group into hotel
Set up and sound check 4–6 PM (rehearse several numbers in their entirety and some partially)
Interview at the radio station 6:30–7 PM
To hotel, strobe evaluation, shower & dress for dinner
Dinner with VIPs 7:30–8 PM
To the club for first 1 hour set of performance 9:00 PM
Three rock and roll numbers
Sign autographs and visit with fans 10:15–10:45 PM
Second set 11:00 PM to 12:15 AM (five loud rock and roll songs, four "rebel yells" and three shouted comments to crowd; three songs were instrumentals or were sung by others in the group)
Greet well-wishers, autograph seekers, and VIPs on the bus 12:15–1:00 AM (one beer, no smoking)
Close out show, load bus, collect money from club and pay commission to club from souvenir sales 1–1:45 AM
To motel, strobe evaluation, telephone manager and make four other calls, eat supper and to bed by 3:00 AM

Day 2:
Up at 8:00 AM for breakfast and pay hotel bill, board bus for trip to next venue
On the bus: 1 hour riding "shotgun" and visiting with the bus driver in estimated ambient noise level of 75 dB, 3 hours in bedroom on bus for bookkeeping activities and sleep
Check-in group at hotel and walk on the beach, visiting with band members, 3–5 PM
Sound check at club, 5:30–6:30 PM
Supper, shower, two phone calls, dress, 6:30–8:30 PM
To club for first set of show, 9–10:15 PM (one beer before show, four shouts to the crowd)
Autographs, 10:15–11:30 PM
Second set, 11:45–12:45 PM (five shouts, six rock-a-billy numbers, one shooter, chug-a-lug of whiskey tossed to him in a "miniature" by a fan)
Close out show. Singer was "worn-out" and hoarse, and the voice clinician handled finalizing of finances with club
Back to hotel, 2:00 AM, for strobe evaluation (no new bleed, but cords were swollen); shower, dress
Private "after-hours" party 3:00–6:00 AM, sang three numbers
Back to hotel, 6:30 AM

Day 3:
Check group out of hotel and board bus 9:30 AM
Bus trip to third venue, 1 hour of talking, most of time spent by self for sleeping, bookkeeping, watching TV, plus 1 hour for song writing
Check group into hotel, 3 PM, sound check (1 hour), supper, strobe evaluation (vocal cords still

swollen, red), shower, dress (one phone call from manager), visit with clinician about previous night's vocal abuse

To venue, dress for show, 8:30–9:00 PM

First set of show, 9:15–10:10 PM, sang all but two numbers, one rebel yell, decreased loudness on most numbers

Autographs, 10:30–11:45 PM, minimal voicing—mostly pantomime

Second set of show 12:00–1:00 AM, hoarse voice, adjusted program to easier numbers, no yells; hoarseness increased by end of set

During close out of show artist stayed on bus with no visitors; voice clinician handled finalizing of finances with club

Back to hotel, 2:00 AM, strobe evaluation showed increase swelling of folds, which were "beefy" and reddened with irregular margins

After 3 days of limited voice rest at home, stroboscopic examination showed recovery of cords to pretour status and hoarseness was not present.

We ask our clients to increase awareness of the times in which unnecessary abusive behaviors might be employed and first to consider their elimination through self-counting of such events during selected portions of those high probability time periods. Charting these behaviors on a chart graphically represents to the client progress in the elimination of these behaviors.

One of the most difficult time periods during which to avoid vocal abuse seems to be immediately after a performance. Usually the performer exits the stage to be greeted by the manager, VIPs who have been promoting and sponsoring the event, as well as the most ardent members of the person's fan club who, because of their position and support, have been given backstage passes to visit with the performer. These participants want to congratulate and to be photographed with the artist. The scene is usually one of great hub-bub and loud vocalizations on everyone's part. The artist therefore is "wooed" into continuing loud vocalizations for some extended time period following the performance. Further encouragement to do so seems to come from the adrenaline rush that persists after the performance.

To counter such influences, clients and their tour managers may be advised to implement a 15 minute time-out immediately after a performance. After the encore, the artist is immediately escorted back to the dressing room to spend time alone. During the first 5 minutes the artist might engage in "cooling down" activities that may be no more than warm-up activities done in reverse order, ending in simple hums and finally silence. During the silent period we recommend that the artist spend at least 5 minutes of sitting down and engaging in relaxation as advocated by Jacobson. Here the performer focuses attention on unnecessary muscle activity and, when recognized, reduces that muscle activity, utilizing skills to do so that have been taught in formal relaxation training sessions. Such a "coasting to a stop" helps the artist come down from a performance without the use of either legal or illegal pharmaceuticals. Some performers have found that progressive relaxation is a formidable substitute to having a cigarette in order to relax. During the remaining 5 minutes of this quiet time, the artist may engage in signing photographs and making preparations to welcome VIPs and fans. As the artist visits with these individuals he or she should focus on the use of quiet conversational voice and to talk to those only in the immediate vicinity. This type of voice may be considered as the telephone voice, "reach out and touch someone." If one could not touch the listener, talking should not be done. Also, encouragement to use pantomime in greeting fans and acknowledging their congratulations helps eliminate unnecessary voice production.

Most artists find that it is necessary to engage in more vocal activity than they would if they were not performers. The amount of time in which vocal artists must use their voices certainly seems to be potentially abusive but sometimes seems absolutely necessary. Thus one must consider ways of modifying what would appear to be necessary vocally abusive behaviors to minimize their potential for damage to the vocal mechanism. One of these considerations involves the use of the telephone. Until an artist has developed a cadre of assistants and managers to field telephone calls, the artist must give special consideration to good vocal production during the use of the telephone. Principles of good voice production can include proper body alignment, which enables the use of good resonance and breath support. Vocal projection and wise intensity production should be another area of concern. Most actors and even some singers understand the use of vocal projection in order to be heard in large performance halls, and many are quite skilled at it. However, when off stage, many performers tend to resort to yelling-type behaviors in order to be heard. Such behaviors are associated with constriction of the throat (hyperfunctional use) and high airflow rates.

Performers first may be reminded to consider how loud their voices really need to be in the speaking situation at hand. Many individuals are unaware of the carrying power of the voice. To create awareness, the clinician and performer can carry on dialogue with ever increasing distance between the speakers. It is surprising to find that even a normal conversational voice can be heard 20 and 30 feet down a noisy hallway. With this revelation individuals are inclined to realize that vocal intensity typically brought to the task of conversing into a telephone microphone may be too loud.

Reduced vocal intensity for nontelephone use also is to be considered. When less intensity is not feasible individuals may be encouraged to employ greater resonance through techniques outlined elsewhere in this volume. One approach found to be particularly helpful is through the use of "yawn postures." The individual is asked to engage in a yawn up to the height of inspiration. This usually is associated with an increasing oral cavity volume by dropping rather than hinging the jaw, a lower tongue position, and a lower larynx position. These behaviors are maintained during exhalation with accompanied voice, and various vowels can be attempted. Then the person can engage with this yawn posture in production of various words and phrases. This is to help develop the idea that vocal projection can come from means other than increased vocal effort (increased vocal intensity derived from increased glottal resistance and increased airflow and air pressures).

Alteration of environmental noise that might mask vocalizations is another way of modifying what seems to be necessary but abusive behaviors. Assuring the performer always is seated in an airplane ahead of the engines would be one simple way of influencing the amount of noise over which the person feels they must talk. The club performer who feels obligated to engage in conversation with individuals when he is not on stage may seek areas away from the effect of highly amplified stage sounds. This may be as simple as going outside or into an adjacent hallway to carry on the conversation.

Many performers feel obligated to visit the club's clientele at the tables to determine how well they are coming across to the audience, to make the members of the audience feel welcome, and to express appreciation for their attendance. If the artist persists in the idea that this is necessary behavior, the clinician may help develop in the performer an understanding that those at the tables at least need not necessarily hear every word that the performer says. Redundancy of the situation and of language assists the listener's comprehension. Thus the performer could use conversational voice that may not always be heard and rely on facial and other body gestures for communicative impact; the listeners may catch a few auditory glimpses of what the person is saying and supplement this with understanding drawn from gestural communication to develop just as much appreciation for that artist as if they had heard every vocal nuance during such conversation. Laughter by the performer may be deemed necessary in such settings, but we point out that the laughter need not be heard and therefore recommend the use of very quiet or silent laughter.

Amplification is another aid to a professional voice user as an attempt to modify what seems to be necessary but vocally abusive behaviors. For example, individuals who use their voice for instructional purposes most often feel it is necessary to use elevated vocal intensity in order for all students to hear them. Most noted might be music teachers, physical education instructors, and tour guides. The use of electronic amplification is recommended. Wireless microphones with receivers and amplifier speaker set-ups may be custom developed for such individuals. The Audio Pack (available from Audio Pack Sound System, 10011 Walford Avenue, Cleveland, OH 44102, 216-651-0066) is a most desirable system for use out of doors. It consists of a headset with a wire that runs to a battery-driven amplifier and speaker system worn as a "fanny pack" around the waist. This allows hands-free operation and complete maneuverability. Professional speakers who typically carry briefcases may find a briefcase amplifier (available from Luminaud, Inc., 8688 Tyler Blvd., Mentor, OH 44060, 216-255-9082) to be very helpful.

There are speakers who believe they must use their voice in ways that are abusive but who have never considered use of substitutes for their voice. These are generally individuals who would use the voice for eliciting someone's attention, for example, coaches or parents calling their children. For these people we suggest using a whistle, light flashes, or some other stimulus to get the listener's attention.

Voice Training

Most voice specialists agree that singing outside of one's "own range" is vocally abusive. Yet, Country–Western and pop singers seem to have less appreciation for this belief. Thus a vocal abuse reduction program might include altering singing range and/or techniques. A voice teacher may be particularly helpful to the speech–language pathologist and the physician in assessing an artist's range as well as evaluating singing technique. A voice teacher also would be indicated for modifying those singing aspects that may be abusive. This specifically includes heightened tongue position and hyperfunction of the pharynx, larynx, neck, and secondary respiratory muscles. The speech–language pathologist's role in helping to assess such techniques includes accessibility to instrumentation for phoneto-gram assessment, airflow assessment, electromyographic assessment, and endoscopic evaluation during vocal performance. Coleman[9] has recently reviewed the use of phoneto-grams and described his methodology. Only a brief overview is presented here. The phonetogram is a display of a singer's very loud vocal productions at increments throughout the pitch range as well as the minimal vocal intensities that can be produced at the same increments. Usually the person's dynamic range between the minimum and maximum intensities at these pitch levels is narrow at the low and high ends of pitch range, and the intensity ranges are greater in the midportion of the pitch range.

Electromyography (EMG) may be used to help the performer recognize and reduce muscular activity that the performer usually believed is necessary but carries risk of vocal abuse. Surface electrode techniques rather than using invasive electrodes can be employed to provide biofeedback in teaching more relaxed vocal productions. If placement over the larynx is not possible due to adipose tissue or other reasons, placement over the frontalis muscle may provide helpful "indices" of laryngeal hyperfunction. We have found informally that frontalis muscle activity is correlated with laryngeal/strap muscle activity.

Through the use of flexible fiberoptics introduced transnasally, videolaryngoscopy has been used successfully in helping the singing teacher alter an artist's appreciation for undesirable tongue postures and laryngeal behaviors that might be considered abusive. Once the performer has developed an appreciation of a correlation between what he or she sees on the screen and what is felt, the visual feedback usually can be withdrawn and vocal training then can be based on kinesthetic awareness only.

Programming Reinstatement of Voice After Voice Rest

Vocal rest, for example that imposed after surgery, may be recommended for varying lengths of time depending on the surgeon's inclinations, which may be influenced by the extent of the surgical manipulation and its location on the folds. Rarely is surgical intervention followed by no voice rest. Some surgeons favor a postoperative recovery period of 3 days before starting to voice again. Others favor a more extended period of up to 2 weeks. The major purpose of postoperative voice rest is to promote healing. The clinician is faced with two major concerns in getting the patient back into normal voice usage: reinstatement of voicing and vocal conditioning.

Reinstatement of Voice

Before lifting the ban on voice production, status of vocal fold healing should be assessed with videoendostroboscopy. No guidelines for determining a patient's readiness for voicing are universally accepted; however, one may consider:

1. An operative site that is not easily observable
2. Absence of recent hemorrhage
3. Presence of no more than minimal swelling or edema
4. Closure of at least one-half the length of the membranous glottis during attempted phonation.

The patient who readily produces voice during the examination generally will have no problems coming off voice rest. When told to say individual words, the person may demonstrate delayed voice onset or, occasionally, miss phonation during production of a word, but this should not be alarming. Once voice is produced during the majority of single words uttered, ranging from single to multiple syllables, phrases, and sentences may be attempted. The gradual use of voice outside the clinical setting for communication and for performance will be addressed later.

The patient who does not produce voice when asked presents a disconcerting situation. Usually the failure results from fear of not being able to produce voice. This inclines the patient to bring so much effort to the task that the folds are not allowed to vibrate. The patient's problem is compounded by "new" vocal fold properties brought about by the surgery and results in the person's attempting old behaviors with an unfamiliar mechanism.

The fear factor can be decreased by eliciting voice from the patient without that person's awareness of being asked to produce voice. Such a method may involve asking the person simply to blow air through the nostrils. After a few trials, the task is modified to include the addition of voice (by the clinician's modeling rather than by verbal instruction). Using an airflow measurement device that also registers voicing simultaneously, one should notice airflow to precede and follow short-term phonation. The patient's attention is focused on the airflow task as a distraction from direct attempts at voice production. After a few successful trials, the patient may be made aware of the fact of successful humming. This may lead into a program we call a *hum-dinger retreat from voice rest*. It embodies four stages: (1) hum, (2) hum and say _____ , (3) think hum and say _____ , and (4) say _____ .

Stage 1: Hum. The first stage includes (a) producing a steady tone for several seconds without pitch change; (b) humming various pitch contours modeled by the clinician (use of the Visi-Pitch is helpful); (c) humming various pitch and loudness contours without a model; and (d) interrupting the hum to produce various time patterns that may resemble slow Morse code.

Stage 2: Hum and Say _____ . The second stage also capitalizes on clinician modeling rather than verbal instruction and focuses on teaching the patient that voice may be sustained independent of various mouth and tongue postures and movements associated with speech units progressing from isolated vowels to sentence production. Each utterance consists of a hum that serves as a "starter" and a slow, smooth-voiced transition to the speech unit. A progression of speech units may include: single vowels, connected vowel sequences, nonsense, and then sensical single syllables featuring first voiced consonants and then multisyllable words, phrases, and sentences without initial mixed consonants.

Stage 3: Think Hum and Say _____ . Stage 3 involves the patient's thinking of a hum (which in reality may be a silent rehearsal of humming) and then giving an utterance. The behaviors should be similar to those in stage 2 with the exception that the hum is inaudible. Usually the patient can quickly be moved through the progression indicated above.

Stage 4: Say _____ . The patient participating in stage 4 is to produce voice in speech units in a spontaneous manner without resorting to hum or mental rehearsal of humming. The success achieved in the previous stages inclines the patient to use voice at the sentence level without the need to experience more elementary units in the progression of earlier stages.

Comments. Whereas the four stages may suggest a laborious process of voice reinstatement, it generally can be covered in less than 15 minutes. This is true particularly if behavioral probes are employed For example, when leaving the level of "Hum and Say multiple-syllable words" the patient may be moved to "Hum and Say sentences" to see if the person can be successful at the new level. If so, one step in the progression will have been skipped. If not successful, the patient can be moved back to the level of "Hum and Say phrases." Once the patient is skillful in producing voice whenever desired, the clinician's attention assumes a new focal point of developing vocal flexibility and durability for professional use and vocal conditioning.

Vocal Conditioning

As is true for any athlete, the vocal athlete who has been "off season" and now wants to get back to performance status must work-out to develop flexibility, agility, and durability.

These characteristics come through practice and drill work often under the guidance of a coach (singing teacher). It is the speech–language pathologist who often helps the patient to get back into good vocal condition in order to benefit from such coaching. Conditioning may involve at least two parts: conditioning tasks and schedule of events. Because of their codependence, however, they cannot be discussed as separate issues. The reader should be alerted that any such discussion is based on a paucity of experimentally and scientifically derived facts and therefore at best reflects dogma developed out of clinical experience. Since few clinicians have identical experiences one may expect wide variance in guidelines for vocal conditioning across clinical programs. With this caveat, a description of the principles of postoperative vocal conditioning as subscribed to at the Vanderbilt Voice Center is presented.

Principle 1: Prescription of Conditioning Tasks and Schedules Is Patient Dependent. Generally speaking, less specificity of what to do and in what time frame is needed for the cautious, compliant, and cognitively astute patient. This is particularly true for the patient who has attained a good understanding of the causes, nature, and implications of the problems leading to the imposed voice rest. For example, it may be sufficient merely to advise such a person that by the end of 1 week soft (low intensity levels) voice may be used for conversation over a period of 6 hours a day and that the person should gradually build up to this by adding a little duration each day.

A patient who is self-directing, overconfident, and who lacks insight about voice and its care may need to be constrained by very specific behavior recommendations. For example, the therapy session in which voice rest was terminated might end with instructions to the patient to use voice in only three sentences that evening. The next day, voice may be used for a total of 5 minutes. Activities for each subsequent day are to be equally detailed.

Principle 2: Vocal Tasks in a Conditioning Program Should Progress From Those That Are Easy to Those That Are More Demanding. Initially, the patient would be expected to use relatively restricted pitch and loudness ranges for just communication purposes. Later, singing-type voice production is used in which attention may be paid to variations in quality as well as pitch and loudness in tessitura and then in other voice ranges. Although a voice teacher may assume major responsibility for decreasing the passaggio, the speech–language pathologist with a background in vocal pedagogy might begin such an endeavor under a conditioning program.

Principle 3: Clinical Policing for Safe Vocal Production Should Accompany Conditioning. The speech–language pathologist guiding the patient's vocal emergence is in a particularly good position to help the patient guard against unnecessary muscular tension. Attention also can be given to use of acceptable abdominal/thoracic respiratory patterns and body alignment. Additionally, it may be necessary to reiterate specific instructions to avoid vocal abuses and to help the patient develop suitable alternatives for behaviors that may incline the person to potential debacles. The conditioning period, then, affords the opportunity to instruct the patient in vocal production, laryngeal hygiene, and preventative measures of dysphonia.

The application of these principles is illustrated in the following cases.

CASE **4**

History: The client is a 43-year-old male professional singer/songwriter of nearly 30 years. He has had some formal voice training. He experienced 3 years of progressive dysphonia that finally ended his performance career. He has an aggressive personality, is self-directing, tends to "push the limits," and usually "marches to his own drumbeat." He is not inclined to follow directions unless they are very specific and consequences for failure to follow them are well spelled out.

Diagnosis: Bilateral intracordal cysts with tethering to lateral aspect of vocal fold ligament and a unilateral vocal fold varix on the medial edge of one vocal fold.

Surgery: June 28, 1991. Bilateral microflap elevation and removal of cysts followed by laser cauterization of vatrix.

Laryngeal videoendostroboscopic examination, July 10, 1991: Incision sites not identifiable. Inflamed vocal folds, bilaterally. No vertical phase difference or mucosal wave appreciated; aperiodic vibration most of the time.

Reinstatement of voice July 10, 1991: Within 15 trials client was able to sustain a hum for up to 10 seconds at one pitch and intensity. He quickly expanded skill to humming various pitches within a three semitone range. Using the hum-dinger approach, he developed spontaneous sentences at subconversational intensities within 10 minutes of instruction.

Program of voice reinstatement: July 10 to 21, use only quiet voice as scheduled below:

July 10:	May use total of five sentences outside the clinic
July 11:	Five 2 minute dialogues
July 12:	Five 5 minute dialogues
July 13:	One hour of accumulated talk time, no dialogue longer than 5 minutes
July 14:	Two hours of accumulated talk time, no dialogue longer than 10 minutes
July 15–17:	Use voice for conversation for only one-half of the day. Otherwise voice rest
July 18:	Talk any time during day
July 19–21:	Talk any time during the day and night

Follow up

July 22:	Video laryngeal endostroboscopic examination: Inflammation decreased; slight mucosal wave except for area of former cysts; glottal incompetence posteriorly. Voice is breathy. After a brief warm-up on three-semitone vocalises, client up to 1.5 octaves using low intensity level
July 29:	Vocal folds still vascular and inflamed. Glottal incompetence is smaller. Vocalized from C3 to A4, but with pitch and aphonic breaks in upper region of range. Did some singing with attention to body alignment. Initiated two 15 minute practice singing sessions per day at home
August 5:	Attended an annual golf tournament with his brothers and joined them in singing one song for President Bush. Same pitch range but had clear tone in head voice; falsetto was quite breathy. Improved mucosal wave. Vocalises done with attention to higher notes. Start four 20 minute practice sessions per day at home, attending to relaxed neck and throat
August 12:	Patient indicated that he sang a solo in church yesterday using full voice. In session today he produced good falsetto at C6 with loud voice. Quieter voice from A5 on up was quite breathy. C3 to G5 is with good quality. Stroboscopy shows improved mucosal wave on left fold in midrange and is normal on right fold. Transferring client to singing teacher for continuation of voice technique training
Sept 15:	Resume touring and singing the lead part with the group.

CASE 5

History: The client is a 33-year-old female, touring Country–Western singer for 10 years with a recent gold record (500,000 sales). She is currently in her 14th year of classical singing lessons. She has an outgoing personality but is compliant in following therapy suggestions. She is a quick learner and is highly insightful.

Diagnosis: Noted to have a bleed on the lateral superior surface of the left true vocal fold approximately 1 year ago. Two weeks of voice rest incompletely resolved the condition, leaving a residual polyp. Polyp later was determined to be an arteriovenous malformation (AVM). This remained stable for 9 months. In the 10th month, coincident with menstruation, an ipsilateral bleed was noted and presumed to be below the superficial layers of the mucosa posterior to the AVM. For two consecutive months bleeding recurred in association with menstruation.

Surgery: Photocoagulation of the AVM and feeding vessel and excision of the residual polyp related to the AVM.

Reinstatement of voice: Two weeks postoperative, operative sites not detectable on laryngeal videoendoscopy, but prominence of new vessels was readily observed (coincident with menstruation). Voice rest extended 1 week. Reexamination showed decrease in prominence of vessels. Residual inflammation from surgery nearly resolved. Voice was easily produced on request. Use of sentences established within 5 minutes.

Program of voice use: June 25 to 31, quiet voice use only as scheduled below:

June 25: Three 5 minute conversations

June 26: Two 30 minute conversations

June 27: Conversational voice for 2 hours in AM and 2 hours in PM

June 28: Unlimited use of quiet conversational voice and 15 minute warm-up singing activities

June 29: Unlimited use of quiet conversational voice and two 15 minute warm-up singing activities

June 30: Unlimited use of quiet conversational voice and two 30 minute warm-up singing activities

Follow up

July 1: Videostroboscopy showed improvement over last examination and suggested vocal activities were not harmful. Transferred to singing teacher for continuation of vocal conditioning and preparation for forthcoming tour

July 5: Return visit. Chief complaints: "lack of strength and breaks in passagio . . . vocal fatigue at end of day but this is improving. . . ." Continue with singing teacher

July 9: Return visit. No complaints. Videoendostroboscopy examination done. Vocal folds appear within normal limits (no prominent vascularity or inflammation) except for decreased mucosal wave over operated vocal fold. Continue preparation for touring and return weekly for re-examination to monitor any vascularity changes as a function of menstruation and/or vocal use. Note: First postoperative concert scheduled for less than 35 days after surgery. May want to go on tour with client to monitor performance and stroboscopically assess its effects on the vocal folds.

CONCLUSION

Behavioral intervention in dysphonia of professional voice users typically involves helping the artist to manage the use of voice to avoid overuse of pitch, intensity, and amount of vocalization. During the formative period of becoming an artist that person is introduced to topics under the rubric of "artist development," which includes managing negotiations, stage presence, and media interviews. Wise management in the use of the voice also should be considered. Such might advocate a schedule that involves performance of no more than 4 days in a row with intervening periods of 3 days of only nonperformance voice use. Principles of good health should be taught, such as proper diet, rest, and physical conditioning, that can be used even when "on the road." Principles of good voice production during performance as well as nonperformance are other worthwhile topics of instruction. Further consideration could be given to early signs and symptoms of impending voice problems, which may help the artist to be a wiser voice manager. When vocal difficulties arise, the artist is well advised to seek early evaluation and treatment which may avoid great financial liabilities associated with prolonged voice rest with or without surgical intervention. Considering voice management as part of "artist development" may be a most significant adjunct to assuring the artist's problem-free pursuit of excellence.

REFERENCES

1. Titze IR: Vocology. *Natl Assoc Teach Sing J* 46:21–22, 1989.
2. Titze IR: Rationale and structure of a curriculum in vocology. *J Voice* 6:1–9, 1992.
3. Gates GA: Coping with dysphonia. *J Voice* 22–26, 1992.
4. Sander EK, Ripich DE: Vocal fatigue. *Am Otol Rhinol Laryngol* 92:141–145, 1983.
5. Stone RE, Sharf DJ: Vocal changes associated with the use of atypical pitch and intensity levels. *Folia Phoniatr* 25:91–103, 1973.
6. Johnson TS: *Vocal Abuse Reduction Program*. San Diego, College Hall Press, 1976.
7. Boone D, McFarlane S: *The Voice and Voice Therapy*. Englewood Cliffs, NJ, Prentice Hall, 1988.
8. Brodnitz F: *Keeping Your Voice Healthy*. San Diego, College Hill Press, 1988, pp 119–123.
9. Coleman R: How I do it: Producing a F_0-SPL profile (phonetogram). *J Voice* (in press).

Appendix 19 A: Diagnosis and ICD-9 Codes Frequently Used at the Vanderbilt Voice Center

CONDITION	SCORE
Larynx related	
Congenital anomalies of larynx, web	748.2
Congenital anomalies of larynx, other	748.3
Atrophy	478.79
Cicatrix	478.79
Contact ulcer	478.8
Edema	478.6
Granuloma	478.79
Hemorrhage	478.5
Imperfect closure (glottis)	748.3
Keratosis/leukoplakia	478.5
Laryngitis, acute	464.1
Laryngitis, chronic	476.0
Movement disorder (spastic dysphonia)	333.8
Muscular incoordination	781.3
Neoplasm, benign	212.1
Neoplasm, malignant	161.9
Papillomatosis	478.5
Paralysis, unilateral partial	478.31
Paralysis, unilateral complete	478.32
Paralysis, bilateral partial	478.33
Paralysis, bilateral complete	478.34
Polyps, nonabuse	478.4
Polyps, abuse	478.5
Sicca	476.0
Speaker's throat	748.2
Laryngectomy related	
Tracheostomy complication and tracheoesophageal fistula	519.0
Late effect	
surgical or medical care	909.3
implant and graft	
Mechanical	96.59
Infection, inflammation	998.69
Stenosis	996.79
Fitting and adjusting prosthetic device	
Other (prosthesis)	V52.8
Other, tracheostomy valve	V52.8
Organ or tissue replacement (A.L.)	V43.8

CONDITION	SCORE
Fitting and adjusting prosthetic device (contd.)	
Attention to artificial opening	V55.9
Attention to artificial opening, trachea	V55.0
History of malignant neoplasm, larynx	V10.21
Problems with head, neck, trunk	V48.8
Velopharyngeal related	
Fitting and adjusting prosthetic device	V52.3
Cleft palate	
Unilateral, complete	749.01
Unilateral, incomplete (cleft uvula)	749.02
Bilateral, complete	749.03
Bilateral, incomplete	749.04
Speech related	
Dysrhythmia (CNS)	333.89
Dysphonia	784.49
Aphonia	785.41
Dyspraxia	784.69
Dysphagia	787.2
Hypernasality	784.49a*
Hyponasality	784.49b*
Articulation disorder (congenital)	315.4

*N.B. Alphabetic designations added by the author and are not part of the official ICD-9 codes.

Appendix 19 B: Procedures Used at the Vanderbilt Voice Center and Their CPT Codes

PROCEDURE	CODE
Medical evaluation of speech	
Voice	31506
Nasality	31506
Speech screening	31506
Comprehensive arctic	31506
Intelligibility	31506
Fluency	31506
Dysphagia, initial 30 min	97700
Dysphagia, additional 15 min	97701
Laryngeal function studies	
Spectrogram	92520
Flo analysis (Visi-Pitch)	92528
Airflow	94010
Vital capacity, total	94150
Respiratory flow volume loop	94375
F_0 profile (phonetogram)	92528
Electroglottography	92528
Electromyography	95867
Electromyography, single fiber, any technique	95872
Intraoperative monitoring/hour	95920
Unlisted otol service, Venti-Voice Evaluation	92599
Unlisted otol service, tracheostoma/TEP evaluation	92599
Laryngoscopy, flexible or rigid with strobe	31579
Laryngoscopy, flexible or rigid	31575
Rhinometry	92512
Pharyngeal videoendoscopy	92511
Complex dynamic pharyngeal and speech evaluation by cine- or video-recording	70371
Interventions	
Initial consultation, brief	90600
Initial consultation, intermediate	90605
Follow-up consultation, brief	90640
Follow-up consultation, limited	90641
Confirmatory consultation, limited	90650
Confirmatory consultation, intermediate	90651
Confirmatory consultation, extended	90652
Medical conference services (electric devices, breathing exercises, symptomatic treatment)	95105

PROCEDURE	CODE
Muscular reeducation, initial 30 min	97112
Muscular reeducation, additional 15 min	97145
Speech therapy, individual, 15 min	92507
Biofeedback, other (computer-assisted tomography)	90915
Biofeedback EMG	90900
Medical conference, 30 min	98900
Medical conference, 60 min	98902
Medical conference, team, 30 min	98910
Medical conference, team, 60 min	98912
Telephone, with patient or family	98920
Telephone, with patient or family, intermediate (new info)	98921
Telephone, with patient or family, lengthy	98922
Prosthesis fitting/training, initial 30 min	31611–55 or 97520
Prosthesis fitting/training, additional 15 min	31611–55 or 97521
Ear protector attenuation measurements	92596
Supplies and materials	
Artificial larynx	99070
Voice prosthesis	99070
Tracheostoma vent	99070
Tracheostomy valve	99070
Catheter	99070
Dilator	99070
Medical testimony	99075
Special reports (insurance)	99078
Analysis of data in computers	99090
Handling, ordering devices	99002
Services in evening	99052
Off-site services	99056
Unusual travel (transport and escort of patient)	99082

20

Multidisciplinary Approach to Treatment

BARBARA H. JACOBSON, PhD
JOHN PAUL WHITE

The comprehensive treatment of the professional voice user dictates that the management process also integrate the expertise and intervention of other professionals. In Chapter 6, the concept of a "voice clinic" was discussed. In such a setting, physicians, speech–language pathologists, voice teachers, psychologists, and representatives from other disciplines participate as needed in the assessment of the professional voice user. In this chapter, we discuss the management of the professional voice user in particular and the singer in more detail. Specifically, we address the ways in which the speech–language pathologist and the voice teacher collaborate to help the patient modify vocal behavior for speaking and/or singing and thus enhance performance.

For the person with a voice disorder, the otolaryngologist is the "case manager" and monitors changes in laryngeal health on a regular basis. Medications are adjusted and surgical options are reconsidered as needed. Other professionals—acting and singing coaches, behaviorists, physician specialists (allergists, pulmonologists)—intervene when necessary. The speech–language pathologist and voice teacher work with the voice professional to manage daily use of the voice. They help singers and speakers to produce the best voice possible and to modify or eliminate unhealthy habits.

There are some very good reasons to coordinate treatment between the voice teacher and the speech–language pathologist. Often, the singer/speaker will exhibit poor vocal behavior that stems from the same physical source or posture, for example, jaw tension. This can result in an inability to focus or project the voice properly for speaking or singing. Treatment from a "dual front" allows for added emphasis and reinforcement for the student. In addition, coordinated priorities for singers and speakers by speech–language pathologists and voice teachers allow for a logical progression toward a united goal. Finally, positive changes in the technique of voice production in either singing or speaking can affect improvement in how the voice is used in the other arena.

While it is common sense for voice teachers and speech–language pathologists to work together when the patient is a professional or strong amateur singer, we would like to suggest that these disciplines consider collaborating when the patient is an "avocational" singer or a professional speaker. In our experience, patients who are able to participate in both voice therapy from a speech–language pathologist and voice lessons from a voice teacher benefit more than might be expected from voice therapy alone.

318

In this chapter, we discuss the vocabulary of the voice teacher and of the speech–language pathologist. We then address common problems seen in both singing and speaking and describe shared treatment and teaching techniques from both disciplines. Finally, we present two case histories that illustrate the collaborative approach to treatment for the speech–language pathologist and the voice teacher. At the end of this chapter are appendices that provide a glossary of terms used commonly in each discipline, terms used in vocal pedagogy to describe voice quality, and singing voice classifications.

THE VOCABULARIES OF SPEECH–LANGUAGE PATHOLOGY AND VOCAL PEDAGOGY

Any discipline, whether it be in science, arts, or humanities, has a particular vocabulary that allows people who work within these areas to communicate with colleagues. Unfortunately, there is rarely a common "dictionary" for people outside the discipline to use as a resource. For speech–language pathologists and otolaryngologists, vocabulary is more reciprocal and communication is generally clear. However, communication between medical and singing disciplines is more difficult. The statement "Your signal-to-noise ratio at your habitual fundamental frequency is abnormal" means nothing to the patient who is a voice student. Or the statement "You need to use more legato as you go through the passaggio" may be incomprehensible to a speech–language pathologist or physician. As our knowledge in the science of the singing voice is improving, so is the sophistication of the vocabulary, and we run the risk of speaking a foreign language to our colleagues in vocal pedagogy, speech–language pathology, and medicine.

At the end of the chapter, we provide a glossary of terms used by speech–language pathologists and by voice teachers. However, we also discuss a few terms that are used commonly by both groups but that may have different connotations for each.

The vocabulary of voice for the speech–language pathologist has grown remarkably in the past 10 years as the inclusion of instrumentation into the assessment process has come about. When diagnosis relied more heavily on perceptual judgments about the quality of a person's voice, it was more common to use terms such as *breathy*, *harsh*, and *hoarse*. Now, words such as *subglottic pressure*, *airflow rate*, and *jitter* have entered the daily lexicon of the speech–language pathologist who specializes in voice and uses objective voice analysis to evaluate and treat patients.

The vocabulary of the vocal teacher, on the other hand, has not changed as much, but is still filled with musical references, often in a foreign language, which may also pertain to vocal technique. Words such as *legato*, *arpeggio*, and *passaggio*, though Italian in origin, are used so commonly that they have been "adopted" into the everyday language of the voice studio.

There are several terms that are used by both speech–language pathologists and voice teachers. Often, they have the same meaning. However, some words carry quite different meanings or have different nuances of meaning. For example, in speech–language pathology, *shimmer* is the term for "intensity perturbation" or the fluctuations in the amplitude of a sound signal from vibratory cycle to vibratory cycle. In vocal pedagogy, *shimmer* is a quality of tone considered to be highly desirable. It generally implies that the voice is being used properly, has a pleasing rate of vibrato (though generally on the faster side), and projects or carries well.

Attack in speech–language pathology generally refers to the onset of phonation and specifically is applied to "easy" and "hard" voice onsets. The voice teacher also would apply this term to the way that sound may be initiated. To the voice teacher, there are three types of attack: a *glottal attack*, an *aspirated attack*, and what may be thought of as being midway between the two, a *coordinated attack*. The glottal attack, the result of a sudden release of subglottic pressure, is neither esthetically pleasant nor vocally healthy. The aspirated attack, the result of air passing through the glottis preceding the onset of tone, is not hard on the voice; however, it is ineffective in singing because of the useless loss of air and the distortion of diction that may occur as a result. The coordinated attack, when the release of air and the onset of sound occur simultaneously, is ideal for singing. It utilizes the breath most effectively, is gentle on the voice, and is esthetically pleasant.

Some terms such as *voice focus*, *resonance*, *articulation*, *hypernasality*, *hyponasality*, *vocal abuse*, and *respiration* have roughly equivalent meanings for both disciplines, although they may have a different emphasis or impact in each area. We have defined those terms conjointly in the glossary.

COMMON PROBLEMS

While the demands placed on the voice for singing and speaking are different, the basic physiology is similar. Thus we expect that methods of voice production for speaking are similarly affected in singing and conversely. Traditionally, speech–language pathologists and voice teachers work independently to identify and change poor habits in speaking and singing. It would seem to be more efficient to coordinate treatment to enhance effectiveness. In the following paragraphs, we identify some common problems that affect both the singing and speaking voice and that often coexist for singers.

Appropriate use of breathing to support the voice has a great deal of importance for the singer. For the speaker, appropriate breath support is generally taken for granted. Historically, in the field of voice therapy, it has received fluctuating emphasis. There is no dispute that adequate airflow from the lungs is crucial to the production of good voice. However, there is a great deal of controversy about the ability of an individual actively to change poor voice merely through altering breathing patterns. It may well be that only people with active lung disease can find voice only affected by impaired breathing patterns. Frequently, however, we see patients who have poor voice focus or excessive glottal fry. Often, these individuals also have excessive laryngeal tension when they speak. They rely on extrinsic laryngeal muscles to produce voice when these muscles were only designed to support the larynx in the neck and not to produce voice. Often a poor awareness of respiratory control can be reflected in the person's ability to achieve good breath support for singing.

Whether a person is breathing effectively in speech or not, learning the almost athletic breathing required for singing is bound to improve the amount of breath available for speech and control of that breath for the average person. Breathing is the cornerstone of singing, and most people find that they are not using anywhere near their available resource of breath in daily speech, nor have they explored the possibilities of breath control that come with learning how to release the air properly.

Laryngeal tension can be present in a number of people with speaking voice disorders. For some individuals, laryngeal musculoskeletal tension is always present. For others, it is situation specific or related to stressful internal states. Persistent laryngeal tension is often difficult for a person to change because he or she has always had tension and has no concept of the contrasting feeling of relaxation. Laryngeal tension has the effect of producing hoarseness or harshness or creating the environment for the development of laryngeal lesions such as vocal nodules or contact ulcers. Another byproduct of laryngeal tension is vocal fatigue as muscles not designed for voice production are called into use for the act of speaking.

Laryngeal tension is one of the biggest stumbling blocks for the singer, and, because of the increased demands on the voice during singing, the problems it creates are intensified. The voice may sound pinched, strained or raspy; potential range is limited; dynamics (the ability to sing soft or loud) are limited; and the voice will fatigue quickly and increase the susceptibility to nodules or contact ulcers. Laryngeal tension may be a result of improper vocal technique, attempting to imitate another singer or singers, or singing in a range that is not suited to the voice. For those whose speaking voices are relatively free, we may approach the singing voice based on speech, hoping to translate the freedom of speaking into the singing voice. For people who experience laryngeal tension in speech this is obviously not an option, and other means must be used.

Vocal resonance or vocal focus is taken for granted by most people. However, one can notice extremes of control when an actor or speaker is able to project the voice to a large audience or when an individual has difficulty being heard or producing voice over noise without strain or hoarseness. The ability to "place" the voice for speaking is related to the ability to keep an open and relaxed vocal tract above the level of the vocal folds. When a constriction occurs—in the neck, throat, or mouth—the optimal transmission of sound is interrupted or thwarted. A tight, muffled, strained voice can result.

Even more for the singer, a focused tone can only be achieved when there is no impairment or constriction, the vocal folds are vibrating properly, and there is a feeling of connection between the breath as the source of the tone, and optimal resonance, which is the final culmination of the fundamental tone. It is the key to projecting the voice, whether loud or soft, with a minimal amount of effort from the throat itself. Like breathing for singing, learning to use the resonators of the laryngo-, oro-, and nasopharynxes to achieve maximum resonance requires exaggeration from the way those resonators are used in everyday speech, but it is important to understand that it is *exaggerated*, not *different*.

Many people *without* voice disorders use a hard glottal attack in speaking. However, we see many people who have voice disorders who produce words with initial vowels (eg, *actor*, *every*, *extra*) with an initial build-up of subglottic pressure that results in a "pop" on release of the breath for production of the vowel sound. After the release of the breath, the vocal folds slam back together. Habitual use of this method of voice initiation can contribute to the development of hoarseness in the speaking voice because of persistent hard wear on the vocal folds, especially at the point of maximum contact. Use of hard glottal attacks in speech also can give the impression of a driving or unpleasant voice.

Glottal attacks can also be a problem for the singer. They may occur consciously in an attempt to exaggerate the diction or mood of a song or unconsciously as a result of improper technique. Glottal attacks may also occur when a singer is trying hard (though incorrectly) to sing carefully in tune and may use a glottal stroke to "nail" the pitch. Furthermore, in singing with the additional breath support required, especially on higher notes, there is the possibility of a glottal termination of the note, a glottal attack in reverse, in which the sound is stopped in the throat as opposed to with the breath.

There is no question that psychological factors play a part in the development of voice disorders. Voice production is an ability that has been present from birth for most people and is tightly bound with behavior and emotions. Aside from the obvious effects of stress, other psychosocial factors can affect how and why a person produces a certain voice. For example, someone who is feeling insecure about his or her ability to project authority may use an inappropriately low-pitched voice to compensate for the perceived inadequacy. An individual who admires another person or even a celebrity may try to imitate that person's voice, even though it is not suited to his or her anatomic structure. A person who has been told to be "seen and not heard" from childhood may have difficulty projecting a voice that is loud enough for normal conversation.

For many individuals who develop voice disorders, stress and anxiety appear to manifest themselves at the larynx. This can result in a situation in which laryngeal musculoskeletal tension creates the environment for the development of a benign vocal fold mass or this tension exacerbates present or emerging lesions. In such an instance, it is important to make the patient aware of the effects, direct or indirect, of laryngeal tension, and to devise treatment methods to change this pattern. For some people, the tension at the larynx has been present for so long that they have accommodated to it and are simply not aware of it.

Personality and related psychological factors affect the singing voice as well; imitation of a certain singer (if that imitation takes one beyond one's own healthy voice) or trying to sound more dramatic than is natural by artificially darkening the tone have psychological roots but physiological results. One's self-esteem can also be a critical factor. There are singers who develop vocal problems because they have placed psychological limitations on their success. Deep-rooted feelings of inadequacy may manifest themselves in such ways as cracking on crucial high notes, always being hoarse for important auditions, or the seemingly inevitable phlegm on opening night. For such people, too much success is at least as fearsome, if not more so, than failure, and they subconsciously cause themselves to fail in order to remain in what they perceive as their comfort zone. If taken to extremes, this phenomenon may lead to more serious and damaging vocal abuse.

Finally, there are some factors in both singing and speaking that can only be alleviated through education. Voice production, in both speaking and singing, are learned in great part through imitation. That can be good or bad, depending on what is imitated and how it is achieved. Placement, timbre, and other related characteristics of the voice are assimilated and then reinforced by repetition. In the same way that speech and voice vary with regional accents and the people of certain geographic areas tend to sound alike, we tend to use, both consciously and subconsciously, the speech and voice patterns we are exposed to everyday. While this does not mean to imply that listening to a great singer or speaker will magically improve the voice, listening does set the stage for healthy voice production as one is hearing healthy voice production. Conversely, people are constantly bombarded with unhealthy vocalism through radio and television. Various programs and advertisements abound with singers and speakers alike who are abusing their voices. An example that is quite prevalent is the "rasp," which sounds like a prolonged throat clearing while maintaining a semblance of pitch. This sound, which likely began as someone's vocal inadequacy, has become an accepted and even sought after vocal singing "style," to the detriment of the vocal health of the performer and indirectly to those who listen to it. The assimilation of voice characteristics in the environment into one's pattern of voice use can be an insidious problem for the singer or speaker.

SHARED TECHNIQUES

The overall goal in voice rehabilitation is to produce the best voice possible with the least effort. This requires development of excellent coordination of function between all the structures and processes involved in voice production for singing and speaking. The processes involved are (1) adequate respiratory support for voice, (2) well-timed and adequate vocal fold closure, (3) appropriate oral tract configuration and resonance, (4) lack of tension in the neck and jaw, and (5) good posture. Problems in voice production generally do not affect just one of the above processes, but cut across several areas.

While it is possible to make changes in the voice while working on one particular behavior, the best results occur when a particular technique addresses several processes simultaneously. In the following paragraphs, we describe some techniques that can assist both singers and speakers in correcting poor voice productions.

Vocal Function Exercises

Vocal function exercises[1] are an adaptation of techniques described by Briess.[2,3] Originally, these exercises were designed to strengthen specific intrinsic laryngeal muscles. However, more recent work has shown that these exercises, when done regularly, can produce improvement in objective measures of voice production. The basic technique is as follows: After "warming up" the voice with a sustained "ee" (/i/) sound and with upward and downward glides, the notes c through g for men and c^1 through g^1 for women are sustained softly and easily on the vowel "oh" (/o/). This corresponds roughly to notes at the middle range for a typical speaker. Times are recorded for each vowel production. These are practiced twice daily. Proper voice focus with a relaxed larynx is maintained throughout the exercises. For the singer, this can be a nontraumatic method to work at problem areas of the singing range or at the extremes of range. The underlying principle is to produce voice that relies on very efficient vocal fold closure with just the right amount of air pressure emerging from the lungs. This delicate balance can be difficult for an individual who has relied on pure respiratory force and/or laryngeal tension to produce voice for speaking or singing and who has developed dysphonia as a result.

The above exercise can be used also for warm-up or cool-down. Warm-up is especially critical to maintain a healthy singing voice. Exercises should begin and stay within a comfortable range and dynamic level, then gradually expand upward and downward and in volume level until the voice is thoroughly warmed up. The time this takes varies from person to person, but 10 to 15 minutes should be a minimum. It is equally as important, though often ignored, to cool down the voice, especially after extended periods of singing. Cool-down is simply the opposite of the warm-up, bringing the voice back to a state of relaxation into a comfortable range and dynamic level. Again, the time may vary, but a good rule of thumb is approximately half the time spent on the warm-up.

Voice Focus

Appropriate voice focus for singing or speaking is crucial for good voice production and voice projection. For speaking, it is usually only possible to achieve this through a combination of a release of tension in the vocal tract, forward tongue placement (for those who use cul-de-sac resonance or a tongue-back placement), and adequate use of the nasal cavity to contribute to forward placement of the tone. Some speech–language pathologists use voice focus techniques to achieve the goal of producing a more appropriate pitch rather than working directly on raising or lowering habitual speaking pitch.

Singers often are asked to practice exercises while observing themselves in a mirror. Often, they have experienced tension for so long that they are no longer aware of it. Though the offending tension may not always be visible to the eye, if they can see it they can begin to feel it, and when they can feel it they can begin to relax it. They can be made much more aware of proper tongue position, jaw and lip relaxation, and any extraneous muscular tension in the neck. Looking in the mirror may also help to focus attention on the so-called mask of the face and thereby aid in achieving more forward placement of the tone. This should be effective when dealing with speaking voice as well.

There are a number of ways to facilitate good voice focus for speaking. These include emphasizing the use of nasal resonance to feel the forward placement of the voice, using sentences "loaded" with voiced continuant sounds (/z/, /r/, /l/, /v/, /m/, /n/, /ŋ/, /z/), and repeating sentences with sounds that use forward tongue placement.

One method of enhancing nasal resonance is to chant a series of sentences that use predominantly nasal sounds (/m/, /n/, and /ŋ/). A pitch is selected that is near the comfortable pitch level. The patient is then asked to chant these sentences, prolonging the nasal sounds to feel the vibration in the "mask" area of the face. Sentences such as "Amy married the mayor" and "Mona's mother has much money" are used to "carry" the voice from the back of the throat to a forward focus. After the patient has mastered this easy mode of voice production, the sentences are repeated in a spoken voice, attempting to maintain the good forward placement of the voice.

Similar exercises can be used in singing by giving such phrases pitch and rhythmic value, whether in scales or simple melodies. Another means of helping singers "find" a more forward placement for the voice is to ask them to hum on a comfortably high note in their range, being aware of the buzzing sensation in the mask of the face, and then, without losing that, gradually opening the mouth to an /a/ (or any other vowel).

For many patients, reduction of muscular tension can be achieved through techniques to enhance appropriate voice focus or through vocal function exercises. However, for some individuals, the tension is so habituated that it is not possible to reduce it through indirect methods. In that instance, it is appropriate to do some direct work on reduction of laryngeal area muscle tension.

First, it is important to assess the areas of tension at the larynx. Aronson[4] has illustrated the predominant areas where muscular tightness can be felt beneath the chin and at the neck. In our experience, many singers and speakers exhibit some degree of muscle "cramping," particularly at the major horn of the hyoid bone and at the superior horn of the thyroid cartilage. Often this is unilateral and may coincide with the presence of a mass lesion on the vocal fold on that side. As Aronson[4] describes it, the technique for assessing tension is to palpate the hyoid bone, thyrohyoid space, and thyroid cartilage along the lateral edge gently, checking for reports of pain, not just pressure, from the patient. In addition, the position of the larynx in the neck, as well as improvements in voice quality, are noted through massage and/or a downward manipulation of the larynx.

Several treatment sessions may be necessary to effect change. Patients can be taught to perform the massage for themselves or at the very least use the palpation technique to check for the status of tension at the larynx. While laryngeal massage is not *the* solution in all cases of dysphonia related to musculoskeletal tension, it certainly contributes to alleviating the problem.

Manipulation and massage should not be attempted by a voice teacher unless that teacher has had specific training related to laryngeal massage or is supervised by a licensed speech–language pathologist or medical professional. Simple touch, on the other hand, can be a useful tool in some cases to call attention to muscular tension or to help a singer note the position of the larynx during singing.

To aid in achieving a more relaxed and open laryngopharynx, an effective tool for many is the "yawn–sigh" exercise. The singer is asked to inhale as though partially yawning, noting the lowering of the larynx during inhalation, and then to attack gently and "sigh" from an easy pitch downward. Later, this exercise can be given pitch and made more directly applicable to singing.

CASE STUDIES

In the following pages, we present two case studies that illustrate the interaction between the speech–language pathologist and the voice teacher. One of these two individuals was singing avocationally at the time of initial assessment. The other person had never sung, but had expressed an interest in pursuing voice lessons.

For the purposes of this chapter, we present a 6 week "window" of concurrent voice therapy and voice lessons, with an initial assessment and a final evaluation at the conclusion of the 6 week time period. The pathologist and the teacher shared goals and mutually observed voice lessons and voice therapy. Both clients were aware that therapy and voice lessons were coordinated and were encouraged to integrate techniques and insights from both.

CASE 1

Case 1 was a 27-year-old male who had begun to experience tightness and soreness in his throat and a harsh voice quality approximately 1 year after giving a particular lecture. Since that time, the symptoms had recurred, always during or after formal presentations. A visit to an otolaryngologist had revealed bilateral contact ulcers.

This person was an analyst of PC-based products. He conducted training sessions two to four times per week for 2 hours each. He estimated that he used his voice 6 to 7 hours each working day. He was involved in Toastmasters, and this added time to his average speaking day. He was also in the process of establishing a music production business and expressed an interest in singing, although he had never pursued it other than casually and had had no previous vocal training.

Evaluation of vocal hygiene revealed that he drank minimal amounts of water daily. Fluid intake consisted primarily of coffee (about 5 cups per day). He did not smoke, and alcohol intake was minimal as he found that it affected his voice adversely. He cleared his throat frequently.

There was an excessive amount of laryngeal area and jaw tension. Perceptually, his voice was moderately dysphonic with hoarseness and harshness. He tended to speak rapidly, which inhibited his ability to take adequate replenishing breaths for speaking. Habitual pitch appeared low. Hard glottal attacks were present in conversation.

Videostroboscopy revealed a slight redness at the posterior commissure at the area of the vocal processes bilaterally. There was a posterior glottic chink. Most notably, there was excessive supraglottic activity on phonation, with evidence of an anteroposterior "press" of the supraglottic structures. Amplitude of vibration was asymmetric and restricted. Taken together, this presented a picture of hyperfunction. Acoustic analysis revealed a low habitual pitch (86.3 Hz). All other parameters were within normal limits. Airflow rates were somewhat elevated at habitual pitch (near 200 ml/sec).

The singing evaluation revealed an average baritone voice, with a total range of less than two octaves (G to d^1), and less than one octave of that (A–g) was produced without sounding strained. His posture was poor, with little rib cage expansion during respiration. He also demonstrated a tendency to jut his chin forward and upward while singing. Inhalation was shallow and gasping with much clavicular movement, and breath support was virtually nonexistent. Due to these and other problems, even the most basic vocal exercises were executed with a great deal of visible muscular interference from the jaw, neck, and tongue. The voice sounded constricted, vowel definition was poor, and the resulting tone was breathy and lacked focus. Attacks were habitually made by means of a glottal scoop (starting tone below the pitch with a glottal onset, and then sliding up to the pitch). The glottal attacks contributed to his overall problems, and the scooping resulted in a tendency to sing flat (under the pitch).

Working with the voice requires working with the personality as well as the body. Most people are somewhat apprehensive in a strange environment. This is especially true in initial voice lessons, because the voice is such an integral part of a person's identity and to make changes in that is unnerving. This person volunteered that he considered himself to be "hyper" and "high strung." One easily observed an extremely "up-tight" personality, as indicated by his body language, his manner of speaking, and his voice quality.

Joint problems in his speaking and singing voice production were a tendency to clench the jaw and neck muscles just preceding the onset of sound, to restrict the free flow of breath, and to produce frequent glottal attacks. The following goals were developed: for speaking, (1) improve voice focus/placement, (2) reduce jaw/neck tension, (3) decrease speech rate, (4) improve vocal hygiene; and for singing, (1) improve breath support, (2) relax tension, especially at jaw hinge to base of neck, and (3) improve placement of the voice.

Voice Lessons

Since this person had never had any vocal instruction, the first voice lesson was devoted to a basic overview of proper vocal production, followed by a discussion of his particular problems. Within the 6 weeks, little more than the most fundamental principles could be covered. Emphasis was placed on more productive breathing, relaxation of tension (especially from the hinge of the jaw to the base of the neck), and the concept of "placing the voice" more beneficially. The voice teacher should always begin with a discussion of the mechanics of the voice and the basics of vocal technique if for no other reason than to make sure that the teacher and student share common terminology. There would also have to be time spent on helping the student to relax in general so as not to approach phonation with the same rigidity and control that he used in everyday life.

Exercises were assigned starting with some relaxation training to help relieve tension in the shoulders, neck, and jaw. He appeared to have been totally unaware of his tension and of the glottal attacks. By helping him to find proper body alignment and to begin to breathe deeply, especially while lying flat on his back, he was immediately able to relax some of the muscular tension in his upper body.

Easy humming exercises in a restricted range were assigned to aid in warming up the voice. These exercises also served to teach the sensations of optimal voice placement, and this concept was discussed as well. He was then given three-part vocal exercises that required pulsation of the lower abdominal muscles while maintaining an expanded rib cage, designed to enable him to feel the beginnings of breath support. Also discussed was what his attitude should be in lessons and in practice: that he must develop an awareness of what he was doing and seek to make improvements in whatever he was working on, but without the self-criticism that usually accompanies that awareness.

In this individual's case, it seemed likely that the problem of glottal attacks and subsequent throat tension was a psychological problem as well as a physical one. One observed in him a very deliberate, controlled personality, and it is not surprising that this rather rigid approach to life carried over to voice production as well. Coincidentally, he had started in therapy with a psychologist about 6 weeks prior to beginning voice study. It was suggested that he explore the feelings and experiences he was going through with his therapist.

By the third session, he was showing signs of relaxing more in his overall approach to singing, and this had a positive result in voice production. He claimed now to be able to identify the sensations of resonance around the eyes and nose where he was seeking to focus his voice (as opposed to the dampened, throaty placement he started with) and did demonstrate a more resonant tone. The glottal attacks were appreciably improved as long as the tone was initiated with a nasal consonant (/m/ or /n/), but when asked to initiate the sound with a vowel the problem returned. Breathing, especially inhalation, was also improved. Again, likely due to being more relaxed, he was able to take much deeper breaths, without involving his throat and shoulders. A key to achieving this in his case was continually to ask for inhalation to be slowed down, to think of it as happening in slow motion. Breath support was somewhat improved by the pulsation exercise, but at this point it was still obvious that he was not able to feel the energy for singing emanating from the breath. There was a small improvement in total range, with the addition of one whole step on the high end, and an overall improvement in vocal quality. He claimed to have made some headway as well in therapy and was beginning to understand that the physical aspects of vocal technique can be either greatly improved or hindered depending on one's psychological and emotional state.

In the fourth and fifth sessions, after reviewing previous exercises, the tension in the area of the head and neck was addressed, specifically, the jaw, the mylohyoid, and extrinsic laryngeal muscles. Many people use the lower jaw and lips far too much in their attempt to provide the extra energy it takes to sing, as opposed to relying on the breath for energy and using the jaw and lips minimally and only to add shape to vowels and articulate consonants. In his case, that problem was heightened because of his overall tension. His larynx rose appreciably with each attack. (This was directly related to the problem of the glottal scooping attacks.) The larynx ascended completely as he ascended in pitch. Using an exercise that requires the singer to inhale as though yawning, then, without altering the position of the mouth or throat, phonate as though sighing, he began undoing the well-learned habit of raising the larynx upon phonation. At a later point, that same exercise would be done on pitch (gliding down the interval of a fifth or an octave) as the transfer was made from speaking to singing. He was also asked to do an arpeggio exercise on /ja ja ja/ while keeping his jaw immobile and absolutely relaxed, using only minimal tongue movement to initiate the /j/. This was used to help achieve jaw relaxation and a flexible tongue and mylohyoid.

Voice Therapy

Initially, the concept of free and easy breathing was introduced to emphasize the sensation of the "source" of the voice. This also served, secondarily, to help decrease his speaking rate. Contrasts were made between the typical speech and singing breathing patterns without sacrificing the concept of support. Using chanting with nasal words/sentences, he was able to "place" his speaking voice appropriately and contrast the difference between that placement and his usual laryngeal focus. This resulted in some decrease in laryngeal tension. Extensive education regarding vocal hygiene was also emphasized.

By the third session, he was able to contrast "good" and "bad" voice placement. He could exert more conscious control over his speech rate. Laryngeal tension was still present, and relaxation techniques (contrasting tension and the warmth of relaxation; muscle stretching, including the "lion" yoga posture; and laryngeal massage) were introduced to direct attention to these areas. His presentation style was videotaped to help him develop an awareness of his body posture and especially his carriage of the head and neck.

At the fifth and final sessions, applications to his work were developed. He audiotaped his presentations and critically reviewed them alone and with the speech–language pathologist. For him, slowing his speech rate gave him the opportunity to concentrate on bringing his voice "up and out." Throughout this course of therapy, hard glottal attacks were noted to be diminishing; however, some direct work was done on easy voice onset, generally after "setting up" with relaxation work. The following comments were excerpted from his diary kept during the six weeks of therapy.

Singing exercises are clearly helping me focus my voice "in front." The MUMs are the most helpful. After I do a twenty minute session [of that exercise] my speaking voice is relaxed and "out." An excellent concept for me was simply to "will the voice up front." I think about this a lot during my practice sessions, and . . . the concept makes sense to me.

Being made aware of my tendency to hold my breath has been very helpful. I can change that pattern when I think about it.

This has been a much better week for consistency. Singing exercises are continuing to help me "see" and "feel" my voice in front of me, and I received a couple of positive comments on my voice.

My [speech] session was particularly helpful this week. I finally understood how to pronounce [attack] the vowel sound "ah" [/a/], "a" [/e/], etc. What did it for me was when Dr. J. explained that I was pushing on my vocal chords at the start of a word like *always*. . . . I guess the insight came when I comprehended the mechanics . . . rather than a concept.

Now here is another occasion where singing has helped my speaking voice. I understand Professor White's explanation of keeping the throat open. I also have a good idea how that feels, so to avoid the hard glottal attacks I simply think of the open throat concept applying the partial yawn idea.

My speaking voice is much better than when I started. The most significant improvement is consistency, and the . . . concentration and discipline has definitely helped me attain that consistency.

By the final session, there had been an appreciable gain in total range (F–g¹), especially in the upper voice, where he sang up to f¹ with relative ease. More importantly, there was marked improvement in vocal quality. The glottal scooping attacks were now under his conscious control, with only occasional lapses. Blending registers (the evenness of quality throughout the range) was also greatly improved, due primarily to the much more stable position of the larynx. Another important factor is that he was much more at ease in general and about his approach to voice in particular.

Reassessment of the speaking voice revealed similar gains. Habitual pitch was much more appropriate and less laryngeally focused. Pitch range was improved. Dysphonia was absent 85% of the time. For this person, episodes of throat pain were now largely nonexistent. Videostroboscopy revealed no redness at the vocal processes, reduction in the size of the posterior glottal chink, increase in amplitude of vibration and vibratory symmetry, and reduction in the amount of the "contribution" of supraglottic structures to phonation. A comparison of acoustic and aerodynamic function is given in Table 20–1.

Positive changes were seen in habitual pitch, maximum frequency range, and airflow rates. These changes indicate increased efficiency of phonation, which corresponded to the perceptual impression of reduced dysphonia.

CASE 2

Case 2 was a 30-year-old woman who had sung for many years in large and small barbershop groups. She also used her voice continually throughout the day at a secretarial job, where she answered the phone and dealt with customers. She claimed to have had some group vocal instruction, but has never had what she termed "formal training." Approximately 9 months prior to assessment, she had "overextended" her voice on a camping trip and since that time had difficulty with voice breaks during singing and changes in her speaking voice. She decided to see an otolaryngologist 6 months after this trip. No specific pathology was diagnosed. She was placed on complete voice rest for 2 weeks with some improvement. Two months later her problems returned, and she had another oto-

Table 20–1   Acoustic and Aerodynamic Analysis Results, Case 1

TCH	INITIAL	FINAL
F_0 (/i/)	107.2 Hz	121.4 Hz*
Jitter	0.125 msec	0.028 msec
Shimmer	3.44%	2.25%
Signal-to-noise ratio	18.45 dB	25.00 dB
Semitone range	26.7	36.6*
Airflow rate (/i/)	266.4 ml/sec	186.3 ml/sec*

*Significant change.

laryngologic assessment at which time bilateral vocal nodules were diagnosed. Voice rest, antihistamines, and a decongestant were prescribed. At the most recent assessment with another otolaryngologist, vocal nodules were still present and voice therapy was recommended.

The voice evaluation revealed no outstanding vocal abuses. Her history indicated that she used her voice extensively during the week; she talked constantly on the phone during the day, occasionally raising her voice to call to someone. She sang three nights per week for approximately 3 hours each time. Performances were generally once a month. Medical and surgical histories were unremarkable. Allergies had been diagnosed but were not felt to be especially problematic. Perceptually, the voice was mildly to moderately dysphonic with voice breaks, dry hoarseness, and breathiness. She was able to sustain /a/ for 8 seconds, and her s/z ratio was 1.5, indicating a significant difficulty in the ability to valve the larynx.

Videostroboscopy revealed small bilateral vocal nodules. There was a large posterior glottic chink. On a glissando maneuver, there was a significant rise of the larynx. Amplitude of vibration was restricted. The nodules appeared pliant on vibration. The open phase of vibration appeared to predominate. Acoustic analysis revealed low fundamental frequency. Other acoustic measures were within normal limits. Airflow rates were elevated at habitual and high pitches and normal at low pitch.

In the initial singing evaluation she indicated that she sang the tenor part in her barbershop quartet. (Though *tenor* normally refers to the highest male voice, in barbershop music it is common to use *tenor* to mean the high voice of the quartet, whether male or female.) She described her range as approximately b flat to a flat^2, but simple scales and arpeggios revealed a total range of e flat to b flat^2, with three distinct and abrupt register changes, the highest register sounding the weakest of the three. There was little evidence of any vocal technique. Though her posture was fairly good, inhalation was shallow and short, and there was no evidence of effective breath support as her relatively large rib cage collapsed quickly after beginning to sing. As is the case with many untrained female voices, she tended to force the lower registers up to the breaking point, delaying the inevitable transition into the next register until the voice would "crack" or "break." The result was a forced and throaty-sounding lower range, an unstable midrange, and a weak, breathy upper range. When asked to try to produce a more focused tone in her upper range, it was easy to see, as well as hear, the strain in her voice as she tried to manipulate the sound with the muscles of her neck and jaw. The larynx was not easily visible, but by touch one could feel it ascend appreciably on the attack and completely by the time she reached e to f^1, a sure indication of laryngeal tension and vocal strain.

The unfortunate result of singing in this manner for a long period of time as she had done was that wrong neuromuscular patterns were established, and the end result was that the more she tried to "correct" the tone, the worse it got.

Subconsciously, and on some level consciously, she associated singing with tension. At what point this originated is unclear, but it seemed obvious that there were underlying personal problems that she was dealing with as well, and it was very possible that her voice problems had psychological origins with physical manifestations. Though her speaking voice displayed similar characteristics, they were not as pronounced. In her case, it seemed wise to use the *relative* freedom of her speaking voice as a point of departure for producing the singing voice with more ease.

It was concluded that, for this individual, her mode of voice production for singing was the origin of her vocal nodules and consequently her dysphonia. The following goals were developed: for singing, (1) establish breath support, (2) improve singing voice placement, and (3) encourage relaxation of laryngeal musculature; for speaking, (1) coordinate respiration and phonation through vocal function exercises, (2) improve voice focus for speech, and (3) improve awareness of muscular tension.

Voice Lessons

After discussing basic information about posture, relaxation, breathing, the concept of resonance, and the sensations of productive vocal placement, she was assigned a simple humming exercise for warming up the voice and the pulsation exercise described previously to aid in establishing support. Since the upper register was weak because of incorrect and infrequent use, and the lower register was forced, she was asked to use only the upper range for 1 week. Vocal exercises were to take place for short periods of time (5 to 10 minutes at the beginning) but frequently throughout the day. In an attempt to incorporate speech into singing, she was given the spoken phrase, "now I know" and asked to repeat it in a nasal, "witchy" (her description) tone, while concentrating on relaxing her throat and jaw. This phrase was chosen because her voice seemed to focus better and with more ease on the vowels /u/ and /o/ and because the /n/ tended to draw the voice forward. Later, pitch was added to the phrase, first in semitones, then whole tones, and finally larger intervals.

It was also recommended that she refrain from performing for the duration of the 6 week study. Her poor vocal habits were so deeply ingrained that under the pressure of performance she would almost certainly revert to old habits.

By the third session there was a decided improvement in quality in the lower range as the voice became more focused and less forced. The pulsation exercise was not achieving results, however, and the upper range showed little improvement. Thus it was changed simply to asking her to sound /b/ first gently, then gradually increasing in intensity while monitoring her lower abdomen with her hand. She claimed that this simple exercise enabled her to feel support for the first time, but there was infrequent continuity into other exercises. This remained one of the main obstacles to her achieving a well-produced voice, and she was made aware that her advancement would be hindered until support was improved. We also addressed the raising of the larynx, and, using the yawn as a starting point, she began the process of learning to relax it down.

In the fourth session, the clinicians continued working with the position of the larynx. In conjunction with that, the client began learning to negotiate a smooth and even transition between the registers. By this time she had made good progress in learning to sing in the lower register without forcing, so dealing with register shifts was made easier. In learning this "blending" most people find it easier at first to descend than to ascend in pitch, but she was an exception, in part because the upper voice was very weak to begin with. Instead, she focused on blending the lower voice into the upper, but beginning the transition at a much lower point in the scale. By doing this, she lengthened the process instead of putting off the change to a higher note, forcing it to happen suddenly. The results were fairly quick, and she was able to produce what was considered her midrange with much more core in the sound and with less effort.

In the last session, the clinicians reviewed briefly what had been covered thus far and dealt further with placement and focus. Using an /u/, she was able to keep much more focus in the high range up to b flat^2, but was not successful with other vowel sounds.

Support remained a problem. There was little improvement in laryngeal movement, as it still raised dramatically in the upper range. In turn, there was only small qualitative improvement in those notes that still sounded airy and unfocused, and there was no improvement in range. The transition between registers was somewhat improved, but the only dramatic improvement was in the quality of the lower range.

Voice Therapy

After some introductory exercises for relaxation, she began by learning the technique for vocal function exercises. She was able only to produce notes b^1 through f^1, even though women are usually able to produce c^1 through g^1. The quality of these notes was quite breathy, and she had difficulty making a soft sound; she tended to begin phonation at a conversational loudness. She was also asked to "think the sound forward" to alleviate tension at the larynx. Initially, she was able to sustain notes for only 13 seconds on average; she rapidly progressed to 20 to 24 seconds.

In the second and third sessions, the clinician worked to broaden the concept of voice placement to her speaking voice. Jaw movement tended to be restricted during speech and, using videotaped samples of automatic speech (counting, days of the week), we provided feedback for attempts to enhance resonance. She did well under such structured conditions, but had difficulty transferring this to spontaneous conversational speech.

By the fourth and fifth sessions, she was beginning to experience some change in her voice outside the clinic. However, she was easily frustrated and felt each setback acutely. Monitoring her voice so closely produced a great deal of anxiety. Consequently, she was "permitted" to monitor her voice production only for restricted periods of time during the day and received praise and reinforcement for successful accomplishment of those goals. Direct attention to relaxation seemed to have the opposite effect for this person, with *increased* tension as a result.

At the sixth session, the videostroboscope was used to help the patient see some of the effects of increased tension (laryngeal rise on pitch elevation, excessive supraglottic "assist" on the initiation of phonation). She found this technique to be useful. During this session, she also worked on contrasting "good" and "bad" voice placement for speech. She was successful at switching between different modes of voice production approximately 70% of the time.

Some quotes from her diary revealed her perspective on her progress:

Had a few good times with my soft tone exercises (average 26 seconds). Tried some new chanting exercises to bring speech more into the mask which put less strain on my throat, but sounded funny.

Worked on breathing and expanding mostly in my middle range. I noticed that expanding . . . helped increase my time on the soft tone exercise.

We worked with the strobe [videostroboscope] at this session. I am still raising my larynx way too much. . . . The nodules are much smaller. . . . I tried to really concentrate on producing the sound with air and not [with] my throat. I could "see" when I was doing it right when I watched the monitor, but I don't "feel" it.

We had a good session this week. . . . I sang up to a B flat with no problem. I sing OK on an "oo" [/u/] vowel, but when I'm singing normal words my voice cuts out. . . . I'm not consistent at anything it seems. I work better in front of a mirror.

In summary, her progress with her singing voice was limited by her inability to grasp several basic and extremely important concepts, among them support and the relaxed, unraised position of the larynx. She was also limited by some problem or problems that were not physical.

Reassessment of her speaking voice at the end of the six week period revealed similar results. She was able to demonstrate some ability to change her voice focus and to relax the larynx consciously. However, this fluctuated and was reflected in her times on the vocal function exercises, which hovered at 23 to 25 seconds throughout this period. She appeared unable to move beyond a certain point. Her dysphonia was reduced, although she continued to have exacerbations on active weekends or after hectic work days.

Videostroboscopy revealed an elimination of vocal nodules, although a "string sign" remained, indicative of some residual swelling in that area. The size of her posterior glottic chink was slightly reduced. Other parameters of vibration remained the same. Her habitual fundamental frequency increased, and airflow rates at habitual and high pitch were diminished to more normal levels. Her frequency range remained essentially the same. A comparison of acoustic and aerodynamic function is given in Table 20–2.

While the person in this case did not demonstrate the dramatic improvement shown in the first case, she was able to change her voice production to a degree. The changes above may be attributed to better voice placement as well as some relaxation at the larynx.

SUMMARY OF CASE EXAMPLES

Both cases illustrate an approach in which the speech–language pathologist and voice teacher worked together to produce a unified impression of each person's targeted areas for improvement. Problems in singing and speaking that at first were thought by each client to be mutually exclusive proved to be interrelated. This became obvious by the observations they made. While the voice teacher and speech–language pathologist did make the association between singing and speaking clear, this concept was not continually stressed. Both clients came to their insights independently.

Within this 6 week "window," the speech-language pathologist and voice teacher were able to help these individuals make some changes in voice production. Each of the clients exhibited varying degrees of ability to hear and feel the initial status of their vocal mechanisms, to establish voluntary control over aspects of their voices, and to carry gains over into "real life"; consequently, they had different degrees of success in making changes and realizing the benefits from those changes.

Table 20–2   Acoustic and Aerodynamic Analysis Results, Case 2

FUNCTIONAL	INITIAL	FINAL
F_0	178.2 Hz	218.4 Hz*
Jitter	.038 msec	.036 msec
Shimmer	3.24%	2.96%
Signal-to-noise ratio	22.45 dB	24.32 dB
Semitone range	34.6	35.4
Airflow rate (/i/)	223.7 ml/sec	157.7 ml/sec*

*Significant change occurred.

The following process is suggested for cooperative treatment between the voice teacher and speech–language pathologist:

1. Jointly assess the patient. If this is not possible, then assess within the same time frame.
2. Compare "problem lists" and create a hierarchy for treatment together.
3. Reevaluate speaking and singing at roughly the same points.
4. Communicate often with each other regarding success and obstacles to progress, with the client's consent.
5. If possible, schedule occasional joint treatment sessions.

In general, a course of voice therapy will be shorter than the time frame for voice lessons. However, this is dependent on the goals the client is expected to achieve for the singing voice.

There are, of course, many different models for coordinating treatment and teaching. At the very least, a mutual familiarity with vocabulary, an understanding of the basic physiology of speaking and singing, and a knowledge of basic therapy techniques and teaching methods contribute to helping the client make changes in the voice.

REFERENCES

1. Stemple JC: *Clinical Voice Pathology: Theory and Management*. Columbus, OH, Merrill, 1984, pp 131–132.
2. Briess B: Identification of specific laryngeal muscle dysfunction by voice testing. *Arch Otol* 66:375–382, 1957.
3. Briess B: Essential treatment phases of specific laryngeal muscle function. *Arch Otol* 69:61–69, 1959.
4. Aronson A: *Clinical Voice Disorders: An Interdisciplinary Approach*. 3rd ed. New York, Thieme, 1990, pp 314–315.
5. Sundberg J: *The Science of the Singing Voice*. DeKalb, IL, Northern Illinois University Press, 1987, p 119.

Appendix 20 A: Glossary

abduction: The action of bringing the vocal folds apart. Vocal folds abduct during the act of inhalation.

acoustic analysis: Evaluation of the sound properties of voice. Measures considered important to acoustic analysis are fundamental frequency (F_0), jitter, shimmer, signal-to-noise ratio, and maximum frequency range.

adduction: The action of bringing the vocal folds together to produce voice. Vocal fold adduction may occur at voice onset, during the production of voiced consonants such as /b/, /d/, /z/, and during coughing or throat clearing. The vocal folds also adduct during swallowing.

aerodynamic analysis: Evaluation of the amount of air and rate of airflow available to set the vocal folds into vibration. Measures include flow or phonation volume, phonation time, and airflow rate. Subglottic pressure, glottic resistance, and glottic efficiency are also measures that can be extracted using equipment designed for aerodynamic analysis. Pulmonary function tests, which measure an individual's amount of lung capacity and use of air for breathing, could also be considered part of aerodynamic analysis.

airflow rate: A measure of the speed of airflow between the vocal folds during voice production. This generally is measured in milliliters per second (ml/sec) or cubic centimeters per second (cc/sec). The value is obtained by dividing the total amount of air expelled, for example, while saying "ah" (/a/) by the amount of time it took to produce that sound. Higher airflow rates (>200 ml/sec) are associated with "breathy" or "weak" voice, and low airflow rates (<80 ml/sec) may indicate tight, strained voice. Trained singers are able to maintain steady airflow rates across various fundamental frequencies.

arpeggio: The notes of a chord sung (or played) in succession. Arpeggio exercises have many uses, but among the more common ones are range extension, flexibility, and legato singing (the negotiation of intervals in a smooth and connected manner).

articulation: In speech–language pathology, the shaping of resonated tones into vowels and consonants by the tongue, lips, and jaw. It is considered to be the "endpoint" of a model of the process of speech production. Musically, *articulation* refers to the way a phrase is executed. In vocal pedagogy, it is the production of consonant sounds. Proper articulation in singing is achieved when the production of consonants is accomplished without tension and the process does not interfere with the production of tone. The result is good tone quality with clear diction.

attack: In speech–language pathology, the onset of sound or the act of bringing the vocal folds together to produce sound. A *hard glottal attack* is a voice onset in which the vocal folds are brought together and pressure is built up beneath them so that on release there is a popping sound. This usually occurs at the beginning of a sentence or breath group and is most noticeable on initial vowels. When used habitually, this is an abusive method of producing voice. An *easy attack* or *easy onset* is a method of voice production in which the vocal folds come together more gently. The coordinated attack (simultaneous release of air and onset of voice) is considered ideal for singing.

bel canto: An Italian term meaning "beautiful singing," which became associated with a vocal style in the 18th century. Bel canto style places an emphasis on the beauty and purity of the voice and considers beautiful tone to be more important than any other aspect of interpretation.

belting: A style of singing used in several types of popular music, generally by female voices, where the chest voice or chest register is pushed upward, often beyond its limits. The effect is a dramatic sound, relatively loud and sounds pushed. A similar manner of production in classical music is referred to as *chesting*.

break: A sudden, audible shift in registration, also referred to as a *crack*.

breathy: In speech–language pathology, this is a vocal quality associated with the release of excessive air during phonation. Breathiness occurs as a result of inadequate or inefficient vocal fold closure. Breathiness can be "functional," meaning produced as a result of inappropriate voice production, or "organic," meaning produced as a result of vocal fold weakness or paralysis or due to a mass interfering with vocal fold closure. In vocal pedagogy, a breathy tone is the opposite of a *focused* tone. It is like a picture out of focus—unclear, lacking definition. It may be used consciously as an interpretive effect, but with that exception it has a negative connotation in the vocal studio. Pathologic causes include edema, nodules, and polyps. When there is no pathology present, the cause is likely to be inefficient *breath support*, inefficient laryngeal control, poor vocal *placement*, or a combination of the above. While breathiness is not harmful to the singing voice, it indicates inefficient use of air and is generally considered to be esthetically unpleasant. It is the lack of breath support that may cause more serious vocal problems.

bridge: The transitional area between vocal registers.

chest voice: Used to describe the lower notes of a vocal range, thus named because of the sympathetic vibrations produced in the chest while singing with the thicker vocal configuration required to produce those tones.

compass: Refers to the total range of a piece of music or to a singer's total range.

covering: A technique of making the transition through vocal registers that aids in maintaining an evenness of vocal quality and color. Used primarily by men, this technique involves vowel modification, generally rounding and darkening the vowel (/a/ to /o/ or /ʌ/, for example) to prevent the sound from becoming "spread" or "white."

crack: See *break*.

crescendo/decrescendo: Increasing/decreasing. Primarily relating to increases and decreases in loudness.

cul de sac resonance: A voice quality in which the tone appears to be "caught" in the back of the mouth. This can occur when there is nasal blockage. Often, tongue retraction can give the voice this muffled quality.

"drinking in the tone": Imagery that conveys the feeling that the tone reverses its direction and comes back to its source. This concept is used by some to aid in sustaining the tone.

dynamics: Varying degrees of loudness and softness, and intensity of a sound.

dysphonia: A disorder of voice production resulting in poor voice quality. Occasionally adjectives are added to this term such as *functional*, *musculoskeletal tension*, or *spasmodic*, which refer to qualities of the dysphonia or to its suspected cause.

edema: A medical term for *swelling*. When referring to the vocal folds, this usually occurs as a result of infection or as a reaction to irritation or vocal abuse.

erythema: A medical term for *redness* occurring in infection and in cases of contact irritation, especially at the vocal processes of the arytenoids or in the posterior commissure of the larynx.

falsetto: The diminutive of the Italian *falso*, "false," this is the lightest and highest vocal register, produced with extremely thin vocal folds. Some voice teachers use the term interchangeably with *head voice*.

flow volume (or phonation volume): The amount of air (in liters or milliliters) expelled during one phonation after a maximum inhalation.

formant: The resonant frequency of a speech sound. It appears as a prominent band of energy on sound spectrography. There are four or five formants in most speech sounds (including fundamental frequency). Researchers have identified a "singer's formant" that is present in Western-style classical singing. This appears as a clustering of energy in the high frequencies. In the male voice this can vary between 2.3 and 3.8 kHz.[5]

full voice: To sing with complete breath support and resonance at a relatively loud volume, as opposed to *half voice*, which implies a lighter, less supported, and often unfocused tone. *Full voice* can indicate either volume level or the technical effort made to produce the tone.

fundamental frequency: The number of times per second that the vocal folds vibrate (in Hertz). While there are several frequencies or harmonics in a sound recorded at the lips, the fundamental frequency (F_0) reflects the tone generated at the vocal folds. For women, average conversational fundamental frequency is approximately 220 Hz. For men, average conversational fundamental frequency is 125 Hz.

glissando: Sliding rapidly up or down a musical scale.

glottal fry: A type of voice production in which the vocal folds are vibrating in a rhythmic, but abnormal fashion. The sound to the ear is one of a popping, bubbling sound. Glottal fry occurs due to a reduction in airflow and subsequent decrease in *subglottic pressure*. It is often heard at the end of a sentence when a speaker runs out of air and drops pitch; however it can be produced over a range of frequencies.

glottis: The area of opening between the vocal folds. Occasionally this term is used to refer to the general area of the vocal folds.

harshness: A quality of voice that is heard as a grating or "hard" sound. There is an aperiodic sound to harshness. Sometimes used interchangeably with *hoarseness*.

head voice: Most voice teachers use this term interchangeably with *falsetto*. Others use it to denote the upper part of the range when produced with relatively light registration, but still fully supported, as differentiated from pure *falsetto*.

hoarseness: A quality of voice that is heard as harshness with breathiness. Hoarseness is often differentiated between *dry*, that generally heard in cases in which some mass lesion is preventing smooth phonation, and *wet*, that present in cases in which the vocal folds are not closing adequately and secretions (eg, saliva) are pooling in the region of the vocal folds.

hooking: A technique that combines vowel modification (usually a more open vowel moving to a more closed one), with pushing lower registration to higher notes. This is generally thought to be esthetically unpleasant and bears a negative connotation in the voice studio.

hypernasal, hyponasal: To the speech–language pathologist, *hypernasality* refers to a disorder of resonance in which too much sound is escaping through the nasal cavity during speech. This is due to velopharyngeal incompetence (the soft palate is too short or too weak to seal off the oral from the nasal cavities). *Hyponasality* refers to a vocal quality in which sounds that should be nasalized (/m/, /n/, and /ŋ/) are not; these sounds become (/b/, /d/, and /g/). There is a great deal of variation in the degree of nasality across the dialects of English. *Excessive nasality* (beyond considerations of dialect) usually denotes a structural, neurologic, or functional abnormality. These terms are not common in the vocal studio, but their meaning is. Hypernasality is often referred to as *nasal twang* or simply *too nasal*, whereas hyponasality or insufficient nasal resonance is often referred to as *too far back* (placement), *too dull, too dark, too covered*. Though what is "right" is as much an esthetic and expressive choice as it is anything else, the singer is generally trying to balance nasal resonance with oral and laryngeal resonance. When control of nasal resonance is primarily a problem with function of the velum, hyper- and hyponasality are regarded as relatively minor vocal problems.

intensity: A measurement of the amplitude of a sound, expressed in decibels (dB). Intensity is the acoustic correlate of loudness. *Dynamic range* refers to the range of intensity an individual can produce, from softest to loudest sound.

jitter: Frequency perturbation or the cycle-to-cycle variation in the frequency of vibration of the vocal folds. There are several ways to measure jitter, and various types of equipment use different methods to extract this value. In general, high jitter values are correlated with a decrease in the quality of the voice.

legato: From the Italian meaning "to tie" or "bind together." As a musical direction, it is one way of performing a musical phrase, meaning to connect the notes smoothly and evenly in a musical line. It is also used conceptually in vocal technique, based on the fact that the voice is an instrument intended to change pitch smoothly, without articulating or punctuating the change with movement of the larynx. It also implies the unbroken connection of breath, vibration, and resonance.

lift: The note at which transition from one register to another register occurs.

manufactured sound: Tone that lacks ease and "naturalness" of production, sounds labored or overly technical.

marking: A rehearsal technique intended to save the voice, marking can be done in a variety of ways, including singing very softly, singing up or down an octave to make the range more accessible, and speaking the words in rhythm.

mask: The area of the face around the nose and eyes where one might wear a mask. This is often used in teaching the concept of *placement*, as a student may be directed to "sing in the mask" or "feel the vibration in the mask."

mean phonation time: The average time to produce a sustained vowel. Often used in assessment as a measure of the "health" of the respiratory and phonatory systems, the average value ranges from 18 to 20 seconds, although this can vary greatly with age.

messa di voce: As a musical direction, the meaning is to *crescendo* and *decrescendo* on a single note. Also used as a vocal exercise. Historically, a singer who could execute *messa di voce* successfully on every note in the range was considered to have complete mastery of vocal technique.

mezza voce: The Italian term for half voice, as contrasted with full voice. This may be a musical directive intended to achieve a certain dramatic effect. It is also a method of singing used in marking.

mixed voice (voix mixte): A tone sung with mixed registration, but with a preponderance of head voice.

optimal pitch: The ideal habitual speaking pitch for a certain individual. Optimal pitch was thought to be located approximately one-fourth from the bottom of one's total range. This concept now is considered to be outdated, and speech–language pathologists tend to help people find their "comfortable" range of habitual pitch.

passaggio: The Italian word for *passage,* which describes the area of the voice between registers where preparation for a change in registration should take place.

phonation: The process of the production of voice. To the speech–language pathologist, it may be described as "breathy," "strained," or "normal." The singer's main concern is to initiate sound so that the vibration of the vocal folds is coordinated exactly with the release of supported air and perceives that the tone is initiated by the air.

placement: A process of the imagination by which the voice is directed to a certain area of the body (usually the head) and the subsequent awareness of resonance in that area.

portamento: A manner of connecting two notes by gently gliding between them, effectively sliding over all of the notes in between.

projection: The quality of vocal production that refers to the ability of the voice to travel through space and be heard over the musical accompaniment.

prosody: The pattern of stress or inflection of a sentence or utterance. Prosody is the contribution of voice to language through the use of pitch, loudness, and duration.

rasp: A tone quality that sounds harsh and gravelly, somewhat like a protracted throat clearing, while maintaining a semblance of pitch. Thought of by some rock singers as a vocal style.

register: A group of notes produced with similar laryngeal function, yielding like quality of sound. Opinions among singers and teachers vary as to how many registers there are (from one to three) and whether to call the lowest *chest* or *pulse*, the middle *middle* or *modal*, and the highest *head* or *loft*.

resonance: The amplification of certain components of the tone produced at the vocal folds along the vocal tract (above the vocal folds and including the oral and nasal cavities). An individual's vocal resonance is determined by the shape of his or her anatomy and by the way this configuration is changed during speaking or singing. Often used mistakenly in the voice studio as interchangeable with such terms as *timbre, tone color,* or *quality of voice*, the singer is concerned with esthetic result of achieving a good balance of resonation among the naso-, oro-, and laryngopharynx.

respiration: The process of breathing. For speaking, we use a relatively small proportion of our available lung capacity to produce voice. People with quite impaired respiration (reduced lung capacity and ability to move air in and out of the lungs) can produce voice without severe difficulty. However, breathing for singing is much more dynamic, more athletic, and more exaggerated than it is for speaking. Breath control is achieved through the development and coordinated interaction of the abdominal and intercostal muscles in an opposite manner from the way they are used in everyday speech. That is, instead of inhalation being active and exhalation passive, the process is conceptually reversed. On inhalation, the abdominal muscles "relax" outward and downward, aiding the contraction of the diaphragm while the rib cage expands. *Breath support* occurs when, as opposed to a passive release of air, exhalation becomes an active and dynamic force by engaging the lower abdominal muscles and moving the air through the expanded rib cage. The rib cage should remain expanded as the process is repeated.

ring: Vibrant tone quality with a predominance of high partials in the frequency range of approximately 2,800 Hz.

s/z ratio: A value obtained by dividing the amount of time an individual produces the sound /s/ on a maximum inhalation by the amount of time to produce the sound /z/ on a maximum inhalation. If the vocal folds are healthy, then the times should be roughly equivalent, or equal to 1.0. The upper limit for "normal" is considered to be below 1.4.

scooping: An upward slur, most often defining an attack that begins below the pitch. Scooping may also occur within a vocal line, and is differentiated from the *portamento* by the fact that it is usually not a conscious act. Generally considered by voice teachers to be unmusical and technically detrimental.

shimmer: For the speech–language pathologist, it is intensity perturbation or the cycle-to-cycle variation in the amplitude of the sound signal. As with jitter, the methods for measuring shimmer vary, and shimmer may be expressed as a percentage, in decibels, or in some other value. Increased shimmer values generally correlate with hoarseness. To the voice teacher, shimmer is a tone quality that is highly desirable. The voice is used properly, has a good vibrato rate, and projects well.

signal-to-noise ratio: The ratio of the periodic signal produced at the vocal folds to the "noise" or aperiodic signal. Someone with a great deal of hoarseness would have a low signal-to-noise ratio; that is, the "signal" and the "noise" might be very similar in loudness.

"sitting on the breath":   A sensation of the voice resting on the supported breath, achieved by maintaining constant breath pressure, a relaxed throat, and an expanded thorax.

spin: Describes tone quality that is free and apparently effortless in production and projects or carries well. Implicit is the presence of true vibrato.

staccato: Italian for "detached," "separate," "short." Notes that are separated by a short amount of space between them.

straight tone: A tone produced without *vibrato*. Since vibrato is normally present in a mature, well-produced voice, a straight tone is considered symptomatic of some constriction in the throat, of a problem with breath support, or both. Straight tone singing can be executed at will and is used by some singers as stylistic effect, and in that case is an esthetic choice.

subglottic pressure: The amount of pressure just below the vocal folds. An adequate amount of subglottic pressure is crucial for the regular vibration of the vocal folds. Subglottic pressure is created by a steady stream of air originating from the lungs and regulated by the amount of tension and mass of the vocal folds. Subglottic pressure is raised to produce increased loudness.

swallowed tone: Tone that is constricted in the throat and therefore lacking high partials and forward placement.

tessitura: Italian for "texture." When referring to a song or role, *tessitura* means that range wherein the majority of pitches lie. When referring to a singer, *comfortable tessitura* describes that portion of the singer's range produced with the greatest ease and beauty.

timbre: The distinctive quality or "color" of a voice produced by the combined effect on the ear of the listener of the fundamental tone and its harmonic overtones.

tremolo: Describes undesirable vibrato, whether too fast, too slow, or too wide.

vibrato: A regular and relatively even pattern of oscillation above and below a pitch, which occurs naturally at a frequency of approximately six to seven times per second in a mature, well-produced voice. Though beauty is subjective, most voice teachers agree that vibrato adds warmth and beauty to tone. It is also one of the measures of the health and function of the voice.

videostroboscopy: A technique to visualize the vocal folds under full light and under "strobed" or flashing light. In stroboscopy a light flashes onto the vocal folds at a rate slightly slower than the rate of vibration of the vocal folds. When seen by the human eye, this gives the illusion of slow motion. The images are recorded on videotape and can be reviewed as often as necessary. An otolaryngologist or speech–language pathologist may use a rigid endoscope or a flexible fiberoptic scope for this procedure.

vital capacity: The maximum amount of air that can be exhaled after a maximum inhalation.

vocal abuse: Encompasses a range of behaviors, from poor vocal hygiene (smoking, inadequate hydration) to misuse and overuse of the voice. For the speaker, this is the etiology of most "benign" voice disorders. For the singer, overuse will become apparent sooner in an untrained or poorly trained voice, but also occurs in well-trained voices that are doing too much: too long, too loud, too high, and so forth. Misuse may be the result of poor vocal technique or the conscious or unconscious imitation of unhealthy vocalism. It may also result from an improper or insufficient warm-up/cool-down period, singing in an inappropriate tessitura (that part of the vocal range within which lies the majority of pitches as opposed to the total range) or singing beyond one's natural range. Unfortunately, some forms of vocal abuse have come to be considered stylistically acceptable, even desirable among certain vocal styles.

vocal focus: *Focus* describes a tone that, through correct production, effectively turns all of the air used to produce it into clear, vibrating singing or speaking sound. Though often used interchangeably in the vocal studio with the term *vocal placement*, focus is better described as the result of good vocal placement and its unencumbered connection to breath support.

voce di capra: Italian for "voice of the goat." Characterized by a quick, bleating pulsation of the tone.

vocalise: A vocal exercise.

whistle register: The female equivalent of male falsetto. The highest notes in a female voice.

wobble: Uneven and unusually slow fluctuation of pitch.

Appendix 20 B: Terms Describing Vocal Quality

The following terms are, for the most part, self-defining, and are used in the voice studio to describe a particular quality of sound. A plus (+) or minus (−) indicates whether the quality is normally considered to be desirable or undesirable.

bell-like (+)	bite (+)	bottled up (−)
bright (+)	buzzy (+)	choked (−)
clutched (−)	driven (−)	edge (+)
edgy (−)	floating (+)	flowing (+)
fuzzy (−)	golden (+)	grainy (−)
hollow (−)	hooty (−)	mellow (+)
metallic (−)	muddy (−)	pear-shaped (+)
ping (+)	pointed (+)	reedy (−)
rich +)	ringing (+)	soaring (+)
spread (−)	strident (−)	toothy (−)
twangy (−)	veiled (+/−)	velvety (+)
vibrant (+)	white (−)	

Appendix 20 C: Voice Classifications

An important part of the language of the vocal studio are those terms used to classify voices. The main factors in determining voice classification are range, timbre, the comfortable tessitura of the voice, the location of the passaggio in the range, and the size of the voice. To a lesser degree, but also relevant in determining a specialized category, are such factors as the singer's temperament, personality, and body type. The main categories into which most voices can be placed are

Female

    Soprano: Highest of the female voices. Brighter timbre.

    Mezzo-soprano: Average female voice. Between soprano and contralto in range and timbre.

    Contralto: Lowest of the female voices. Darker timbre.

Male

    Counter-tenor: A male voice singing mostly in falsetto.

    Tenor: Highest of the male voices (with the exception of counter-tenor). Brighter timbre.

    Baritone: The average male voice with a range and timbre between tenor and bass.

    Bass-baritone: Between bass and baritone in range and timbre.

    Bass: The lowest of the male voices. Darker timbre.

Within these main categories are many more descriptive subcategories, most of them used only in classical music, specifically, opera. Most of the main categories above can be divided into at least two subcategories: lyric, which implies a lighter voice both in size and color, and dramatic, a darker and heavier voice. Further divisions include spinto (thrust or pushed), cantante (singing), and helden (heroic). Then there are those categories that are descriptive more of what the voice *does* as opposed to how it *sounds*. *Coloratura*, for example, usually implies soprano, but can describe any voice that is very agile and specializes in singing florid music. Such terms as *buffo* (comic) or *soubrette* (coquette) refer to the character of the singers and their roles in the opera as well as their voices. When a voice seems to be between categories or overlap in another category, both are used, and the voice is called a *between type* (in German, *Zwischen Fach*).

21

Phonosurgery

CHARLES N. FORD, MD

DEFINITION OF PHONOSURGERY

Phonosurgery can be defined as any surgical procedure designed to improve voice. For years laryngologists have engaged in surgical alteration of the vocal folds by removing benign and malignant growths of the vocal tract, and often voice improvement was achieved. Although voice improvement is an incidental effect of some cancer surgeries, it has become the primary goal in the management of most benign vocal fold lesions. Surgical techniques have advanced rapidly with increasing ability to assess results. Although it is not yet possible to fine tune the voice in a manner comparable to most musical instruments, phonosurgery provides a variety of approaches to improve many voice disorders.

Evolution

The evolution of phonosurgical techniques can be attributed to the emergence of microlaryngoscopy and the clinic-based voice laboratory that allows surgeons to appreciate abnormal vocal fold function and to quantify pathology in dysphonic patients. Problems of magnification, binocular vision, and suitable anesthesia had to be overcome before effective microlaryngeal surgery could be performed. Laryngeal videostroboscopy has afforded laryngologists an opportunity to see the effect of surgery on vocal fold vibration. This in turn has allowed the surgeon to refine techniques and achieve more predictable results. Improved outcomes makes phonosurgery an option in managing dysphonias in professional voice users.

Scope of Phonosurgery

Any surgical alteration of the vocal tract can affect the voice, but in a practical sense phonosurgery is limited to surgery of the vocal folds. Such surgery may alter the physical characteristics, placement, contour, and function of the vocal fold. Marangos[1] has suggested a classification of phonosurgery based on four broad categories: (1) vocal fold surgery, (2) laryngeal structure surgery, (3) neurolaryngeal surgery, and (4) substitute phonation surgery. For the purposes of this book, we will limit our discussion to vocal fold surgery and address those techniques most applicable to the professional voice patient. Although conservation and reconstructive surgery subsequent to the removal of a cancer

344

may aid voice preservation or improvement, the primary goal of these procedures is the removal of life-threatening disease. Such procedures do not fall within the scope of phonosurgery.

Preoperative Assessment

The goal of phonosurgery is to detect and treat the appropriate pathology so that voice improvement results. Recognition of pathology and selection of surgical indications is just as important in phonosurgery as in other surgical endeavors. A thorough preoperative assessment should include laryngeal videostroboscopy, which affords the surgeon an opportunity to observe the vocal fold pathology and how it affects vibration. Subtle changes such as focal scarring, cysts, and sulci are often missed with indirect laryngoscopy. Videostroboscopy is helpful in identifying adynamic areas in the vocal fold associated with such lesions and may reveal occult lesions.

The close collaboration of a speech pathologist trained to recognize structural and functional voice disorders will result in better patient management, surgical planning, and postoperative care. The proper identification and localization of pathology is essential to successful surgery. It is helpful preoperatively to determine those components of a patient's dysphonia that are due to the presence of vocal fold lesions and those factors that are due to compensatory mechanisms. For example, a patient may have very minimal glottic insufficiency and have severe dysphonia due to laryngeal hyperfunction; such a patient might respond well to voice therapy alone. Conversely, a patient may have a vocal fold cyst that is undetected by indirect laryngoscopy and therefore may be referred for unnecessary voice therapy when surgery is indicated. Consequently it is important that the laryngologist have access to a voice laboratory and establish a good working relationship with a speech pathologist. Some otolaryngologists most skilled in laryngeal microsurgery collaborate with a speech pathologist or phoniatrician throughout the perioperative period.

Historically, voice results from laryngeal surgery have been subjectively assessed and dependent on the clinical experience of the laryngologist and speech pathologist. These subjective judgments have caused several problems in evaluating the efficacy of various phonosurgical techniques. Moreover, subjective judgments frequently have not been based on the anatomic and physiologic status of the vocal apparatus. This subjectivity may result in erroneous judgments about the physiologic abilities of the speaker and inappropriate recommendations for phonosurgery. Combining subjective and perceptual judgments with objective voice assessment and videostroboscopy has increased the clinician's ability to recognize disease, plan surgery, and assess phonosurgical results.[2]

GENERAL PRINCIPLES OF PHONOSURGERY

Applied Anatomy

The surgeon must appreciate the functional anatomy of the vocal fold so that essential membranous vocal fold structures are preserved. It is important to remove diseased tissue with minimal alteration of the remaining histoarchitecture of the vocal fold, and it is essential to avoid secondary intention healing. Histologically, the vocal fold is composed of five layers of increasing density. These layers comprise two mechanical layers, the body and the cover.[3] The *body* is chiefly composed of the vocalis muscle, and the *cover* includes the epithelium and three layers of lamina propria. The body is generally stiff relative to the loosely coupled cover so that the cover moves around the body in a predictable way. During sound productions at normal pitch and loudness, the cover is considerably displaced, both vertically and laterally. These displacements are smaller during high-pitch productions and larger during loud productions. In cases of vocal pathology, the body may be flaccid or the cover may be stiff; either condition will change the predictable pattern of movement and tell the clinician something about the underlying pathology and the need for treatment.

An awareness of functional anatomy requires the operator to appreciate the plane of superficial lamina propria (Reinke's space). Normal vibration necessitates the free movement of the epithelium and superficial lamina propria (cover) over the underlying vocalis muscle (body). The intervening connective tissue (*transition*) consisting of the intermediate and deep layers of lamina propria (vocal ligament) is composed of increasingly dense collagen and is rich in fibroblasts. Iatrogenic injury at this level may result in fibroblastic proliferation and scarring that impairs normal vocal fold vibration. It is generally unnecessary to damage tissue at this level, because most benign pathology of the vocal fold occurs at a more superficial plane. By confining benign excisions to the plane of the superficial lamina propria, which consists of sparse collagen and elastic fibers, the surgeon avoids extensive fibroblastic activity and promotes healing without scar formation.

Surgical Principles

Surgery performed on the vocal folds using direct laryngoscopy and magnification provided by an operating microscope affords an opportunity to alter the vibratory properties of the vocal fold. The results of surgery depend on the pathology and surgical techniques. Although techniques vary, and all surgeons do not have the same level of technical ability, there are certain general principles that apply[4]: (1) Patient selection is a key to successful surgery. It is imperative to make an accurate preoperative diagnosis and to have a good concept of the location of the pathology. (2) The surgeon should limit excisions to pathologic tissue and avoid excising normal adjacent tissue in order to preserve the functional integrity of the membranous vocal fold. (3) After lesions are excised, the remaining tissues should be carefully coapted to avoid secondary intention healing that is functionally detrimental. This may require undermining and always requires care during excision to ensure adequate residual mucosa.

Specific principles relevant to vocal fold microsurgery include a constant awareness of the underlying functional anatomy of the vocal fold. The surgeon should avoid unnecessary stripping of mucosa for benign disease. Although there are many otolaryngologists skilled in the use of cupped forceps avulsion, the technique involves an element of chance and lacks precision; it is possible to strip away normal, functionally important mucosa. Mucosa should be sharply incised, and when possible vocal fold lesions should be approached through incisions on the superior surface away from the medial vibrating edge. It is always inadvisable to denude mucosa on opposed sides of the anterior commissure to avoid web formation. The key to dissecting benign lesions is to confine the dissection to the plane of the superficial lamina propria. This should be easy in phonosurgery because most benign pathology is confined to more superficial planes. The vocal ligament must not be violated if one is to preserve normal vocal fold vibration and voice.

PHONOSURGICAL MANAGEMENT OF BENIGN LESIONS

Nodules

Vocal nodules are one of the most dreaded and common causes of dysphonia among professional voice users. Nodules are most often the result of faulty or excessive voice use. Vocal excesses, such as inappropriate loudness and excessively high pitch, increase the mechanical trauma to the vibrating vocal folds; this may alter the epithelium and sub-epithelial tissues leading to nodule formation. It is important to diagnose nodules accurately so that appropriate voice therapy can be initiated when indicated. One should distinguish other lesions, such as cysts and tumors of the anterior-to-middle one-third of the vocal folds. It is not uncommon that a unilateral vocal fold lesion induces a contralateral opposed nodular lesion in response to chronic irritation.

All nodules are not alike, and there is a spectrum of nodular changes from functional nodal diathesis during phonation to discrete anatomic nodules with epithelial thickening, parakeratosis, and occasional dyskeratosis. The underlying subepithelial tissue may exhibit a range of reactions from simple inflammation and edema to angiogenesis and thrombosis. Some nodules may appear as fusiform mucosal thickening, while others may be discrete exophytic hyperkeratotic lesions. Occasionally, nodular pseudocysts occur at the midmembranous vocal fold, and it may induce nodular changes in the contralateral folds so that typical nodules are simulated. This condition calls for surgery, and early recognition can save the patient unnecessary voice therapy.

Once it is clear that surgical intervention is warranted, careful microscopic examination is needed to rule out the possibility of underlying cysts, sulci, or other vocal fold pathology. Excision should be very precise and can best be done with sharp microexcision technique (Fig. 21–1). The forceful traction of the vocal fold during excision could result in too deep an excision and the unnecessary sacrifice of adjacent normal mucosa and should be avoided. After the lesion is excised, the edges of remaining mucosa can be trimmed to produce a smooth vocal fold edge. Uninvolved mucosa should be preserved and adjacent tissue destruction avoided by using cold microexcision techniques.

Polyps and Edema

Diffuse edema manifested by distention of Reinke's space and circumscribed polypoid lesions may be addressed by similar microsurgical approaches. Surgery should be precise, and sharp dissection is preferred to avulsion techniques. Microsurgery is preferred to the use of a laser, although the laser (or microcautery) can be used to coagulate prominent vessels on the mucosal surface of polyps. Incisions should be made laterally on the superior surface and parallel to the vocal fold (Fig. 21–2). This is the routine approach for cordotomy and affords maximum preservation of the membranous vocal fold. In cases of Reinke's edema, it is often possible to suction the viscous liquid or gelatinous material from Reinke's

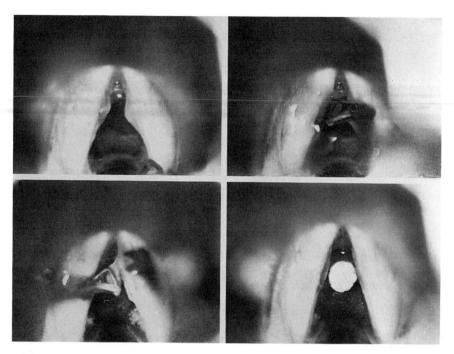

Figure 21–1. Operative photo of vocal nodules being excised with sharp, microscopically guided resection technique and angle scissors. An associated microweb is also managed by lysis.

space. If the material is more organized and cannot be readily suctioned, the surrounding tissues may be bluntly dissected to facilitate the blunt extraction and suction of the residual fibrinous material. If the mucosa has been distended from the pathologic edema over time, redundant mucosa will be present. This should be redraped over the vocal fold and the redundancy resected with a microscissors. The technique of resection is similar to face-lift surgery in that the redundant medial flap of mucosa is draped laterally over the site of incision and resected sharply along the line of the initial incision.

Polypoid degeneration and discrete polypoid lesions are handled similarly. Isolated polyps can be gently grasped and resected with a sharp microscissors in a fashion similar to that described for management of nodules. Resection should be carefully controlled, and stripping techniques with blunt avulsion is not indicated. Microsurgical methods are preferred to gross excisional biopsy without magnification or attempts to excise such lesions with indirect laryngoscopy. Special care should be taken at the anterior commissure to avoid injury to opposing epithelial edges and secondary web formation. The mucosal edges should be carefully coapted after the lesion is excised. This can be facilitated by bluntly compressing the tissues with angled alligator forceps, with adrenalin-saturated cotton, or with blunt dissectors. The mucosal margins can be undermined in the superficial lamina propria plane to afford relaxation and to facilitate closure where the tissues appear under tension or the wound is gaping. The use of fibrin glue may be helpful, especially if the adjacent mucosa is damaged or if the passive coaptation of the tissues is incomplete.

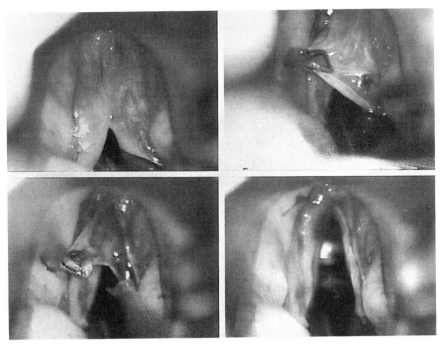

Figure 21–2. Operative photo showing Reinke's edema with extensive degenerative changes in both vocal folds. Surgical technique includes lateral superior incisions, aspiration, resection of redundant mucosa, and redraping.

Vocal Fold Cysts and Related Problems

Two types of vocal fold cysts are encountered: mucous retention cysts (Fig. 21–3) and epidermoid cysts (Fig. 21–4). Other conditions, such as sulcus vocalis and mucosal bridges, often occur in patients with underlying epidermoid cysts, and they may be important in the pathogenesis of these lesions.[5] Epidermoid cysts cause regional vocal fold stiffness manifested by the loss of mucosal wave on videostroboscopy. These cysts are histologically similar to cholesteatoma and consist of a multilayered, stratified squamous epithelial matrix filled with keratotic material. The wall may be fragile and require gentle dissection from attachments to mucosa and vocal ligament. The lesion may be dissected much like a cholesteatoma, but there is often a fibrous layer adjacent to the matrix that may necessitate piecemeal excision, particularly when the cyst has ruptured into the vocal ligament.[6,7]

Typically a pore is found that opens from the cyst at the medial edge of the vocal fold. The dissection must incorporate this pore, and incision should be made near the medial edge of the vocal fold. A medial flap is developed first, separating the cyst from the mucosa and allowing the attachments to the vocal ligament to supply helpful countertraction. The medial flap is very fragile because the cyst is in the plane of the superficial lamina propria. Dissection here can result in mucosal tears so patience and precision are necessary. Next it is dissected free of the vocal ligament. The ligament is easily identified, and the plane of

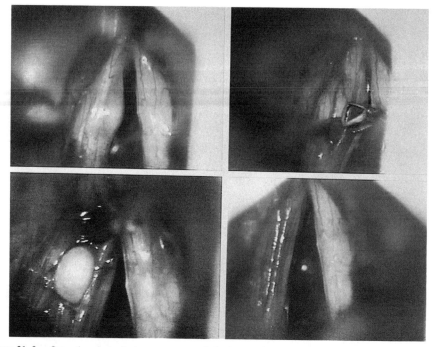

Figure 21–3.   Operative photo depicts exposure and dissection of a mucous retention cyst.

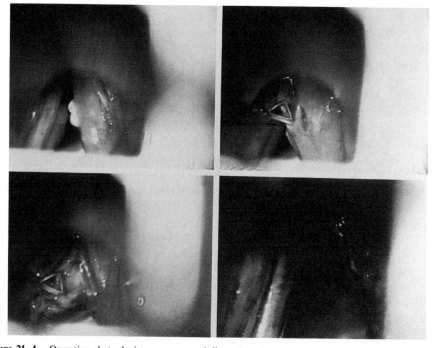

Figure 21–4.   Operative photo depicts exposure and dissection of a ruptured epidermoid inclusion cyst.

dissection on the lateral surface is relatively easy to identify and follow. If the cyst has ruptured into the vocal ligament, the collagenous fibers must be spread and the cystic contents bluntly teased out. The lesion is typically clumpy and amorphous compared with the well-defined vocal ligament from which it must be distinguished. The cyst may be freed posteriorly and anteriorly with semisharp dissection. Blunt dissection is time consuming, but it is important to avoid sacrificing normal tissues because these patients have a paucity of normal mucosa, and, in contrast to polypoid edema patients, mucosal excision is not advocated.

Hirano[8] described a useful approach for well-circumscribed lesions that have an intact medial edge. An incision is placed on the superior mucosal surface immediately posterior to the lesion and then extended anteriorly over the cyst by gently spreading the edges apart. This approach avoids the risk of entering the cyst during the incision and lessens the chance of rupture. Cysts are bilateral in more than 50% of patients, and a careful search for a contralateral lesion should be made at the time of surgery. Associated sulci and mucosal bridges also should be managed. The sulcus can be excised in a manner similar to that used for the cyst. Mucosal bridges consist of only a thin bipedicled strip of mucosa. These need only be sharply excised.

Sulcus vocalis is a term that has been applied to any condition with a sulcus or groove running along the medial edge of the vocal fold. Some furrows or grooves occur with vocal fold atrophy, for example, in patients with tenth cranial nerve paralysis or presbylaryngis, where the mucosal edge is intact and pliable. These cases do not necessitate excision, but they can be successfully handled with collagen augmentation or other techniques. Sulcus vocalis may result from the rupture of congenital epidermal cysts along the medial edge of the vocal fold. Typically sulcus vocalis is associated with dense scar tissue attached to the vocal ligament, and the vocal fold is stiff. Excision of sulcus vocalis defects does not address the problem of tissue deficit, and it is important to spare all available adjacent mucosa and attempt to coapt edges by careful undermining. Fibrin glue may be helpful. Residual glottic insufficiency may be addressed with other techniques such as collagen injection or thyroplasty.

OTHER TECHNIQUES IN PHONOSURGERY

Laser Techniques

The basic principles of microsurgery are also applicable for laser surgery. The essential point is to respect the functional anatomy and to limit the area of tissue destruction when treating a benign disease of the vocal fold. An inadequate understanding of anatomy or a lack of appreciation of the zone of tissue damage induced by the laser can cause scar formation and disabling dysphonia. Conventional lasers have been overused in treating benign vocal fold lesions. Laser ablation is the preferred method of treating laryngeal papillomata and some hemangiomas, granulomas, and selected early T1 cancers of the vocal fold. As a precision tool for incisions, the use of microspot technology may afford a greater role for the laser in managing other benign vocal fold lesions by limiting the zone of adjacent tissue destruction.

In general, the laser beam destroys more tissue than is immediately apparent to the surgeon, so it is necessary to take precautions and be conservative. It is possible to treat most benign lesions with power settings between 4 and 10 W and to limit exposure settings to 0.1 second in the repeat mode. The microspot micromanipulator provides improved focus by eliminating parallax error; this makes it possible to incise vocal fold mucosa precisely with minimal laser-induced damage to adjacent tissues. Basic principles of tissue diagnosis should be used, and specimens should be histologically studied. Dissection is facilitated by the traction-assisted dissection of lesions rather than by complete vaporization. The center of the laser beam should not be focused along the line of projected incision because that would result in normal tissue being destroyed beyond the desired line of excision. Instead, the aiming beam should be centered on the lesion, or a small lesion should be shaved down with the edge of the beam by centering the beam on a platform medial to the lesion. The removal of charred debris will reduce postoperative inflammatory reaction and fibrosis and thereby decrease functional damage.

Injection Techniques

Injection techniques are most commonly used for vocal fold augmentation. Other applications include the treatment of spasmodic dysphonia by injecting botulinum toxin and the injection of steroids or other medicines into the larynx. Polytef (Teflon) was first injected into vocal folds by Arnold,[9] and it remains the most common material used for augmentation.[10] Cross-linked bovine collagen (GAX-collagen, Phonagel, Zyplast) and autogenous fat offer some unique advantages, and these methods are currently under investigation. Gelfoam paste and silicone are also used but have not been approved for such use in the United States.

The primary goal of vocal fold augmentation is to improve voice by reducing glottic incompetency. Positive changes include reduced transglottic airflow, increased vocal intensity, improved signal-to-noise ratio, and increased phonation time. Injection techniques accomplish this by (1) displacing the medial edge of one vocal fold toward the midline to facilitate glottic closure, (2) limiting displacement to the plane of the true vocal fold, (3) restoring or maintaining a smooth vocal fold edge with proper contour, and (4) preserving the viscoelastic properties of the vocal fold to allow normal vibration. All of this should be accomplished without substantially compromising the airway.

Polytef must be injected into a deep muscular plane laterally in the thyroarytenoid muscle. Placement adjacent to the lateral end of the vocal process of the arytenoid may allow some medial displacement of the vocal process. The tip of the needle should be placed in the plane where maximum displacement is desired. Guarded needles on the Bruening injector are no guarantee of correct placement; it is important to visualize the point of insertion and to observe carefully the contour changes achieved during slow injection. The most common error is to inject too far inferior to the glottic plane so that the subglottic space balloons medial to the vocal fold and results in a brassy voice with continued breathy dysphonia. Attempts to improve the situation by additional injection have resulted in severe dysphonia and dyspnea. Injections that are not sufficiently lateral may cause symptomatic granulomas and seromas with vocal fold stiffness and voice deterioration.

In contrast, collagen must be injected in a relatively superficial plane.[11,12] The vocal fold is entered on the superior surface at the point of greatest concavity or atrophy. In the midmembranous portion of the vocal fold, the first resistance encountered after the epithelium is punctured is the vocal ligament. Injection in this plane affords an easy diffusion of the collagen in an anteroposterior axis, and the medial edge can be monitored closely for appropriate displacement. If the injection is too deep, the implant will be rapidly resorbed in the thyroarytenoid muscle. If the injection is too superficial, a bleb may begin to form; this should be recognized, and the bleb should be dispersed by gently rubbing with the edge of the needle. With the currently available cross-linked collagen, less than 0.6 cm^3 is usually required; overcorrection is not necessary. Skin testing with observation for 4 to 6 weeks is suggested, as with other injectable foreign proteins. Other substances are injected into the larynx, including silicone, Gelfoam, fat, steroids, and botulinum toxin. For augmentation, the preferred method of exposure is by indirect mirror laryngoscopy or direct laryngoscopy. The microscope may be used with either approach. Another approach that can be used in patients in whom laryngoscopy is not feasible is transcutaneous needle placement with fiberoptic nasopharyngoscopic guidance.[13] Transcutaneous placement of needles through the cricothyroid membrane can also be guided with electromyographic signals to localize the thryroarytenoid muscle.[14]

LARYNGEAL FRAMEWORK SURGERY

For the professional voice user, the risk of vocal fold damage is often so threatening that even individuals with vocal fold paralysis might not feel that the potential benefits warrant surgical intervention. Surgical modification of the laryngeal framework has been proposed as an effective method of treating voice disorders, and recent reports advocate type I thyroplasty (Mediaization Laryngoplasty With Silastic, in the 1993 Phonosurgery Classification of the American Academy of Otolaryngology-Head and Neck Surgery), as described by Isshiki et al,[15,16] for primary management of glottic insufficiency. Investigators report excellent results and argue that framework modification is preferable to Teflon injection.[17] The major advantages of thyroplasty relate to preservation of membranous vocal fold integrity. In this procedure, a window is placed in the thyroid cartilage and displaced medially sufficient to move the vocal fold toward the midline. Medialization is adjusted until good apposition with the opposite vocal fold occurs during phonation and the voice is improved. Unlike Teflon injection, thyroplasty affords delicate intraoperative adjustment, does not alter the vocal fold structure, and may be totally reversible.

ENHANCING PHONOSURGICAL RESULTS

Phonosurgery in the Professional Voice Patient

Patients who use their voice professionally need special consideration and the greatest degree of conservatism in surgical management. Usually, acquired lesions should be treated by voice rest, medical management, and voice therapy before surgery is considered. Normal-appearing vocal folds do not preclude underlying pathology, just as a normal tympanic membrane does not rule out significant otopathology. Voice symptoms are crucial in assessing the appropriateness of phonosurgery. A professional singer often can compensate for a small lesion and thus produce a natural-sounding voice, but these compensatory strategies may lead to pain and severe dysfunction. Small acquired lesions, such as nodules, and even some congenital lesions may be well tolerated by some professional voice users; indeed, the timbre of some popular and folk singers may depend on these lesions. Even though these patients may complain of a change in voice, the solution is not necessarily the removal of an obvious but benign lesion. Hasty phonosurgical intervention could impair or ruin a musical career, and initial conservative management is always indicated for these patients. When there is a question about the diagnosis and the patient fails to respond to conservative measures, diagnostic microlaryngoscopy may be necessary to confirm the diagnosis.

General Precautions

Patients should be well informed about the proposed surgery, and the procedure should not be trivialized by being labeled "minor surgery." Current trends in the United States dictate that many phonosurgical procedures be performed on an outpatient or ambulatory basis. This tendency is unfortunate and exists in part because some surgeons in fact do consider the surgery minor. It is often easier to monitor and control vocal abuse, straining, humidity, and anxiety during the immediate postoperative period if the patient is hospitalized.

Phonosurgery is elective and should not be performed on patients with active upper respiratory infection or allergies. During active infection or the immediate postinfection period, the vocal folds are engorged, bleeding may pose some problem, and postoperative healing may be complicated. Allergic edema may complicate surgery and produce postoperative coughing. The allergy may produce or contribute to postoperative dysphonia and may make an assessment of the surgery more difficult. The surgery should not be done during the active season if the patient has a known seasonal atopic disease; when necessary, allergic patients should be appropriately treated before surgery. Adequate nutrition and hydration will make anesthesia safer and contribute to good surgical results.

There is no evidence that postoperative voice rest is helpful to phonosurgical patients. Whispering may be harmful. A short period of relative voice rest seems reasonable. Longer periods of voice rest, as much as 1 week after the operation, should be followed by voice therapy to ensure a smooth transition from a limited use of the structure to the demands of normal speaking. Voice rest beyond 1 week will be counterproductive for most patients and should be avoided.

Ongoing Assessment and Modification

The most important measure to enhance phonosurgical results is a careful evaluation of surgical results by both the surgeon and the speech pathologist. By studying the results of surgery and comparing the functional results with the particular procedure performed, the surgeon can continually modify surgical techniques to achieve optimal results. In the past, it may have been sufficient to note that the lesion was removed and that the vocal cords appeared "normal." It is now obvious that normal-appearing vocal folds in fact can be very abnormal: they may contain stiff areas, undergo aperiodic vibration, produce a loss of tone, and show subtle defects that are only apparent during stroboscopic or microscopic examination. Objective measures of acoustics, glottic waveforms, and aerodynamics allow the surgeon to compare different modes of treatment. Comprehensive assessment requires both subjective and objective measures. In the professional voice patient, the voice is obviously the essential end product, but the voice must be produced with appropriate effort and without secondary symptoms.

REFERENCES

1. Marangos NE: Phonosurgery—a classification. *Otolaryngol-HNS* 104:282–283, 1991.
2. Hirano M: Objective evaluation of human voice: clinical aspects. *Folia Phoniatr* 41:89–144, 1989.
3. Hirano M: *Clinical Examination of Voice*. New York, Springer-Verlag, 1981.
4. Ford CN, Bless DM, Blaugrund SM: Phonosurgery, Johnson JT, Blitzer A, Ossoff R, Thomas JR (eds): in *AAO-HNS Instructional Courses*, vol 3. St. Louis, CV Mosby, 1990, pp 293–306.
5. Bouchayer M, Cornut G, Witzig E et al: Epidermoid cysts, sulci, and mucosal bridges of the true vocal cord: a report of 157 cases. *Laryngoscope* 95:1087–1094, 1985.
6. Bouchayer M, Cornut G: Microsurgery for benign lesions of the vocal folds. *ENT J* 67:446–466, 1988.
7. Bouchayer M, Cornut G: Instrumental microsurgery of benign vocal fold lesions, Ford CN, Bless DM (eds): in *Phonosurgery: Assessment and Surgical Management of Voice Disorders*. New York, Raven Press, 1991, pp 143–166.
8. Hirano M, Yoshida T, Hirade V, Sanada T: Improved surgical technique for epidermoid cysts of the vocal fold. *Ann Otol Rhinol Laryngol* 98:791–795, 1989.
9. Arnold GE: Vocal rehabilitation of paralytic dysphonia. *Arch Otol* 76:358–368, 1962.
10. Dedo HH, Urrea RD, Lawson L: Intracordal injection of Teflon in the treatment of 135 patients with dysphonia. Laryngoscope 83:1293–1299, 1973.
11. Ford CN, Bless DM: A preliminary study of injectable collagen in human vocal fold augmentation. *Otolaryngol-HNS* 94:104–112, 1986.
12. Ford CN, Bless DM: Clinical experience with injectable collagen for vocal fold augmentation. *Laryngoscope* 96:863–869, 1986.
13. McCaffrey TB, Lipton R: Transcutaneous Teflon injection for paralytic dysphonia. *Laryngoscope* 99:497–499, 1989.
14. Blitzer A, Brin MF, Fahn S, Lovelace RE: Localized injection of botulinum toxin for the treatment of focal laryngeal dysphonia (spastic dysphonia). *Laryngoscope* 98:193–197, 1988.
15. Isshiki N, Morita H, Okamura H, Hiramot M: Thyroplasty as a new phonosurgical technique. *Acta Otolaryngol* 78:451–457, 1974.
16. Isshiki N: Recent advances in phonosurgery. *Folia Phoniatr* 32:119–154, 1980.
17. Koufman JA: Laryngoplasty for vocal cord medialization: An alternative to Teflon. *Laryngoscope* 96:726–731, 1986.

Appendix A: Patient History Questionnaire for the Professional Voice User

HENRY FORD HOSPITAL
DIVISION OF SPEECH–LANGUAGE SCIENCES & DISORDERS
PROFESSIONAL VOICE CLINIC

PATIENT HISTORY FORM

Name _____   Age _____

Date _____   Occupation: _____

Referring Physician: _____

Description of the Problem:

1. Please describe your voice problem: _____

    _____

    _____

2. When did you first notice the problem: _____

    _____

    _____

3. How did the problem begin? _____ suddenly   _____ gradually

    _____ intermittently

4. How has the voice problem changed since the onset? _____ improved

    _____ worsened   _____ no change   _____ fluctuates

Past Voice History:

5. Have you had any of the following voice symptoms?

_____ hoarseness lasting more than 2 days

_____ tired voice after lengthy talk

_____ neck muscle tension

_____ pain in neck muscles

_____ constant throat clearing

_____ excessive coughing

_____ dry throat or mouth

_____ lump in throat feeling

_____ loss of voice

_____ change in pitch

_____ difficulty maintaining a loud voice

_____ sore throat

_____ fullness in nose and throat

_____ tightness in nose and throat

_____ shortness of breath while speaking or singing

_____ scratchy throat

6. Have you seen a physician for your voice? _____ yes _____ no

If yes, for what reason? _____

7. Have you ever seen a speech–language pathologist? _____ yes _____ no

If yes, for what reason? _____

8. If you have received advice or treatment for a voice problem, please check the recommendations given:

_____voice rest

_____ humidification

_____ surgery

_____ voice therapy

_____ medications

_____ antireflux program

_____ voice instruction

_____ reduce throat clearing, loud talking

9. When is your voice the best? _____ early morning _____ afternoon

_____ evening _____ night

10. When is your voice the worst? _____ early morning _____ afternoon

_____ evening _____ night

Past Medical History:

11. List any major illnesses and their approximate dates. _____

_____

12. List any major surgeries and their approximate dates. _____

_____

13. Do you have allergies? _____ yes _____ no   If yes, please describe._____
_____

14. List any medications that you currently take (prescribed and nonprescribed)

_____ _____ _____

_____

Personal/Lifestyle:

15. Do you smoke currently? _____ yes _____ no

16. Did you ever smoke? _____ yes _____ no

17. If you answered yes to either item 15 or 16:

    a. How many packs per day? _____

    b. How many years of smoking? _____

    c. If you used to smoke, when did you stop? _____

18. Indicate your consumption of the following beverages:

    a. alcohol _____ yes _____ no   If yes, how much _____

    b. caffeinated coffee or tea _____ yes _____ no   If yes, how much _____

    c. caffeinated soda _____ yes _____ no   If yes, how much _____

19. In what types of physical activities (e.g., exercise) do you participate regularly?

_____

20. What time do you usually eat your last meal or snack? _____

21. Do you play any musical instruments? _____ yes _____ no   If so, what instrument? _____

Voice Use:

22. Does your occupation require you to use your voice frequently? _____ yes _____ no

23. Are you involved in any of the following activities?

_____ long telephone conversations _____ never _____ occasionally _____ frequently

_____ teaching to groups of people _____ never _____ occasionally _____ frequently

_____ speaking in large rooms _____ never _____ occasionally _____ frequently

_____ singing before a group _____ never _____ occasionally _____ frequently

_____ choral singing _____ never _____ occasionally _____ frequently

_____ teaching instrumental or vocal music _____ never _____ occasionally

    _____ frequently

_____ preaching _____ never _____ occasionally _____ frequently

_____ taking voice instruction _____ never _____ occasionally _____ frequently

_____ taking acting instruction _____ never _____ occasionally _____ frequently

_____ speaking on television or radio _____ never _____ occasionally _____ frequently

_____ acting in plays _____ never _____ occasionally _____ frequently

_____ coaching a sport _____ never _____ occasionally _____ frequently

_____ public speaking (eg, sales presentations) _____ never _____ occasionally

 _____ frequently

_____ aerobics or gymnastics instruction _____ never _____ occasionally

 _____ frequently

_____ excessively long conversations _____ never _____ occasionally _____ frequently

_____ cheerleading _____ never _____ occasionally _____ frequently

_____ leading meetings _____ never _____ occasionally _____ frequently

24.   Do you currently take voice or acting instruction? _____ yes _____ no

25.   Please complete the following chart, indicating your use of voice in *speaking* activities. For each day of the week and time of day indicate the "average" amount of time (i.e., hours) you spend talking in one of the activities above (or in another vocally demanding activity).

	Sunday	Monday	Tuesday	Wednesday	Thursday	Friday	Saturday
morning							
afternoon							
evening							
night							

26.   Please complete the following chart, indicating your use of voice in *singing* activities. For each day of the week and time of day indicate the "average" amount of time (i.e., hours) you spend talking in one of the activities above (or in another vocally demanding activity).

	Sunday	Monday	Tuesday	Wednesday	Thursday	Friday	Saturday
morning							
afternoon							
evening							
night							

27. If you sing, what type of music? _____

28. If you sing, what is your range? _____ bass   _____ baritone   _____ tenor

     _____ alto   _____ soprano

29. Do you warm up before performing? _____ yes   _____ no

30. Do you cool down after performing? _____ yes   _____ no

Appendix B: Common Laryngeal Positions

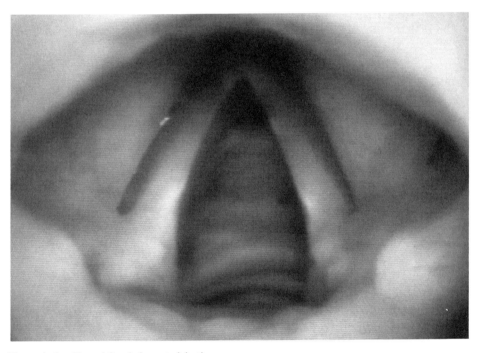

Figure A–1.   Normal female larynx, abduction.

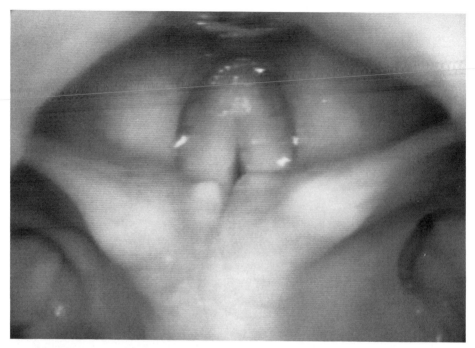

Figure A–2.   Normal female larynx, adduction.

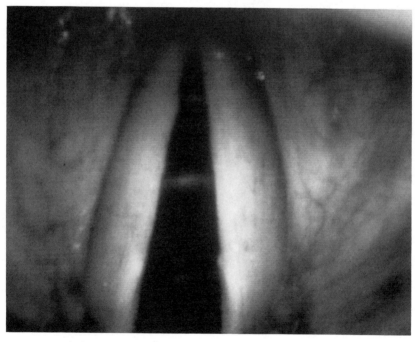

Figure A–3.   Normal male larynx, abduction.

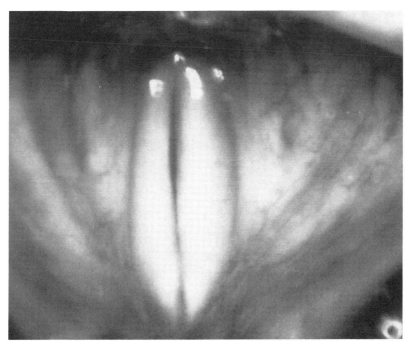

Figure A–4. Normal male larynx, adduction.

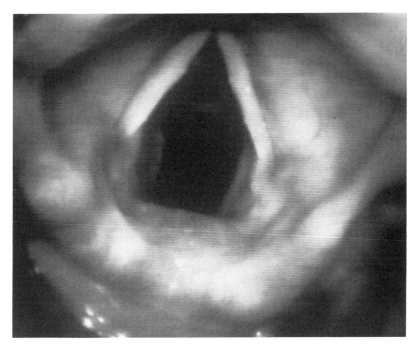

Figure A–5. Vocal nodules, early.

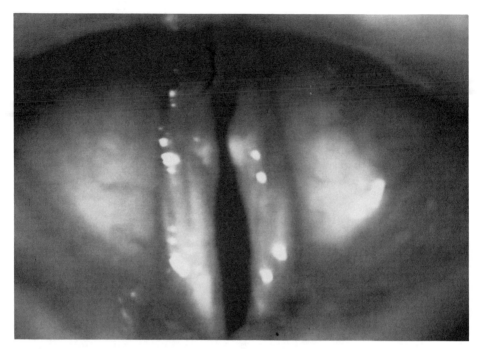

Figure A–6. Vocal nodules.

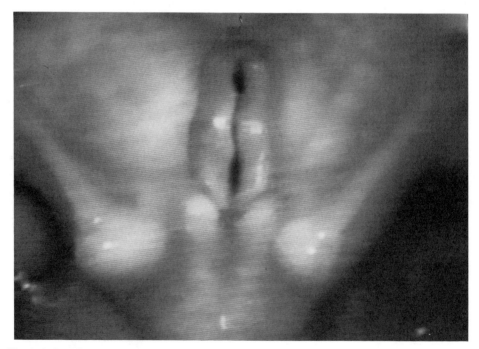

Figure A–7. Vocal nodules, chronic.

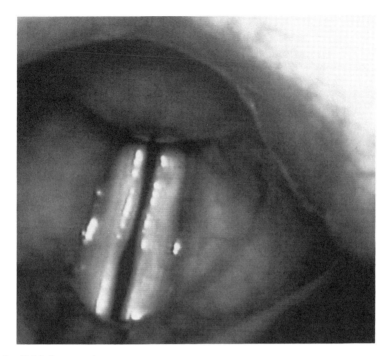

Figure A–8. Reinke's space edema.

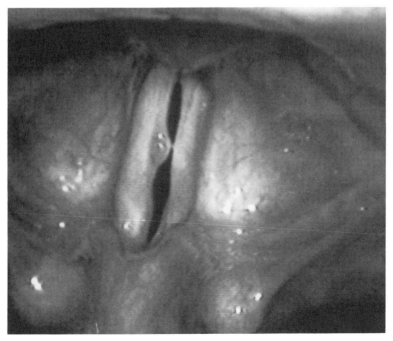

Figure A–9. Unilateral vocal polyp.

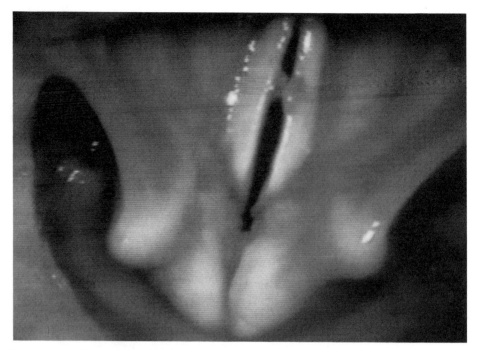

Figure A–10.   Bilateral vocal polyps.

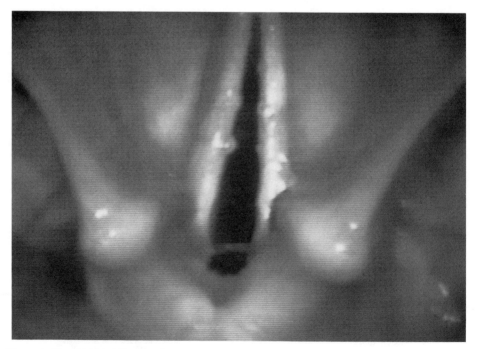

Figure A–11.   Multiple bilateral polyps.

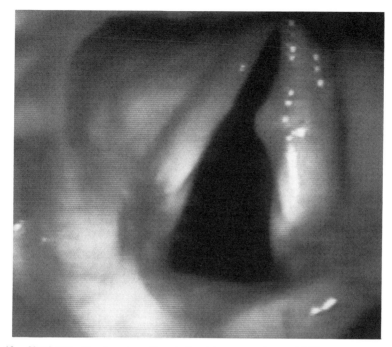

Figure A–12. Vocal cyst with adjacent small contact nodule on opposite vocal fold.

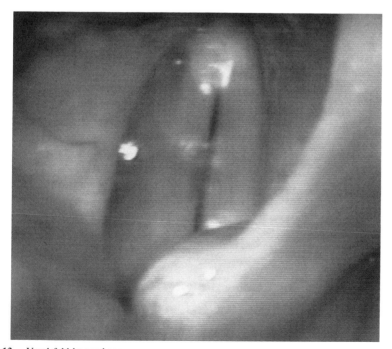

Figure A–13. Vocal fold hemorrhage.

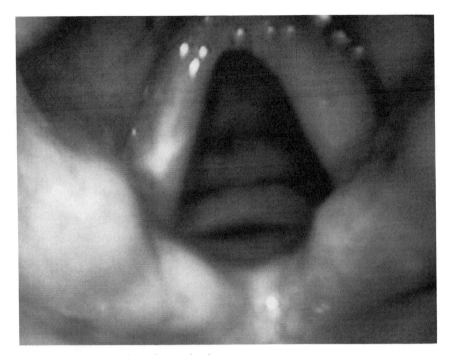

Figure A–14. Anterior commissure laryngeal web.

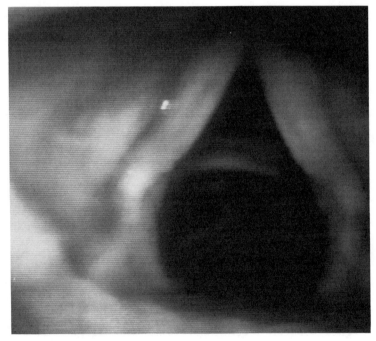

Figure A–15. Sulcus vocalis.

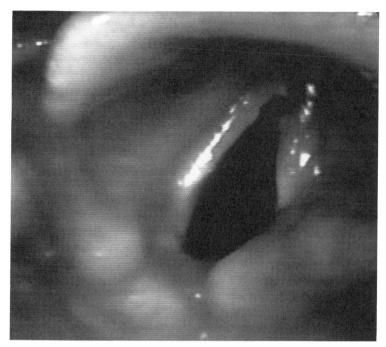

Figure A–16. Unilateral (right) vocal fold paralysis.

Index

370